A HISTORY OF MEDICINE

In Two Volumes

VOLUME TWO

A HISTORY OF MEDICINE

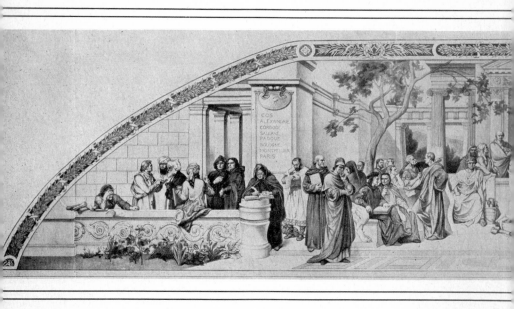

CHARLES C THOMAS • PUBLISHER

By RALPH H. MAJOR, M.D.

Professor of Medicine and of the History of Medicine
The University of Kansas
The School of Medicine
Kansas City, Kansas

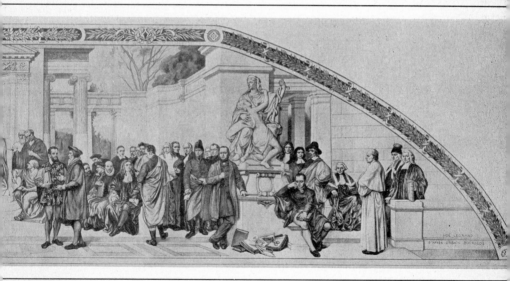

SPRINGFIELD · ILLINOIS · U.S.A.

Charles C Thomas · Publisher
Bannerstone House
301-327 East Lawrence Avenue, Springfield, Illinois, U.S.A.

Published simultaneously in the British Commonwealth of Nations by
Blackwell Scientific Publications, Ltd., Oxford, England

Published simultaneously in Canada by
The Ryerson Press, Toronto

Library of Congress Catalog Card Number: 54-6571

Printed in the United States of America

TITLE PAGE ILLUSTRATION

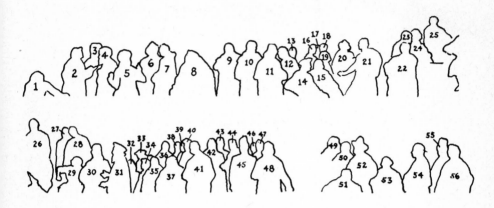

Histoire de la Médecine

DECORATION DU GRAND AMPHITHEATRE DE LA FACULTÉ DE MÉDECINE
DE PARIS*

1. Bachtischua	17. Alex de Tralles	37. J. L. Petit
2. Aaron d'Alexandrie	18. Dioscoride	38. M. Servet
	19. Thémison	39. Van Helmont
3. Albucasis	20. Pline L'Ancien	40. Rabelais
4. Rhazès	21. Celse	41. Laennec
5. Avicenne	22. Galien	42. La Peyronnie
6. Gariopontus	23. Érasistrate	43. Broussais
7. Jean de Milan	24. Hérophile	44. Corvisart
8. Constantin l'Africain	25. Aristote	45. Larrey
	26. Hippocrate	46. Desault
9. Paul D'Egine	27. Pythagore	47. Dupuytren
10. Guillaume de Salicet	28. Alcmæon	48. Claude Bernard
	29. Asclépiade	49. Mauriceau
11. Guy de Chauliac	30. Vésale	50. Sydenham
12. Mondino	31. A·Paré	51. Bichat
13. Aétius	32. Fallopio	52. Harvey
14. Jacques Desparts	33. J. Dubois	53. Barthez
15. Arnaud de Villeneuve	34. Fernel	54. Frère Cóme
	35. Baillou	55. Bordeu
16. Arétée	36. Riolan	56. Ant. Louis

* Printed through the courtesy of Faculté de Médecine de Paris, and from a wall picture given to Mr. Charles C Thomas by Dr. Martin Fischer.

Contents

List of Illustrations

A HISTORY OF MEDICINE

The Eighteenth Century

THE EIGHTEENTH CENTURY in medicine has been described as an age of "theorists and system-makers" (Garrison). Some of these system-makers, following a suggestion of Sydenham that the natural history of disease should be studied in the same spirit that natural objects were studied, felt impelled to classify diseases as plants and animals were classified—into classes, orders and genera. François Boissier de Sauvages initiated the movement by the publication of his *Nosologia methodica,* 1760, closely followed by Carl von Linné, a physician and later famed as a botanist, whose *Genera morborum,* published in 1763, gave a great impetus to the movement; by Rudolf Vogel in 1764; and by William Cullen, the eminent clinician of Edinburgh, whose *Synopsis nosologiae* appeared in 1769. This penchant for the minute classification of disease continued into the following century with Pinel and Schönlein as its outstanding proponents.

Before the century had passed, pathology had been founded as a science, physical diagnosis had been placed on a firm basis by the discovery of percussion, chemistry had witnessed one of its great triumphs in the discovery of oxygen, and medical science had learned how to prevent one of the worst scourges of the human race—smallpox. Clinical medicine also did not lag behind but developed an imposing array of clinicians whose careful observation of disease and study of various methods of treatment mark an epoch in the history of the healing art. It was a great century in the history of medicine and the harbinger of greater triumphs yet to come.

Natural science—chemistry, physics, biology and botany—were beginning to interest large segments of people as never before. The old schools of Iatro-physicists and Iatro-chemists were revived by the newer discoveries in physics and in chemistry. Philosophy, too, was pursued with an intensity reminiscent of Hellenic antiquity. Its devotees asserted anew that all knowledge was the domain of philosophy, that they sought a synthesis of all existing knowledge.

The views of the philosophers exerted great influence, especially in Germany, where there was a great renaissance in philosophy, beginning with Leibnitz and passing down through Kant, Fichte, Schelling and Hegel. Indeed, this was a golden age of philosophy.

At the beginning of the century, it was Gottfried Wilhelm Leibnitz (1646-1716), whose influence was particularly felt. Leibnitz was
a man of prodigious energy and of unusual mental activity. His
early studies were in mathematics, which resulted in the discovery
of differential and of integral calculus. He next turned to other
fields and wrote books on diplomacy, international law, civil law,
politics, physics, and finally philosophy. Mysticism, the supernatu-
ral, and the accidental were all excluded from his system which was
based on logic, natural law, and experiment. Over a period of many
years, he formulated his doctrine of the universe, which, in its ulti-
mate essence, consisted of individual centers of force, or monads.
"Monads," he wrote, "are the very atoms of nature," but, as centers of force, have neither parts, extension in space, nor shapes—
qualities which distinguish them from the atoms of Demokritos and
the materialists.

Among the leaders in medical thought, particularly in Germany,
a fusion of Iatro-chemical and Iatro-physical concepts with philosophical speculation is quite evident. One of the leaders of this new
synthesis was Georg Ernst Stahl, who was born in Ansbach in 1660
and studied at Jena under G. W. Wedel, a well-known adherent of
the Iatro-chemical School. Stahl's early interest was largely in chemistry; he is remembered in the history of that science as the pro-
mulgator of the phlogiston theory. This theory, first proposed by
Becher and reminiscent of the Arabian alchemist, Jabir, held that
combustible substances lose something when they are burned.
Metals, according to this theory, are composed of a *calx,* different
for each metal, and *phlogiston* (from the Greek φλογιστός = burnt),
which is common to all combustible substances. When a metal,
such as lead or tin, is calcined in the air, *phlogiston* is set free and
the *calx* is left behind. This theory dominated chemical thinking
until it was demolished by Lavoisier in 1777.

Dozent in Jena for a time, Stahl was called to Halle as professor
in 1694. Here he had as colleague, Friedrich Hoffmann, with whom
he violently disagreed. Because of this disagreement and his growing unpopularity, Stahl resigned in 1716 to become court physician
in Berlin. He died in 1734.

Stahl's system, "Animism," was expounded in his *Theoria medica
vera,* published in 1708. Disagreeing with Descartes, who distinguished sharply between the life of the soul and that of the body,
Stahl taught the all important role of the "anima," the supreme life
principle, which in health regulates all the functions of the body
but which disappears at death. This "anima" he identified with the

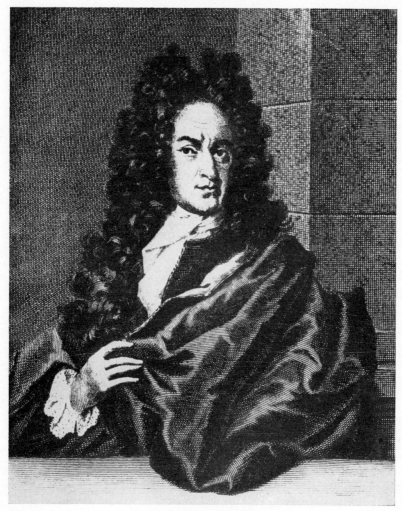

GEORG ERNST STAHL
From an engraving in the Académie de Médecine, Paris.

Hippocratic *physis* (φύσις), stating, "Man has his physician within him, and nature is the physician of disease." The role of the physician is to support the *anima*, which regulates the health of the body. He taught that fever was due to the increased activity of the *anima* in attempting to restore health and, therefore, should not be combated. In the causation of disease, he laid great stress upon "full bloodedness" *(Vollblütigkeit)*, which the *anima* combated with nose-bleeding, menses and hemorrhoidal bleeding. When the *anima* was not entirely successful, the physician should assist with vene-section, cathartics, emetics and methods to produce profuse sweat-ing. He was a strong opponent of the employment of opium and quinine, which he considered harmful to the *anima*.

Stahl's theories, which he thought were derived from Hippocrates, really have more in common with the doctrines of Paracelsus and of van Helmont. He was not able to establish a school of "Animism" although the later school of "Vitalism" at Montpellier represented by Théophile Bordeu was based largely on the theories of Stahl. While Stahl's theories seem in many ways to be a retrogression to the older mystical teachings of Paracelsus and of van Helmont, yet they had a very beneficial effect upon medical thinking in that they emphasized the unity of the living organism and combated the one-sided materialism of the period.

Friedrich Hoffmann, Stahl's great rival and one-time colleague, was a very different type of man. Unlike the envious, sensitive and unpopular Stahl, Hoffmann possessed tact, charm, and abundant good nature. He was born in Halle in 1660, studied, as did Stahl, with Wedel at Jena, and then proceeded to England, where he worked with Robert Boyle. He practiced medicine for a time at Halberstadt and, in 1694, was appointed professor at the newly founded University of Halle, sharing the chair of medicine with Stahl. Hoffmann, a learned man and a gifted teacher, drew large numbers of students and physicians to his courses. In 1709, he was called to Berlin as physician to King Frederick I, but, disliking court life with its intrigues, he returned to Halle in 1712 and was warmly received by the faculty, students and townspeople. He taught and practiced with great success until his death in 1742.

Hoffmann was a voluminous writer; his chief work, *Medicina rationalis systematica,* in nine volumes, was published in 1718-1740. Hoffmann's system seemed clear and logical. Our knowledge is limited, he taught, and based upon what we perceive through our senses. All energy and all properties of matter we perceive as move-ment, as force and counterforce, as contraction and extension. Life is movement, especially of the heart and of the blood; death is cessation of movement. Health is normal movement; disease, dis-turbed movement. The normal movement of the blood keeps diges-tion active and evacuations normal. The body is like an hydraulic

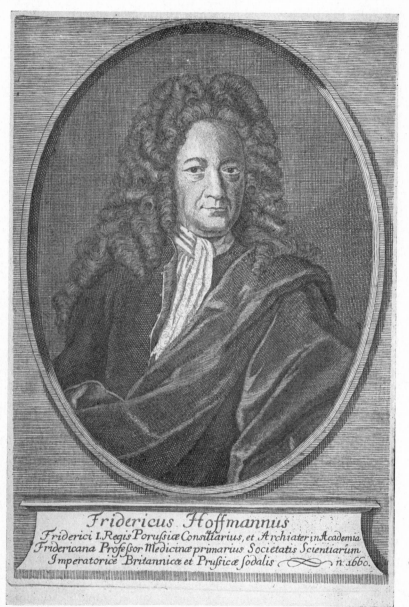

Fridericus Hoffmannus
Friderici I. Regis Porussiæ Consiliarius, et Archiater in Academia
Fridericana Professor Medicinæ primarius Societatis Scientiarum
Imperatoriæ Britannicæ et Prussicæ sodalis n. 1660.

FRIEDRICH HOFFMANN

machine, the activity of which stems from a kind of nervous fluid —like the ether. This is secreted by the brain and distributed by the nerves and the blood. It regulates the "tonus" of the tissues. If too great an amount of nervous fluid flows to a part, a spasm results; if too little, atony. The treatment is relatively simple as soon as we establish whether the disease is due to spasm or to atony. Local inflammations, hemorrhage, catarrh and neuralgia belong to the spastic group; chronic diseases to atony. Where there is spasm, the physician should employ relaxing antispasmodics, sedatives, laxatives, soothing and evacuating methods; when atony, irritating and stimulating remedies, such as wine, camphor, quinine and ether. Hoffmann laid great stress on diet, mineral waters and venesection. Many observers have pointed out the resemblance of Hoffmann's teachings to those of the ancient Methodists with their *status strictus* and *status laxus*.

The therapy employed by Hoffmann was simple and logical, his prescriptions particularly being by their simplicity in marked contrast to the prevalent polypharmacy. His simple prescriptions, his good clinical judgment, combined with an agreeable and sympathetic personality, explain his phenomenal success as a physician. His name is still applied to Hoffmann's anodyne. As a clinical observer, he was one of the first to describe rubella and to write excellent accounts of chlorosis and typhus fever.

While Hoffmann was at the height of his fame in Halle, there appeared in the Netherlands a physician whose great reputation added such luster to the University of Leyden that it became to eighteenth century medicine what Padua had been to medicine two centuries earlier. This physician was Hermann Boerhaave.

HERMANN BOERHAAVE

Boerhaave, the son of a clergyman, was born at Voorhout, near Leyden, in 1668 and, destined for the church, studied theology at Leyden, taking courses also in philosophy, mathematics and medicine. In 1690, he received his doctor's degree in philosophy at Leyden, but, deciding later to become a physician, he obtained a doctor's degree in medicine at the University of Harderwyk in 1693. He then located in Leyden, began the practice of medicine, and, in 1701, became a lecturer in the theory of medicine at the university and, in 1709, professor of medicine and botany.

His renown as physician and teacher spread rapidly, students from all over Europe flocking to his lectures and demonstrations. His most famous pupil, Haller, described him as *"communis totius*

Europae praeceptor" (the general teacher of all Europe). Leyden still keeps his memory green. He is buried in St. Pieterskerk; a statue of him stands before the old hospital; the new medical center is called Boerhaave Kwartier; and no medical congress meets in Leyden without laying a wreath on his grave.

Boerhaave wrote comparatively little: two large works, *Institutiones medicae* (Medical Institutions) and *Aphorismi de cognoscendis et curandis morbis* (Aphorisms on the diagnosis and treatment of diseases), together with some botanical and chemical writings. The *Institutiones medicae,* first published in 1708, went through 15 Latin editions and a translation into French. The *Aphorismi,* which appeared in 1709, went through 10 Latin editions, one English translation, and two French translations. Widely read by physicians and students, the most quoted works of their time, these books are now largely forgotten.

In the theory of medicine, Boerhaave has been described as an eclectic, taking some theories from the Iatro-physicists, others from the Iatro-chemists. All life, he taught, was the result of movement of the "solids" and of the "fluids" of the body; disease was a disturbance of this movement either in the solids or in the fluids. Disease, when its cause was in the solids, was produced by organic maldevelopment or changes in the size, number or position of the tissue constituents; when in the fluids, disease was due to plethora, or improper mixtures, which he termed "Acrimonia" and could be salty, sour, sharp, aromatic, fatty, alkaline or viscous.

Boerhaave, for all his theories, never allowed them to conflict with his treatment of patients. He placed Sydenham, who certainly was never addicted to medical theorizing, on almost the same eminence as Hippocrates himself, calling him, "the light of England, the Apollo of the art, whose name I would blush to mention without a title of honor."

The numerous students drawn to Leyden by the fame of Boerhaave were attracted by his genial and charming personality, by the grace and clearness of his lectures on botany and chemistry, and, especially, by his bedside teaching. In the old hospital by the Vrouwen Kerk, two wards, one for men and the other for women, each with six beds, were turned over to this master for teaching students. Each day when he made rounds with his students, the history of the patient was carefully read and discussed, the patient inspected, his urine examined. Boerhaave employed a thermometer to take the temperature and used a hand lens to study the patient's excretions. The examination was not along anatomical lines, the condition of

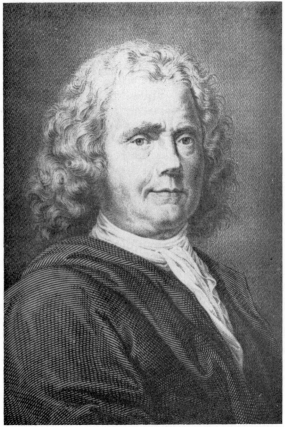

Sigerist, *Grosse Ärzte*, München, 1932

HERMANN BOERHAAVE

the individual organs not being studied since percussion and auscultation were unknown and microscopic examinations of the blood
and urine still poorly understood. The students studied the general
state of the patient, the severity and prognosis of the disease, together with the treatment indicated. "On 12 beds half the physicians
of Europe were trained!" (Sigerist).

About 1725, Boerhaave developed gout, which became so painful
that, in 1729, he gave up his courses in botany and chemistry but
continued his bedside teaching until his death nine years later.

Boerhaave made no great discoveries in medicine, as did some of
his contemporaries. His writings, which had a great vogue in their

day, show little originality, are largely forgotten, and do not number among the eighteenth century books still read with interest and profit. Yet, his influence on medicine was lasting. The methods of instruction he introduced at Leyden became a model for all Europe, the foundation of modern clinical teaching. Equally important was his influence through the illustrious pupils he trained.

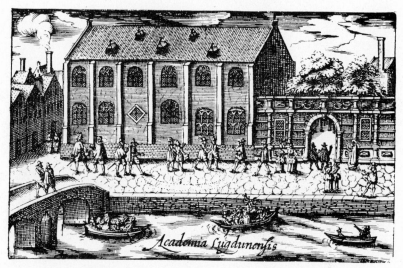

THE UNIVERSITY OF LEYDEN IN THE SEVENTEENTH CENTURY
From Meurs, Joannes, *Athenae Batavae*, Leyden, Elsivir, 1625.

ALBRECHT VON HALLER

The most eminent of Boerhaave's pupils was Albrecht von Haller, called by Garrison "the greatest systematist after Galen and one of the most imposing figures in all medical history." Like Galen, he came upon the medical scene at a period when rival sects, the Iatro-physicists and Iatro-chemists, like the Dogmatists, Empiricists and Methodists of Galen's time, were trying to dominate medical science. Like Galen, Haller refused to follow the theories of any one school but based his medicine upon the foundations of anatomic and physiologic observations and experiments. Again, there is a similarity in the reverence with which many of his followers regarded his work, which they considered as so complete and so nearly perfect that further progress was scarcely possible.

Haller was born at Bern in 1708 and early showed unmistakable

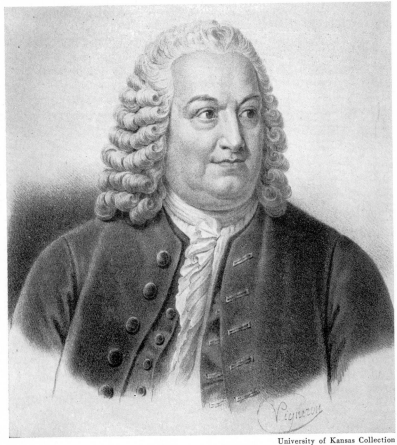

ALBRECHT VON HALLER

Lithograph by Vigneron after the well-known engraving of Bause, 1773.

signs of great intellectual capacity. At the age of nine, he wrote Latin verses, composed a Greek and Hebrew dictionary, wrote brief biographies of more than 2,000 persons, and showed great talent as a poet. He began the study of medicine at Tübingen at the age of 15 and then went to Leyden, where he studied under Albinus and Boerhaave. The latter he almost worshipped and never ceased to eulogize. He received his doctor's degree at the age of 19, writing a dissertation in which he disproved the contention of Professor von Coschwitz of Halle that the lingual vein was a salivary duct.

After graduation, he went to London and, later, to Paris, where he studied under Winslow. In 1728, he went to Basel, where he studied under the mathematician Bernoulli and, the following year, returned to Bern, and began the practice of medicine. He was not very successful as a practitioner, however, because the good burghers of his native city seemed skeptical that such a learned man could be a good doctor. He had much leisure time, which he used in anatomical and physiological researches, in collecting botanical specimens, and in writing poetry. In 1732, he published anonymously his first poetical work, *Versuch Schweizerischer Gedichte*. This was received by the public with great enthusiasm and established his place in the history of German literature.

In 1736, Haller's fame as anatomist, physiologist and botanist had grown so great that he was called to the newly founded University of Göttingen as professor of anatomy, botany and medicine. He accepted the offer and remained at Göttingen for 17 years, teaching all branches of medicine, establishing botanical gardens, carrying on innumerable anatomical and physiological researches, working on medical and scientific bibliography, and writing some 1300 scientific papers. Various universities, including Berlin and Oxford, extended calls to him. In 1753, he felt unequal to the increasing duties of his position, possibly because of "homesickness, which sooner or later attacks every Swiss in a foreign country" (Sigerist), resigned his position at Göttingen, to the astonishment of the learned world, and returned to Bern. Here he spent the rest of his days, not as he had hoped in retirement and leisure, but as public health officer of Bern and a great savant. He carried on one of the most gigantic correspondences in the history of science, the letters of his correspondents, now bound, filling several shelves in the Library of Bern. He died in 1777.

"One really does not know, Sudhoff remarks,

what one should marvel at more in Haller, his genius as an investigator who revealed new truths to us, his erudition which made him familiar with not only all branches of natural science, but with the literature of esthetics and belles-lettres, or his unbelievable productivity.

Wilhelm Scherer, author of a notable history of German literature, comments, "He was equally distinguished as a man of learning, a critic and a poet." He was equally eminent as an anatomist, physiologist, botanist, medical historian, and poet.

It is very difficult even to approximate the number of Haller's writings. As editor of the *Göttinger gelehrten Anzeigen*, he wrote more than 1,200 reviews. Snebier, in his *Eloge historique d'Albert de Haller,* lists 576 items. Haller himself, in his *Bibliotheca anatomica,* summarizes 195 of his treatises on anatomical and physiological topics. Haeser lists his "important" works to the number of 49. They include two encyclopedic works, four works on anatomy, 12 on physiology, seven on botany, five on bibliography, one book of poetry, four historical novels, and two books on theology.

The first scientific medical work done by Haller was in anatomy, his interest in this field having been stimulated by his old teacher Albinus. His chief works in this field were his *Icones anatomicae,* Göttingen, 1756, and his *Opera minora anatomici,* Lausanne, 1762. Not only were these books models of clear, concise and accurate description, but the illustrations, as Choulant remarked, "are very clear, vivid, highly exact, and artistic . . . emphasizing perfect pictorial representation of anatomic subjects." Choulant praises the *Icones* very highly noting, "This work will always remain the main source of information for accurate anatomic studies, especially of the arteries and the viscera."

The study made by Haller in embryology was noteworthy, being the most important contribution to that subject from the time of Malpighi, the first to employ the microscope extensively in embryology, to that of von Baer, who described the mammalian ovum in 1827. Haller, who began his work as an embryologist, believing in epigenesis—that organs are successively formed out of the indifferent matter in the egg—decided, from his own researches, in favor of preformation and made the remarkable statement, "The ovary of an ancestress will contain not only her daughter, but also her granddaughter, her great-granddaughter, and her great-great-granddaughter." His most valuable work in embryology was his investigation of the growth rate of the embryo, an entirely original line of research, which remains one of the most fundamental contributions to the science of embryology.

Haller's physiological works number 12, the most important of which was his *Elementa physiologiae corporis humani,* in eight volumes, first published in Lausanne, 1757-1766. "When we turn from any of the preceding writers on physiology . . . ," as Foster observed, "and open the pages of Haller's *Elementa,* we feel that we have passed into modern times." All the phenomena of the body are studied, each section describing the anatomy of the parts with data on their minute structure, physical properties, and chemical composition. In this work, we find many physiologic discoveries later forgotten and rediscovered, two notable examples being the myogenic theory of the heart beat and the role of bile in the digestion of fat.

The greatest contribution made by Haller to physiology was his demonstration that irritability is a specific property of all muscular tissues and that sensibility is the exclusive property of nervous tissue. "This classic research, based on 567 experiments, of which he himself performed 190, was made at Göttingen in 1757" (Garrison).

Haller's botanical works, while limited to a study of the plants he collected in Switzerland and at Göttingen, bore the stamp of his remarkable mind and raised him to the rank of one of the greatest botanists of his time, surpassed only by Linné. He had the conception of new "natural" classification of plants based on the habitat, the composition of fruits and seeds, rather than along the somewhat artificial lines upon which Linné based his classification. He planned an elaborate botanical work with his system as its basis, but the press of other work was too great, and he could never find sufficient time to carry out this project.

His work on medical bibliography was an ambitious undertaking, which he did not live to finish. The first of these works was the *Bibliotheca botanica,* 1771-1772, followed by the *Bibliotheca medicae pars botanica,* 1771; *Bibliotheca anatomica,* 1774-1777; *Bibliotheca chirurgica,* 1774-1775, each work in two volumes; and the *Bibliotheca medicinae practicae,* 1776-1788, in four volumes, the fourth volume appearing after his death. These books contain an exhaustive summary of the important works in each field, with a biographical sketch of the author, all written with the clarity, judiciousness and accuracy so characteristic of Haller. This *Bibliotheca,* as the work of a single author, still remains the most impressive monument of scholarship in the history of medicine. At the time of his death, the manuscript of a history of medicine was found but has never been published.

GERHARD VAN SWIETEN

Another famous pupil of Boerhaave was Gerhard van Swieten, a Hollander, who was born at Leyden in 1700, studied first at Louvain and then at Leyden, where he received his doctor's degree in 1725. He was a favorite pupil of Boerhaave, who employed him as an assistant in the chemical laboratory and saw patients with him. Van Swieten had become expert in the Ramsay system of shorthand and took down, word for word, Booerhaave's commentaries on patients, which he later published in his *Commentaria.*

In 1744, van Swieten was called in consultation to see the Empress Maria Theresa's sister, who was ill in Brussels. He was unable

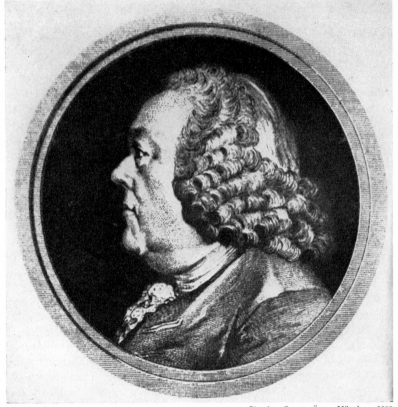

Sigerist, *Grosse Ärzte*, München, 1932

GERHARD VAN SWIETEN

to save the life of the patient but made such a deep impression that th Empress offered him the post of her personal physician in 1745. Van Swieten was already recognized as the ablest of Boerhaave's assistants and as the logical successor to Boerhaave's chair. He was, however, a Roman Catholic, which seemed an insurmountable barrier in strongly Protestant Leyden. After some deliberation, he accepted the post as physician to the Empress in Vienna. Here he began to lecture on anatomy, physiology, pathology and medicine, not in the University since he was not a professor, but in the Court Library, the director of which he had become. His lectures attracted large numbers of medical students, who spread his fame as an inspiring teacher and a skillful clinician.

Three years later, Maria Theresa appointed van Swieten *"Praeses,"* or president of the medical faculty, and charged him with the task of reforming the school of medicine. The University of Vienna, although, next to Prague, the oldest German university, had not, from the date of its founding in 1365, played any role in the development of medicine. Anatomy was poorly taught; there was no botanical garden, no chemical laboratory, no clinic. The professors were poorly paid and of mediocre caliber.

The reorganization of the medical school carried out by van Swieten was drastic. The school was placed under the direct control of the state with van Swieten as representative. The professors were appointed, not by the faculty, but by the Empress on nomination by van Swieten. The salaries of the professors were paid by the state; the dean's appointment had to be confirmed by the state; and the licenses to practice medicine were to be granted by the state. These changes, as can well be imagined, called forth the bitter opposition of the medical faculty, who saw their old prerogatives abolished and their former influence greatly reduced. However, the opposition was unable to checkmate the plans of van Swieten, for behind him stood the powerful empress.

Van Swieten proceeded next to establish a botanical garden, a chemical laboratory, and a new institute of anatomy, and to separate the department of anatomy from that of surgery. New professors were appointed. Dr. Laugier of Nancy was appointed to the chair of botany and chemistry, and later, Nicholas Jacquin, a Hollander from Leyden, succeeded him. To assist in clinical teaching, Anton de Haen, an old colleague of van Swieten's in Leyden, was appointed professor of practical medicine. In the Bürgerspital, two wards, one for men and one for women, each containing six beds, was set aside for clinical teaching on the exact model of Leyden. Indeed, the whole reform of medical education was a transplantation of the Leyden plan to Vienna. The plan succeeded admirably. Vienna now took her rank as a first class medical school. The school created by van Swieten has since been called by history the First Vienna School, or the Old Vienna School.

The reformation of the medical school had its effect upon the entire university, and a reorganization of the philosophical and theological faculties took place. The changes in the theological faculty were fought bitterly, especially by the Jesuits, who became van Swieten's bitter enemies. Van Swieten, in turn, hoped to accomplish the dissolution of the Jesuit order, but in this he was unsuccessful. Nevertheless, he was successful in his attempt to alter the dominant

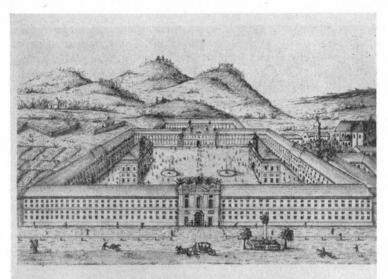

Das „Große Armenhaus" in der Alservorstadt (1695)

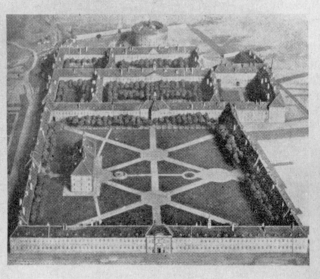

Allgemeines Krankenhaus 1784

Schönbauer, *Das Medizinische Wien*, Vienna, 1947

THE UPPER ILLUSTRATION SHOWS THE *GROSSES ARMENHAUS* OF VIENNA
IN 1695, WHICH, IN 1784, BECAME THE WORLD FAMOUS
ALLGEMEINES KRANKENHAUS

clerical tone of the medical school; and following his suggestion, the conferring of degrees took place in the halls of the University instead of in St. Stephen's Cathedral, where they had previously been held with religious ceremonies, which included an oath of the candidates that they believed in the teachings of the Catholic Church and in the Immaculate Conception of the Virgin. Despite van Swieten's hostility to the Church hierarchy, he remained a good Catholic, went to mass daily, and, in 1759, was appointed president of the Commission for the Censorship of Books. The library at Vienna contains a list of the books reviewed by van Swieten—3,120 books, 595 of which he marked *"damnatur"*—condemned. Among these books are works by Lessing and Voltaire.

These manifold activities of van Swieten left him little time for writing, and his only medical work of note was his *Commentaria in Hermani Boerhaave aphorisomos,* 1754-1775, in five volumes. This work is written in a Hippocratic manner, describing cases and avoiding all speculation. The chapters on fevers, syphilis, rheumatic fever and exanthemata are masterpieces. In addition to being an excellent clinician, he was a man of deep sympathies and innate kindliness, whose services to the poor and unfortunate were proverbial. He was a bitter opponent of the Rosicrucians, alchemists, quacks and charlatans, "whose ovens he destroyed, whose books he burned and whom he wished to chase out of the country." In 1758, the grateful Empress Maria Theresa created him a baron. He died in 1772, to the great grief of the Empress.

Although primarily an organizer, van Swieten was also an outstanding student and a man of tremendous industry. In addition to his native Dutch, he spoke Latin, Greek, French, German, Italian, Spanish, English and Hungarian. He found Vienna a disorganized, poorly equipped and second rate medical school and raised it, mainly by his own efforts, to the rank of one of the leading schools of Europe.

ANTON DE HAEN

Anton de Haen, who succeeded van Swieten, was born in The Hague in 1704. He was another pupil of Boerhaave and, on van Swieten's recommendation, had been appointed professor of practical medicine at Vienna in 1756. De Haen was an excellent physician and teacher. He developed clinical teaching to a perfection previously unknown. Very careful, meticulous histories were taken of each patient, the patient was carefully inspected, the urine and blood were examined, and then all the evidence was reviewed in

These variations depend on the cause which can diminish or increase the volume of air commonly in the thoracic cavity.

Such a cause whether it be in a solid or a liquid mass produces what we observe for example in casks, which, when they are empty, resound at all points; but, when filled, lose just so much of this resonance as the volume of air which they contain has been diminished.

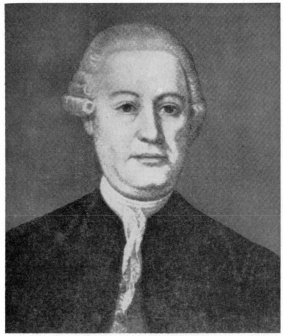

University of Kansas Collection

LEOPOLD AUENBRUGGER

Oil portrait in the possession of the Gesellschaft der Ärzte in Vienna.

In this work, Auenbrugger describes the technique of percussion, which he performed "slowly and gently with the tips of the fingers brought close together and extended." He describes the sounds given by the normal chest as well as in hydrothorax, in cavities, in hydro-pericardium, and in cardiac enlargement. His great discovery attracted little attention. His chief and revered teacher, van Swieten, wrote not a syllable on the subject, and his colleague, de Haen, like-wise said nothing. Maximilian Stoll, who succeeded de Haen as di-rector of the medical clinic, tried out the new method and praised it in his work, *Praelectiones in diversos morbos chronicos,* Vienna, 1788. Then we hear no more of it for a time. Haller praised it, and Prof. Christian G. Ludwig of Leipzig spoke of it as "a torch which would bring light into the darkness of chest diseases." In 1770, Rogières de la Chassagnac translated it into French and published it as a supplement to his own *Manuel des pulmoniques,* but remarked that he himself had never tried the new method.

Near the end of the eighteenth century, Jean Nicolas Corvisart, studying the works of Stoll, found a reference to Auenbrugger's discovery and began practicing the new method of percussion. In 1808, he published a French translation of Auenbrugger, stating in the preface:

I could have raised myself to the rank of author by revamping the work of Auenbrugger, and by publishing a work on percussion. But by that, I should sacrifice the name of Auenbrugger to my own vanity. I have not wished that; it is he, it is his beautiful and legitimate discovery (*inventum novum,* as he says justly) which I have wished to make live again.

The fame of Corvisart and the excellence of his translation carried the news of the discovery, now 47 years old, and the name of Auenbrugger throughout the medical world. Auenbrugger died the following year.

GIOVANNI BATTISTA MORGAGNI

The same year that Auenbrugger's *Inventum Novum* appeared, another work was published, destined also to have a profound influence on medicine. This work, *De sedibus et causis morborum* (The Seats and Causes of Diseases), by Giovanni Battista Morgagni did not, however, wait 47 years for approval and recognition.

Giovanni Battista Morgagni was born in Forli in 1682. He was a precocious youth and, at the early age of 14, wrote poetry and essays and discussed publicly problems of philosophy. In 1701, at the age of 19, he received his medical degree at Bologna, where he was a favorite pupil of Valsalva. He devoted himself to anatomy and, at the age of 24, published his first work, *Adversaria anatomica prima,* 1706, which contained an excellent description of the larynx and corrected many previous anatomical errors. In 1711, he was appointed professor of practical medicine at Padua, and, four years later, the university authorities, on the advice of Lancisi, appointed him professor of anatomy. In an address made after receiving this appointment, he remarked that he was overwhelmed by the thought of holding the same chair that had been filled by Vesalius, Realdo

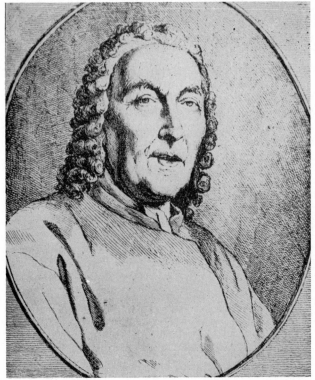

GIOVANNI BATTISTA MORGAGNI
Engraving by Angela Kauffman.

Colombo, Falloppio, Fabrizi, Vesling and Molinetti. He proved
himself worthy of his illustrious predecessors.

He soon became a popular teacher, attracting not only Italian
students but also foreigners, particularly Germans, who came in
large numbers to attend his lectures and his demonstrations. The
second volume of his *Adversaria anatomica* appeared in 1717, and
his *Adversaria anatomica omnia* came out in 1719. These works
established his reputation as an anatomist, as a scholar of great intellectual capacity, and as a master of Latin prose. It was, however, his
De sedibus et causis morborum, a work first published in 1761, when
the author was 79 years of age, that inscribed his name among the
greatest in the history of medicine. He has justly received the title of
the "Father of Pathology."

The *De sedibus* was begun, so Morgagni tells us, with the idea of correcting and improving Bonet's *Sepulchretum* by the addition of his own material and that of Valsalva. Bonet's work he found poorly arranged, repetitious, lacking a satisfactory index, and, worst of all, inaccurate, as he discovered on looking up the original sources. Encouraged by a young friend, whose name he fails to mention, he began writing his own observations, which he circulated among his colleagues in the form of letters. Encouraged further by the enthusiastic reception they found, he decided to write his own treatise.

Morgagni's *De sedibus et causis morborum per anatomen indagatis*, translated by Benjamin Alexander in 1769 with the title, *The Seats and Causes of Diseases investigated by Anatomy*, remains one of the imperishable books of medical literature. Many authors previously had recorded the results of autopsy findings in an attempt to explain the cause of death. But here, for the first time, we find a vast array of pathological findings, well arranged and indexed, each preceded by a minute history of the disease, the symptoms present, the treatment employed, and finally a discussion of the relationship between the clinical picture and the autopsy findings. Morgagni's knowledge of the literature of the subject is apparent on every page, where he discusses previous articles on the subject and meticulously gives each author due credit for his own observations. He often begins with Aristotle and reviews the entire literature down to his own time. These reviews demonstrate Morgagni's ability as a historian.

The number of pathological states described by Morgagni, many of them for the first time, is enormous. He described syphilitic aneurysms, acute yellow atrophy of the liver, pneumonia with consolidation of the lungs, meningitis due to acute otitis, hyperostosis frontalis, cancer of the stomach, gastric ulcer, gall stones, endocarditis, mitral stenosis, aortic insufficiency, pulmonary stenosis, coronary sclerosis, the tetralogy of Fallot, coarctation of the aorta, and regional ileitis. He gives the first description of cerebral gummata and of heart block, which he speaks of as "epilepsy with a slow pulse." Here also we gain an insight into his theory of medicine. In most instances, he follows the Iatro-mechanical theories of Borelli although at times he speaks of chemical changes and sometimes suggests that mechanical and chemical causes act synergistically. He also believed in contagion, refused to dissect the bodies of persons who had died of tuberculosis or of smallpox, and, in the case of rabies, recognized clearly the presence of a specific agent or, as he termed it, "a peculiar species of poison." His greatest contribution of all was that he, as Virchow remarked, introduced the "anatomical concept" into medical practice. He pursued the investigation of disease from its symptoms to the organ from which the symptom arose and then demonstrated the disease in the organ concerned. "With him," said Virchow, "begins modern medicine."

It would be a mistake, however, to consider Morgagni solely as a pathologist who spent his entire professional career in the autopsy room seeking the causes of death. In addition to being a true scholar, a historian, and a philosopher, he carried out a large number of physiological experiments and was also active as a practitioner of medicine and as a clinical consultant. In 1935, for the first time, his *Consulti Medici* was published in Bologna by Enrico Benassi, who found twelve large volumes of unpublished manuscript written by Morgagni in the library at Parma. The consultations, one hundred in number, record Morgagni's advice on the diagnosis and treatment of patients referred to him by other physicians or often advice based on the physician's letters regarding patients he did not see personally. These consultations reveal Morgagni as a clear and cogent reasoner, but, when placed by the side of his *De sedibus,* they pale and suffer by comparison. It is his *De sedibus* that places him among the greatest physicians of all times. He died in 1771 at the age of 89.

The University of Leyden, with Boerhaave as its chief luminary, was by common consent the leading medical center at the beginning of the eighteenth century. Boerhaave's famous pupils had spread his reputation far and wide. Haller's influence on medicine knew neither national nor geographical boundaries; van Swieten and de Haen had re-founded the medical school of Vienna. Leyden attracted many students from the British Isles, among them Richard Mead, William Hillary, and John Huxham. With Edinburgh and its newly founded medical school, its relations were particularly close.

THE EDINBURGH MEDICAL SCHOOL

The Medical School of the University of Edinburgh was established in 1685, Dr. Archibald Pitcairne (1652-1713) being regarded as its founder. He was one of the original members of the Royal College of Physicians of Edinburgh, which was incorporated in 1681, and, four years later, he was made professor of medicine in Town's College, which now began to be called the University of Edinburgh. In 1692, he was called to Leyden as professor of medicine and, while a teacher there, taught the celebrated Boerhaave himself. Later he returned to Edinburgh.

Much of the early fame of the Edinburgh Medical School was

linked with the names of the three Alexander Monros. Alexander Monro *primus* (1697-1767) was the son of John Monro, an old army surgeon, who had been a pupil of Pitcairne's at Leyden. Alexander Monro *primus*, who was a pupil of Boerhaave, was appointed professor of anatomy in 1720 at the age of 22 and held the chair until he was succeeded by his son, Alexander Monro *secundus* (1733-1817) in 1758. Alexander Monro *secundus* was succeeded by his son, Alexander Monro *tertius* in 1808, who held the chair until 1846. Thus, the Monro dynasty held the chair of anatomy at Edinburgh from 1714 until 1846, a period of 126 years. During the tenure of Monro *primus* and *secundus,* some 13,000 medical students had been taught by either father or son. Monro *primus* was a gifted teacher and a skillful anatomist. Monro *secundus* was also an excellent teacher and carried out many anatomical investigations on the lymphatics and the nervous system. He described the connection between the lateral and third ventricles, since called the foramen of Monro. Monro *tertius* was less successful either as an anatomist or as a teacher. Charles Darwin, a student of this Alexander at Edinburgh, remarked that he "made his lectures on human anatomy as dull as he was himself."

William Cullen, a colleague of Monro *primus* and Monro *secundus,* was an outstanding teacher at Edinburgh and, according to Bostock writing in 1834, "contributed, in no small degree, to raise Edinburgh to the rank, which it long held, of the first medical school in Europe." Cullen was born in Hamilton in 1710 and, after studying at the University of Glasgow, which had no medical school at the time, was apprenticed to a surgeon in Glasgow for two years. Following this, he went to sea for two years, practiced for a time in Scotland and northern England, studied at the new Edinburgh Medical School for two years, and then began practice at Hamilton, where he took as an apprentice a youth who became later the celebrated Dr. William Hunter. Determined to obtain an M.D. degree, Cullen presently went to Glasgow, where he received his degree in 1740. He settled in Glasgow and became professor of medicine but, in 1755, went to Edinburgh as professor of chemistry. He finally became co-professor of medicine and, in 1773, sole professor. He was at this time 63 years of age and had already built up a large, lucrative, and aristocratic consulting practice in Edinburgh.

Cullen was an excellent teacher, clear, forceful, logical, vivacious and interesting. He not only interested his students but inspired them with enthusiasm to study and learn. He drew students to Edinburgh, particularly English-speaking students from England

and the Colonies, as Boerhaave had once drawn them to Leyden.
His first work that brought him fame was his *Synopsis nosologiae
methodicae,* 1769, a rigid classification of diseases by their symptoms
on the same arbitrary principle Linné had adopted for classifying
plants. All diseases are arranged by classes, orders, genera and species

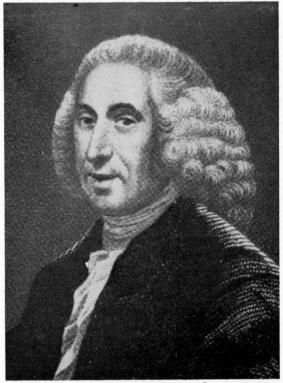

Sigerist, *Grosse Ärzte*, München, 1932

WILLIAM CULLEN

and regarded as fixed entities. While this system is unnatural, it
seemed logical at the time, greatly simplified medicine, and established Cullen's reputation during his life time. His *First Lines on
the Practice of Physick,* 1776-1789, which was subsequently translated into French and German, exerted a profound influence not
only in England and in the Colonies but on the Continent as well.
    The point of view adopted by Cullen stood midway between
Stahl's conception of the *anima,* or "sentient soul," and Boerhaave's

more materialistic Iatro-mechanical views. He also accepted Haller's views on irritability and, at times, his teaching showed a resemblance to Hoffmann's doctrine of increased and decreased tonus. According to Cullen, the nervous system is the source of life, the regulator of all vital phenomena. The diseased nervous system can be either too strong—spasm—or too weak—atony.

Cullen was considered an authority on fevers. Pyrexiae, or febrile diseases, he stated "form a class which may be subdivided into the five orders of Fevers, Inflammations, Eruptions, Hemorrhagies and Fluxes." He divided fevers into "Synocha," fever with a strong inflammatory reaction; "Typhus," fever with a weak reaction; and "the most common form of continued fevers . . . a combination of the two genera mentioned . . . and we have therefore given such a genus a place in our Nosology, under the title of Synochus." When the fever has a strong reaction, he employs antispasmodics; when the fever is due to "the weaker energy of the brain," he advises stimulants.

The views held by Cullen on the cause and treatment of the gout attracted much attention and were considered almost oracular. He denied the presence of any "morbific matter." "Gout," he states, "is manifestly an affection of the nervous system," and "the stomach and other internal parts relapse into the state of atony." For the treatment, he advocates bodily exercise, "abstinence from animal food and fermented liquors," blood-letting, antiplogistics, blistering, Peruvian bark, Portland powder (birthwort and gentian) and opiates.

Cullen died in 1790, famous as a teacher and consultant, beloved as a man. John Bostock, whose father had been a favorite pupil of Cullen and who himself had graduated at Edinburgh, wrote, "No one produced a more powerful and lasting effect upon the state of medicine, in all its branches, both theoretical and practical, than Cullen." As a delineator of disease, he was considered by Bostock "as rivalling Sydenham or any of his distinguished predecessors." Modern students of medicine understand with difficulty why Cullen was such a towering figure in his age. His *Nosology*, which he regarded as his masterpiece, was soon forgotten after his death; his theories of disease soon had only an antiquarian interest. Most historians agree with the verdict of Sir William Hamilton, "Cullen did not add a single new fact to medical science" (Garrison).

While Cullen loved theories to illustrate his remarks, he never was a slave even to his own system and was wont to say, "There must be a tub to amuse the whale." His pupil and secretary, John Brown, was of a very different temperament.

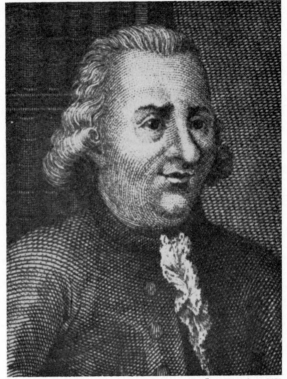

Sigerist, *Grosse Ärzte*, München, 1932

JOHN BROWN

JOHN BROWN AND THE BRUNONIANS

John Brown was born in 1735-36 of poor parents and was apprenticed early to a weaver. Later, showing signs of much mental ability, he was sent to the grammar school at Dunse, where he studied the classics and theology. He entered the University of Edinburgh destined for the ministry but later studied medicine, supporting himself, it was said, by translating the medical theses of the graduates and the writings of the professors into Latin. He also became well known as a teacher of Latin. He soon made a most favorable impression on Cullen, who gave him employment as a private instructor in his own family. He afterwards quarreled with Cullen, wrote a rival treatise on medicine, his *Elementa Medicinae*, 1778, in which he announced a new theory of medicine, and began to lecture on his system.

This theory of Brown was essentially that of Asklepiades and of the ancient medical sect, the Methodists, to which he added some ideas of his own and some obviously derived from Haller. The quality or principle, he taught, on which the phenomena of life depend is excitability. The "exciting powers," or stimuli, may be divided into two classes—the external stimuli, "heat, diet and other substances taken into the stomach, the blood, the fluids secreted from the blood, and air"; the internal stimuli, "muscular contraction, sense or perception, and the energy of the brain in thinking and in exciting passion and emotion." Furthermore, these "stimuli are either universal or local." *"Life is a forced state;* if the exciting powers are withdrawn, death ensues as certainly as when the excitability is gone." Health is a condition of moderate excitability. Disease results from a local or general increase or decrease of excitability. Diseases fall into two main groups—"sthenic," where there is increased excitability; "asthenic," where there is decreased excitability. Therapy was relatively simple: sedatives for "sthenic" diseases, stimulants for "asthenic" diseases.

This theory was simple and direct and soon had many adherents, as well as a greater number of bitter enemies. The Brunonians, as Brown's followers were called, like their leader, were noisy, argumentative, and not averse to brawls. Brown, who gave lectures while still a student of medicine, after attending 10 sessions of medicine at Edinburgh, went to the University of St. Andrews, which awarded him a degree although he had never studied there. He was at this time 44 years of age. As a lecturer, he attracted many students, but his biographer, Beddoes, says:

His voice was in general hoarse and almost croaking. . . . Before he began his lecture, he would take 40 or 50 drops of laudanum in a glass of whisky; repeating the dose four or five times during the lecture. Between the effects of these stimulants and voluntary exertion, he soon waxed warm, and by degrees his imagination was exalted into phrenzy.

Brown's favorite remedies were laudanum and whisky. He presently became addicted to both and was "committed to prison for debt, where his pupils attended his lectures." He gave up whisky in 1775, and, as Beddoes relates, "after some perseverance in this experiment of abstemiousness, he returned to the bottle and never afterward relinquished it." In 1786, Brown left Edinburgh for London, where he hoped to establish himself as a physician and also lecture to students. Two years later during the night, he died, after having taken a very large dose of laudanum.

The Brunonian system aroused the passions of the medical profession in a way they had not been aroused since the days of Paracelsus. While Brown himself lectured in Edinburgh, there was constant warfare between the Brunonians and the Cullenites. They fought with tongues, fists and cudgels and, at times, challenged each other to duels until the University decreed expulsion for fighting a duel. With the departure of Brown, the tumult subsided. Brown made relatively few converts in Great Britain although, in the Colonies, Benjamin Rush of Philadelphia accepted some of his theories. In France, he found few adherents, but, in Germany "in the famous land of theories . . . the new system found its second home" (Baas). At the University of Göttingen, the Brunonians, led by a young professor, staged a revolt against the authorities, seized the town hall, and were dispersed only by a troop of Hanoverian horses.

Two Scotchmen of this period, both identified with Edinburgh, made important contributions to medical progress of more lasting value than either Cullen or Brown. They were Sir John Pringle and James Lind.

John Pringle was born in Roxburghshire in 1707, studied first at St. Andrews and then at Edinburgh but, being intended for a commercial career, went to Amsterdam to enter business. During a casual visit to Leyden, he heard a lecture by Boerhaave and was so deeply impressed that he decided to study medicine. He entered the Medical School at Leyden, graduated in 1730, and settled in Edinburgh. In 1742, he went to Flanders with the British Army and was placed in charge of a military hospital and served with the army until the Treaty of Aix-la-Chapelle in 1748. He then settled in London, where he became a Fellow of the College of Physicians and president of the Royal Society, was created a baronet, and was appointed physician to the king.

"Few members of our profession," wrote Munk, "have obtained a wider reputation than did Sir John Pringle." Posterity remembers him as the author of *Observations on the Diseases of the Army,* London, 1752, in which he laid down the true principles of military sanitation and stressed the importance of proper ventilation. This work has earned for him the title of "the founder of modern military medicine." He mentions the historic suggestion of the Earl of Stair to the French general, the Duke of Noailles, "that the hospitals on both sides should be considered as sanctuaries for the sick. . . . This agreement was strictly observed on both sides all that campaign." He also recognized the value of antisepsis, and, in his paper, *Experiments and Observations upon Septic and Aseptic Substance,*

published as an appendix to the *Observations,* he described the effect
of various chemicals in checking putrefaction. He gave an excellent
description of typhus fever, proving that jail fever and hospital
fever are the same; i.e., typhus fever, and described accurately the
various forms of dysentery. Scurvy, a disease of which he saw much
in the army, he found, however, "more peculiar to marshy countries
and arising "from a putrid cause."

Scurvy had been the enemy of soldiers and seamen for untold
centuries. The soldiers in the Fifth Crusade at the siege of Damietta
(1219) suffered severely from the ravages of scurvy. In the sixteenth
century (1536), the intrepid explorer and navigator, Jacques Cartier,

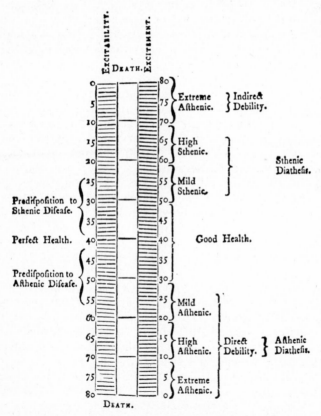

BROWN'S CHART OF STHENIC AND ASTHENIC STATES
From John Brown's, *Elements of Medicine,* Philadelphia, Spottswood, 1791.

landed on the Gaspé Peninsula in Canada, discovered and navigated the St. Lawrence River, but was almost compelled to abandon his expedition because of an outbreak of scurvy among his men. Hearing that the Indians cured this disease with a decoction of the "Ameda" tree (probably sassafras or spruce), he employed that remedy with great success and wrote enthusiastically, "If all the physicians of Louvain and of Montpellier had been there, with all the drugs of Alexandria, they could not have done as much in a year as that tree did in six days." Later medical authors described the disease in great detail, some believing it due to climate and faulty diet, others considering it a contagious disease. It was reported in Flanders, Holland, Germany, England, and throughout Europe. Sir Richard Hawkins (1562-1622) of the British Navy wrote that "in 20 years, during which he used the sea, he could give an account of 10,000 mariners who had been consumed by the scurvy alone." With good reason, this disease became known among seafaring men as the "calamity of sailors."

The true nature of scurvy, which scourged the King's Army and Navy, was discovered by James Lind. Lind was born in Edinburgh in 1716, became apprenticed to a surgeon at the age of 15 and, at the age of 23, entered the navy, serving as a surgeon for nine years and seeing service in the English Channel, in the Mediterranean, off the Guinea Coast, and in the West Indies. During these voyages, he saw many tropical diseases and became interested in naval hygiene. He left the navy in 1748, received the M.D. degree from the University of Edinburgh the same year, and began the practice of medicine in Edinburgh. In 1758, he left there to become physician to the Haslar Hospital, a naval hospital near Portsmouth, where he worked for 25 years, resigning in 1783. He died in 1794.

Three noteworthy books were written by Lind. They are *A Treatise of the Scurvy*, Edinburgh, 1753; *An Essay on the most Effectual Means of Preserving the Health of Seamen in the Royal Navy*, London, 1757; and *An Essay on Diseases incidental to Europeans in Hot Climates*, London, 1768—three classics in the literature of scurvy, naval hygiene, and tropical diseases. His work on scurvy recommended the use of lemon juice in its prevention and cure, a method of treatment which he later used with great success at the Haslar Hospital, where he usually had 300 to 400 cases of scurvy under his care and often 1,000 at a time. *Lind died 41 years after the publication of his A Treatise of the Scurvy, without seeing any of his suggestions officially adopted by the British Navy. The year*

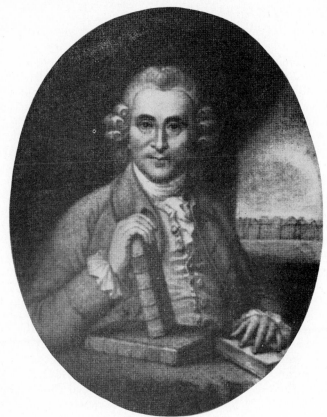

Edinburgh Medical Journal, 1926

JAMES LIND
Portrait by Sir George Chalmers.

of his death, a small squadron sailing for the East Indies was given an adequate supply of lemon juice and arrived at Madras 23 weeks later without a single case of scurvy on board. Two years thereafter, lemon juice was added to the rations of the sailors, and scurvy disappeared from the British Navy.

Lind's *Essay on the Jail Distemper,* which is included in his work on naval hygiene, recommends the destruction of clothing and bedding of patients suffering from typhus fever. He cites several incidents to prove his contention that typhus fever is transmitted by fomites.

BRITISH PHYSICIANS AND SURGEONS

In England there were at this period several outstanding physicians and surgeons who, leaving theories to the Cullenites and to the Brunonians, studied disease at the bedside and wrote down their observations and conclusions in the true Hippocratic spirit. William Heberden (1710-1801), a graduate of Cambridge and one of the best Latin and Hebrew scholars of his time, was a man of wide learning and culture. Dr. Samuel Johnson called him, "Dr. Heberden, *ultimus Romanorum,* the last of our learned physicians." His *Commentaries on the History and Cure of Diseases,* written in Latin and translated into English by his son, William Heberden, Jr., appeared simultaneously in Latin and in English in 1802, the year after the author's death. This work contains the first clear description of angina pectoris, one of the earliest accounts of chickenpox in English, a description of "Heberden's nodes" and of nyctalopia. Herberden's writings are distinguished by their clarity of diction, their accurate delineation of disease pictures, and their sanity in treatment, all in marked contrast to the vague verbosity which characterizes so many medical works of this period.

Sir George Baker (1722-1809), a graduate of Cambridge, successful practitioner in London, physician to the royal household, and nine times president of the Royal College, was a keen clinician and a scholar who "had few equals and no superior" (Munk). "If it was desired," said Macmichael, "to know all that had ever been said or written on the subject from the most remote antiquity down to the case in question, a consultation was proposed with Sir George Baker. From his erudition everything was expected." In 1767, he read his famous *Inquiry concerning the cause of the Endemial Colic of Devonshire* before the Royal College of Physicians. He noted that the colic was very common in Devon but rare in Hereford, that the farmers in Devon used lead-lined cider presses, that he could extract lead from the cider of Devon, but none from the cider of Hereford. He was fiercely attacked by his old friends in Devon and assailed from the pulpit as a faithless son of Devon; but the practical farmers removed the lead lining from their cider presses, and the Devonshire colic disappeared.

William Withering (1741-1799), a native of Shropshire, graduated at Edinburgh in 1766 and practiced medicine in Birmingham. His practice became so extensive that he traveled much both by day and by night, and, during these trips, he read and wrote. His carriage was equipped with a light so that he could study while traveling along the countryside at night. An ardent student of botany, his

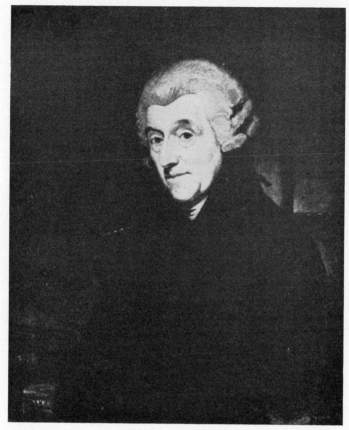

WILLIAM HEBERDEN
From the portrait by Sir William Beechey belonging to the
Royal College of Physicians.

first published work was on this subject, *A Botanical Arrangement
of all the Vegetables naturally growing in Great Britain,* 1766.
Hearing that an old woman in Shropshire had a secret remedy for
the cure of dropsy, he obtained the recipe. "This medicine," he says,
"was composed of 20 or more different herbs, but it was not very
difficult for one conversant with these subjects to perceive that
the active herb could be no other than the Foxglove." He began
to use the Foxglove in his practice and, after 10 years of experience,
published in 1785 *An Account of the Foxglove and Some of its
Medical Uses,* with a beautiful colored plate of the *Digitalis pur-*

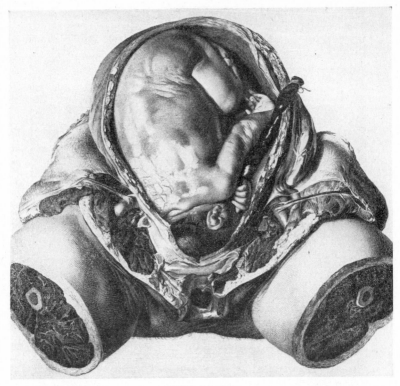

FETUS IN SITU

Illustration from Hunter, William, *The Anatomy of the
Gravid Uterus,* 1774.

purea, outlining his method of administration "proper or improper,
successful or otherwise." "Time," he writes, "will fix the real value
upon this discovery, and determine whether I have imposed upon
myself and others, or contributed to the benefit of science and mankind." Time has long since given its verdict, and digitalis remains
a sheet anchor in the treatment of cardiac disease.

Caleb Hilliard Parry (1755-1822), a native of Gloucestershire, England, graduated in medicine at Edinburgh in 1777 and had a long
and successful career as a practitioner in Bath. He wrote one of
the earliest accounts of angina pectoris, which he attributed to
disease of the coronary arteries. His *Unpublished Medical Writings,*
which appeared three years after his death, contains the first clear
account of exophthalmic goitre, describing eight cases, the first of
which he observed in 1786.

WILLIAM AND JOHN HUNTER

William Hunter, who served three years in Hamilton as the apprentice of William Cullen, when the latter was beginning his medical practice, gravitated towards London, where he achieved as great a reputation as his friend Cullen achieved in Edinburgh.

William Hunter was born at Long Calderwood, Lanarkshire, Scotland, in 1718. In 1731, he went to Glasgow to study for the ministry. He remained there five years, but, having changed his mind, he worked for Cullen and, in 1740, attended Alexander Monro's lectures at Edinburgh. The following year, he went to London, where he lived for a time with Dr. Smellie of Lanark, another Scotchman, who was just beginning his career as an obstetrician. Presently, he became assistant to Dr. John Douglas, an excellent anatomist, and, as a surgical pupil, entered St. George's hospital, where he became an expert dissector. In 1746, he gave lectures in anatomy, which were very popular, and, in 1748, began to practice as an obstetrician, having been appointed one of the "Surgeon-men-midwives" at the Middlesex Hospital. His rise as an obstetrician was rapid, and, in 1762, he delivered Queen Charlotte of a son who afterwards became George IV. He did not, however, give up his anatomical work and, as early as 1746, taught that the lymphatics were an absorbent system and not continuations of the arteries. In 1747, he demonstrated the lachrymal ducts and, in 1752, being now assisted by his brother John, demonstrated the *tubuli seminiferi*. In 1768, he built a house in Great Windmill Street, containing a lecture theatre, dissecting rooms, and a museum. Here he lived until he died in 1783, dissecting, lecturing, and collecting specimens and preparations. He assembled a remarkable collection of pictures, portraits, engravings, books, manuscripts, coins, medals, gems, minerals, corals, shells, and specimens of natural history. This collection he left to the University of Glasgow. Although he had an enormous practice and spent huge sums on his art collection, anatomy, rather than practice or art, was the ruling passion of his life.

The greatest scientific achievement of William Hunter was unquestionably his monumental work, *The Anatomy of the Gravid Uterus*, a labor of 30 years, which appeared in 1774. This work, published by the famous printer, John Baskerville, of Birmingham, contains 34 copperplates, which, to quote Choulant, "represent the gravid uterus and its contents in life-size, anatomically exact and artistically perfect."

However, William Hunter's great achievements were overshad-

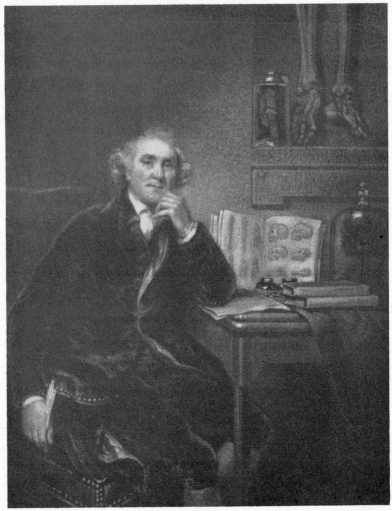

JOHN HUNTER

Engraving from portrait by Sir Joshua Reynolds.

owed by those of his brother, John Hunter, 10 years his junior.
John Hunter was born in 1728, the youngest of 10 children, his
father being 70 years of age at the time and dying when John
was only 10 years of age. As a youth, he was described as indolent
and lazy, spoiled by his indulgent mother, and receiving a very im-

perfect education. Meanwhile, his elder brother, William, had become a renowned anatomist and practitioner in London, so, in 1748, when John was 20, he went to London to work in his brother's dissection room. He soon showed great skill in dissection and for 11 successive winters worked in this dissection room, becoming a more skillful anatomist than William Hunter himself. He made many discoveries, including a demonstration of the branches of the olfactory nerves, the branches of the fifth nerve, previously unknown, the course of the arteries in the gravid uterus, and the presence of lymphatic vessels in birds. Meanwhile, he became a surgeon's pupil in St. George's Hospital and, in 1756, house surgeon.

In 1755, John Hunter went to Oxford but remained there only two months. Speaking later of this experience, he remarked, "They wanted to make an old woman of me, or that I should stuff Latin and Greek at the University; but these schemes I cracked like so many vermin as they came before me." He returned to London and worked once more with his brother in the dissection room, assisted in William's anatomical lectures, and gave some lectures himself. Although William Hunter always mentioned in his lectures the discoveries of John, the younger brother felt that he had not received due credit for his work, and hard feeling developed between the two brothers, which eventually led to a complete estrangement.

The younger man joined the army in 1760, took part in the expedition to Belle Isle, and served in Portugal. This experience gave him "an abundance of surgery; like Ambroise Paré, he began his practice with gunshot wounds" (Paget). He also carried out some physiological experiments, introducing food into a lizard's stomach and finding it did not digest during hibernation. He also tested the hearing of fishes by observing the effects of firing a gun.

On his return to London in 1763, he began practice as a surgeon and lectured on anatomy and surgery. These lectures were not so remunerative as the lectures of his brother William. John was a poor speaker and suffered from serious defects of style and expression, due largely to his inadequate general education. He was very nervous and, at the beginning of each course, "composed himself by a draught of laudanum" (Bettany). He found it extremely difficult to express himself either clearly or elegantly, and, on one occasion while lecturing on gunshot wounds, he remarked that a bullet "having gone into the man's belly and hit his guts such a damned thump that they mortified." Despite his limitations, he was a great teacher and attracted a group of brilliant pupils who later achieved fame, among them Matthew Baillie, Everard Home, Astley Cooper, John Abernethy, Philip Syng Physick, and Edward Jenner, who lived two years in Hunter's house. His pupils were deeply attached to their master and invariably referred to him as "the dear man."

John Hunter's progress in surgery was slow. His yearly income for the first 11 years never reached 1000 pounds, but, with the years, it steadily increased and eventually reached 6000 pounds, a very large sum for those times. Yet, his chief interest in life was not the size of his practice but the museum of natural history which he was collecting. His brother-in-law, Everard Home, says that he always purchased some addition to his collection as soon as he had saved 10 guineas in fees. Eventually, Hunter spent more than 70,000 pounds on his museum. The museum was at first housed in his home but later grew to such proportions that he built a separate building for it. Since he wished to study living animals, to experiment on them, and to observe their habits, he purchased two acres of land about two miles from London, where he built a small house. Here he kept fishes, frogs, leeches, eels, fowls, opossums, hedgehogs, a jackal, a zebra, an ostrich, buffaloes and leopards.

One of the most famous specimens of his museum was the skeleton of the Irish giant, Byrne, or O'Brien, who, learning that Hunter coveted his body, had left instructions that, after death, his body should be placed in a leaden coffin and sunk at sea. Hunter bribed the watchers and finally obtained the body at a cost of 500 pounds although he had to borrow the money to pay the men. Hunter's passion for his museum and his dissection room is illustrated by his oft-quoted remark when he was called, while engaged in a dissection, to see a patient. Dropping his scalpel, he turned to his pupil, Ottley, and said, "Well, Lynn, I must go and earn this damned guinea, or I shall be sure to want it tomorrow."

John Hunter's reputation as an anatomist, naturalist and investigator spread rapidly so that, in 1767, he was elected Fellow of the Royal Society although he had never read a paper before that body. Subsequently, he read papers on digestion of the stomach after death, the torpedo, the production of heat by animals and vegetables, the organ of hearing in fishes, and upon several other topics. In 1768, he was elected surgeon to St. George's Hospital, 20 years after he had first come to London. In 1776, he was appointed surgeon-extraordinary to the king and, in 1789, was appointed Surgeon-General of the army.

In 1767, Hunter inoculated himself with pus from a patient with gonorrhoea to determine whether the poison of gonorrhoea was identical with that producing syphilis. He developed gonorrhoea and also a chancre, whose appearance he described in such a graphic manner that the lesion has since been called "a Hunterian chancre." This lesion was followed by the appearance of inguinal buboes, copper colored spots on the skin, and, Hunter, realizing that he had syphilis, took mercury for three years and considered himself cured. The patient from whom Hunter inoculated himself obviously had both gonorrhoea and syphilis. He had a severe attack of epigastric angina in 1773, and, for the next 20 years, had severe attacks of angina pectoris, brought on many times by anger so that he often remarked that his life was in the hands of any rascal who chose to annoy or tease him. The end came in 1793 at a meeting of the board of St. George's Hospital, when, during a violent dispute, Hunter ceased speaking suddenly and, struggling to control his temper, hurried into an adjoining room, where he uttered a deep groan and fell lifeless into the arms of Dr. Robertson, one of the hospital physicians.

Hunter's four masterpieces were *The Natural History of the Human Teeth,* 1771; *A Treatise on the Venereal Disease,* 1786; *Observations on Certain Parts of the Animal Oeconomy,* 1786; and his *Treatise on the Blood Inflammation and Gun Shot Wounds,* 1794. The book on teeth was the first thoroughly scientific treatise on dentistry in English, and in it he made a careful study of the anatomy and physiology of the teeth. He described diseases of the dental pulp and insisted that the diseased pulp must be removed be-

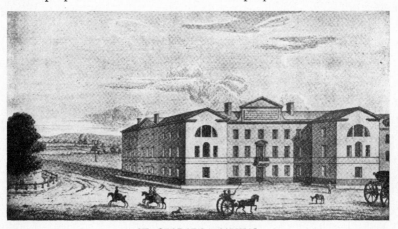

ST. GEORGE'S HOSPITAL
From an engraving by Isaac Ware, probable date, 1736.

fore filling. His statement, "Probably a Tooth might by slow degrees be moved to any part of the mouth by pressure," remains a leading maxim of the orthodontist. His work on venereal disease contains a wealth of clinical observations but is marred by his maxim, "Of the Poison being the same in Gonorrhea and in Chancre," a pardonable mistake perhaps in the light of his own unfortunate self-inoculation. The third book on Animal Oeconomy was a reprint of papers read before the Royal Society with some additions. In his last work, he drew on his experience with gunshot wounds during his service with the army some 30 years previously, discussed the physiology of the blood, and recorded numerous clinical observations on different types of inflammation, together with experiments he had carried out.

He was a student and an investigator in a wide range of science— a naturalist, anatomist, physiologist, pathologist, geologist, plant physiologist, and a great practical surgeon. A keen and acute observer, he, nevertheless, often made mistakes, but his inquiring mind was always open. To one of his pupils who asked him if he had written so-and-so, he answered, "Never ask me what I have said, or what I have written; but, if you will ask me what my present opinions are, I will tell you." In a letter to Jenner, Hunter remarked, "Why think—why not try the experiment?" This advice, paraphrased to "Don't think, but try," was Hunter's own attitude towards biological investigation.

Hunter carried out innumerable experiments in an attempt to solve problems that he constantly encountered in his practice. When he first tied the femoral artery in a case of popliteal aneurysm, this operation was suggested by an experiment he had made on the growth of a deer's antlers. He tied one of the external carotid arteries supplying a half grown antler and noted that it became quite cold but, a week later, had become quite warm and was growing again, thanks to the collateral circulation. Hunter found surgery an operative science; *he made it a physiological science as well.*

JENNER AND THE DISCOVERY OF VACCINATION

Edward Jenner, one of Hunter's favorite pupils, was born in Berkeley in 1749, the son of the vicar of Berkeley. After a thorough grounding in the classics, he decided, at the age of 13, to become a physician and was apprenticed to Mr. Ludlow, a surgeon of Sodbury, near Bristol, with whom he remained six years. During this apprenticeship, a young woman came for medical advice, and, when smallpox was mentioned she exclaimed, "I cannot take it, for I have had cow-pox." This chance remarks seems to have made a deep impression on young Jenner, who never forgot the incident and apparently resolved to study at some future time the truth of this statement.

After reaching the age of 21, he went to London as the pupil of John Hunter, then 42 years of age, in whose home he lived for two years. Between these two men grew up a deep and lasting friendship, which lasted until Hunter's death. Jenner is said to have discussed cowpox with his master, but there is no mention of the subject in any of Hunter's letters although they kept up an active correspondence for 20 years. Hunter's last letter to Jenner was written only two months before Hunter's sudden death.

Jenner soon tired of life in London and returned to Berkeley, where he settled down as a country practitioner. Here, in the midst of a busy practice, he carried out experiments on hedge hogs, foxes and lizards, studied birds, and made observations on the cuckoo. These observations, later reported to the Royal Society of London, led to his election as Fellow.

In 1777, Jenner saw his old teacher, John Hunter, in Bath and was much disturbed by his appearance, fearing that he was "affected with symptoms of the Angina Pectoris." These fears were expressed in a letter written in 1778 to Dr. Heberden, who had described angina pectoris in 1768. Jenner in this letter also described the heart of a patient who had died of angina pectoris, this heart showing thickening of the coronary arteries and "a kind of firm, fleshy tube, formed within the vessel, with a considerable quantity of ossific matter dispersed irregularly through it." He continued to make observations on angina pectoris and read a paper on the subject before the "Medico-Convivial Society" of Rodborough, an association he had been instrumental in forming. He did not publish his paper, however, for fear that John Hunter might read it and "his fears excited by its truly formidable nature" (Baron).

Jenner was active in forming another society, the "Convivo-Medical Society" of Alveston, where he often spoke on the reputed value of cow-pox inoculation as a preventative of smallpox and urged his medical colleagues to test the method. His suggestions fell on deaf ears. In 1796, cox-pox appeared on a farm near Berkeley. Jenner obtained some pus from a sore on a dairy maid's hand and inserted it by means of superficial incisions in the arm of James Phipps, a healthy boy of eight. The inoculation succeeded, and the boy developed a small pustular sore, followed by scabs and a small scar. Six weeks later, Jenner inoculated the boy with variolous lymph, but no smallpox followed.

The following year, Jenner inoculated three more patients successfully and resolved to publish a paper on the subject. He submitted the paper to the Council of the Royal Society, who returned it to him with the "friendly admonition that, as he had gained some reputation by his former papers to the Royal Society, it was advisable not to present this, lest it should injure his established credit" (Moore). Undaunted, Jenner determined to publish it himself, and, in 1798, the *Inquiry into the Causes and Effects of the Variolae Vaccinae* was published in London.

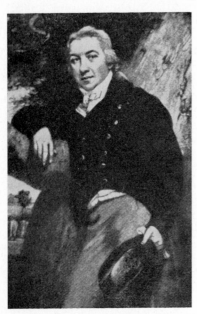

EDWARD JENNER
Portrait by J. R. Smith, 1801.

Jenner's discovery aroused much controversy in London, some physicians attacking his views, others attempting to appropriate them as their own. In America, the idea was enthusiastically supported by Dr. Benjamin Waterhouse of Cambridge, Massachusetts, who vaccinated his own son, and by Thomas Jefferson, President of the United States, who had several members of his family vaccinated. In France, Napoleon ordered all his soldiers vaccinated, and the Empress of Russia urged all her subjects to be vaccinated. Soon the method spread to Austria, Germany and Italy, where it gained the support of the leading physicians of those countries.

Jenner's fame soon was world wide. The English Parliament in 1802 voted him 10,000 pounds and in 1807 an additional 20,000 pounds. In 1808, the National Vaccine Establishment was formed by the government and placed under his direction. Five years later, during the war with France, Captain Milman, a relative of Jenner's, was captured by the French and imprisoned at Verdun. Jenner wrote a letter to Napoleon requesting his release. Napoleon, on reading the letter, exclaimed, "Ah! C'est Jenner, je ne puis rien refuser à Jenner."

After the first parliamentary grant in 1802, Jenner took a house in London, with the plan of practicing there. But, after a year's experience, he wrote a friend, "I have now completely made up my mind respecting London. I have done with it, and have again commenced village-doctor." He returned to Berkeley, to his old life in the country, treating his patients, vaccinating all who wished, and enjoying the company of his friends. He died of apoplexy in 1823 and was buried in the chancel of the parish church at Berkeley.

Jenner's discovery ranks among the greatest discoveries in medicine, and no one will dispute his title as a benefactor to the human race. The disfigurement from smallpox, a commonplace in the eighteenth century, has become a rarity. In countries enforcing compulsory vaccination, the death rate from smallpox approaches zero. During the first World War in the United States Army, which numbered more than four million vaccinated soldiers, there were only 853 cases of smallpox with 14 deaths.

DISCOVERIES IN PHYSIOLOGY AND CHEMISTRY

While the eighteenth century produced no physiologists in England as outstanding as Boyle, Lower and Mayow, the spirit of inquiry initiated by the Oxford physiologists and the Royal Society continued to be a potent ferment. The outstanding English physiologist of the eighteenth century, however, was not closely identified with any academic seat of learning but was a clergyman, the Rev. Stephen Hales (1677-1761), the "perpetual curate" of Teddington, at that time a country village of less than 500 inhabitants 15 miles from London.

Stephen Hales was born at Bekesbourne in Kent and, at the age of 18, entered Bene't College, Cambridge, later known as Corpus Christi College. Here Hales became interested in physical science, in biology, in chemistry, and in astronomy. Here also he became the close friend of William Stukeley, a medical student, who carried out dissections in anatomy and experiments in physiology with Hales's assistance. However, Hales, as a divinity student and intended for the Church, was ordained in 1703 and, in 1709, was appointed to the parish of Teddington, where he remained until his death at the age of 84. Soon after settling in Teddington, he began his experiments, carrying them out in the parsonage alone and unaided. In addition, he was quite active as a parish priest, became a trustee of the new colony in Georgia, was active in improving the health of seamen, in improving the ventilation of prisons, and in combating gin drinking and drunkenness, both so widespread in his day.

The first research carried out by Hales was on the physiology of

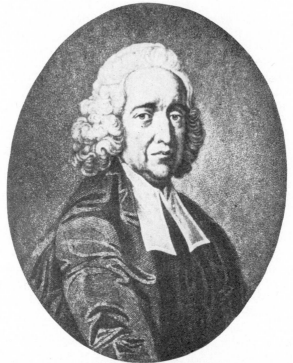

Stirling, *Some Apostles of Physiology*, London, 1902

STEPHEN HALES

From a portrait by F. Coates.

the circulation of the blood. In his classic experiment, performed about 1711, he tied a brass tube into the crural artery of a horse, attached a glass tube nine feet in length to the brass tube, and, on "untying the ligature on the artery, the blood rose in the tube eight feet, three inches perpendicular above the level of the left ventricle of the heart"—the first recorded estimation of the blood pressure! He also found that the pulse rate is more rapid in small animals than in large and that the blood pressure is more or less proportional to the size of the animal. He then studied the output of the heart per minute, estimating the capacity of the left ventricle by pouring melted wax into the ventricle through the pulmonary vein and allowing it to harden. Although his method of estimating the capacity of the ventricle was crude, he showed that the ventricular output per beat is proportional to the size of the animal and that the heart of a small animal, because of a more rapid pulse, expels a weight of blood equal to its own body weight in less time than a large animal. He next studied the resistance offered to the blood flow through the arteries, veins and capillaries, noted that hot water, when introduced, produced relaxation of the vessels and increased the rate of flow; whereas, cold water, quinine, cinnamon, and also alcohol constricted the vessels. These remarkable experiments came to the attention of the Royal Society which elected him Fellow in 1718. This notable work on cardiovascular physiology was not published until 22 years later.

From human physiology, Hales turned his interest to plant physiology, and, in 1718, a few days after his election to the Royal Society, he read before that body a paper, "Upon the Effect of ye Sun's warmth in raising ye Sap in trees." This initial paper was followed by a series of interesting experiments which stamp him in the words of Harvey-Gibson as "the first genuine plant physiologist we meet with in the history of the science." Having previously measured the blood pressure in animals, he now proceeded to measure the sap pressure of plants and the velocity of the flow of the sap, which he found most rapid in the stem, intermediate in the roots, and slowest in the leaves, corresponding to the velocity of the blood flow in the arteries, veins and capillaries. He next turned his attention to the larger subject of the flow of sap, which some had believed circulated in the plant just as blood circulated in animals. He found that the leaves "perspired" or, as we say now, transpired and that transpiration on the surface of the leaf promoted a continuous flow of sap, that the upward flow of sap was due to transpiration capillarity and root pressure, and that there was no circulation of the sap similar to that of the blood—conclusions as valid today as when he announced them. Hales next devoted his attention to a study of the gaseous content of solid substances, arriving at the conclusion that "air" could exist in two states—an "elastic" or gaseous state and a "fixed" or solid state. He gave a clear account of the existence of gases in a free and combined state, and showed that air ascended with the sap and that substances apparently solid contained air.

These experiments on plant physiology were published by Hales in his book, *Vegetable Staticks,* 1727. In 1733, this work appeared as volume one of *Statical Essays,* while volume two consisted of *Haemastatics,* the first appearance of his work on blood pressure, which had been done 22 years before. Hales's reputation had grown steadily with the years. In 1733, Oxford conferred upon him the degree of Doctor of Divinity, and the publication of his *Essays*

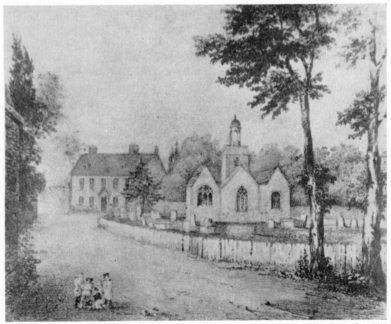

Clark-Kennedy, *Stephen Hales*, Cambridge, 1929

TEDDINGTON PARISH CHURCH IN THE EIGHTEENTH CENTURY

The parsonage is seen on the left. Here Hales carried out his experiments.

increased his fame, having been translated into German, Dutch and Italian. In 1755, on the death of Sir Hans Sloane, he was elected to his place as one of the eight foreign members of the *Académie Royal des Sciences* in Paris.

Hales published in 1758 his last book, *A Treatise on Ventilators,* describing his method of improving the air supply of vessels and prisons. Three years later, he died at the age of 84.

In the course of his experiments on distillation and fermentation, Hales prepared a great number of gases, including probably hydrogen, carbon dioxide, sulphur dioxide, ammonia, and nitrous oxide. He did not, however, study them further since he was not interested in the properties of the different gases but in the gaseous content of solid substances. Other investigators, stimulated by his observations, became interested in the properties of these gases, and their investigations ushered in a new era of chemistry as well as of medicine. Prominent among these investigators were Black, Cavendish, Priestley, Scheele and Lavoisier.

Chemical thought was still dominated by the phlogiston theory of Stahl, who taught that combustible substances and metals capable of calcination contain phlogiston as a common constituent, this escaping on combustion or calcination. The outstanding chemists at the end of the eighteenth century unwittingly demolished the phlogiston theory with their experiments, although some of them remained champions of that theory.

Joseph Black (1728-1799), born at Bordeaux and educated at Belfast, Glasgow and Edinburgh, became professor of chemistry at Glasgow in succession to William Cullen and later succeeded Cullen as professor of chemistry at Edinburgh. Black, in the thesis he presented for his doctor's degree in 1754, showed that lime when burned into caustic or quick-lime lost weight, a discovery which contradicted the phlogiston theory since lime, according to that theory, became caustic by taking up phlogiston and, therefore, should have become heavier. He also showed that the loss of weight was due to the loss of a specific gas which he called "fixed air," which he identified with the *gas silvestre* of van Helmont. Black found, too, that this gas was given off in fermentation, was produced by burning charcoal, and was present in expired air. "Fixed air" we now call *carbon dioxide*. In addition, Black made important observations on heat, introduced the doctrine of latent heat, and was the "founder of calorimetry, the measurement of heat" (Lenard).

Henry Cavendish (1731-1810), an eccentric English nobleman, nephew of the Duke of Devonshire and grandson of the Duke of Kent, one of the wealthiest men of his time, made a number of very impressive discoveries. He had been a student at Cambridge for four years but left without taking a degree; then, after spending some time in France, settled down in London, where he attended the meetings of the Royal Society and devoted himself to the study of mathematics, physics and chemistry. He had little intercourse with his relatives, ordered his dinner daily by a note on his hall table, and instructed his female servants to keep out of his sight on pain of dismissal. In 1766, Cavendish prepared hydrogen, or "inflammable air," by treating iron with acids and, in 1781, demonstrated that, when hydrogen and oxygen are burned, water is formed. He also proved that atmospheric air is a mixture of nitrogen and oxygen in constant proportions. Some of his papers were read before the Royal Society and published by them in the Transactions, but many of his experiments were not published until years after his death. His collected works were first published in 1921. Even though his investigations undermined the phlogiston theory, he continued to be a champion of this theory and tried to harmonize his results with it.

An even more zealous champion of the phlogiston theory was Joseph Priestley, well known to his generation as a theologian, politician, and man of science. Priestley was born at Fieldhead, Yorkshire, in 1733, and had a thorough training in theology and in classical languages, learning Latin, Greek, Hebrew, Syriac and Arabic as well as French, German and Italian. He became a dissenting minister, served first at Needham Market and later at Nantwich, where he founded a school and gave an elementary course in natural science. This experience aroused in him a passion for natural sciences, and, although he was entirely untrained in the methods of science, he soon developed an unusual gift for experimenting. From Nantwich, he went to Warrington, where he taught classical languages but spent his leisure in experiments on electricity. Encouraged by Benjamin Franklin, whom he had met in London, he wrote a *History of Electricity,* which contained, in addition to a history of the subject, an account of his own investigations. This work was first published in 1767, the same year in which he was elected a Fellow of the Royal Society.

From Warrington, Priestley went to Leeds as minister of a dissenting chapel and began to experiment on airs. "This," he says, "I was led into in consequence of inhabiting a house adjoining a public brewery, where I at first amused myself with making experiments on the fixed air, which I found ready made in the process of fermentation." He adds, "When I began these experiments I knew very little of *chemistry,* and had in a manner no idea on the subject before I attended a course of chemical lectures delivered in the academy at Warrington by Dr. Turner of Liverpool."

Priestley reported his experiments in his *Observations on different kinds of air,* first published in 1772. This work described his tests with fixed air (carbon dioxide), inflammable air (hydrogen), nitrous air (nitrous oxide), which he discovered, and hydrochloric acid gas, also his own discovery. He made the interesting finding "concerning the restoration of air, in which candles had burned out, by plants growing in it." His greatest discovery came in 1774, when he heated mercuric oxide with a burning glass and obtained a gas which was not inflammable but was exceedingly favorable for combustion so that "a candle burned in this air with a remarkably vigorous flame." He had discovered oxygen, which he, true to the phlogiston theory, called "dephlogisticated air." Air supported combustion, according to this theory, because it takes up the phlogiston given off by the burning body. When a candle burns out in a closed jar, it is because the air in the jar becomes saturated with phlogiston and can take up no more. Common air is partly dephlogisticated or a part of it contains no phlogiston and thus supports combustion. This new air was completely dephlogisticated, contained no phlogiston, and thus increased the intensity of the combustion.

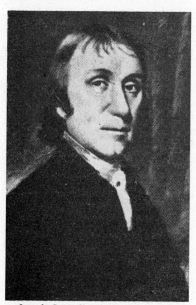

Lenard, *Grosse Naturforscher*, München, 1932

JOSEPH PRIESTLEY

The later events in Priestley's life are well known. He went to Birmingham as junior minister to a Unitarian chapel, where he became very unpopular because of his religious and political views. On July 14, 1791, a group assembled in Birmingham to celebrate with a dinner the anniversary of the fall of the Bastille. This celebration enraged certain inhabitants of the town, who turned their wrath against Priestley, whose sympathies with the French Revolution were notorious. His chapel was burned, his house sacked, his manuscripts and scientific apparatus destroyed and Priestley himself fled to London for safety. In 1794, he emigrated to America and settled in Northumberland, Pennsylvania, where he died in 1804.

Another devoted follower of the phlogiston theory was the Swedish apothecary, Karl Wilhelm Scheele (1742-1786). Scheele, after being apprenticed to an apothecary in Gothenburg, became proprietor of a pharmacy in Köping, a small town on Lake Malar some 70 miles from Stockholm. Here he found time for an extraordinary amount of original research. His record as a discover of new substances is probably unequalled in the history of chemistry. In 1772, Scheele obtained oxygen by heating red oxide of mercury and from black oxide of manganese and saltpeter. Since this oxygen increased combustion, he called it "fire air." This discovery was two years before Priestley described "dephlogisticated air." Scheele explained combustion in the terms of the phlogiston theory and apparently considered hydrogen as pure phlogiston. Both Priestley and Scheele noted that, when a candle was burned in a closed vessel, exactly as much "fixed air," or carbon dioxide, was formed as oxygen had disappeared. Thus, both observers, while ardent champions of the phlogiston theory, had in reality destroyed that theory without recognizing the true import of their discoveries.

The death blow to the phlogiston theory was administered by Antoine Laurent Lavoisier, whose work marks a new era in chemistry and had a profound effect upon physiology and medicine.

Antoine Laurent Lavoisier was born in Paris in 1743, the son of a wealthy merchant, who gave him a careful education. He studied at the Collège Mazarin, where he was a brilliant student, then studied botany at the Jardin des Plantes, astronomy at the Observatoire, and, at the age of 24, submitted a thesis on lighting the streets to the *Académie des Sciences* and received the gold medal. Following this, he read several papers before the Academy on geological and physical subjects and, at the age of 25, was elected member of the Academy.

Encouraged by this recognition, Lavoisier began to devote his entire time to the pursuit of science and fitted up his own laboratory, where he carried out numerous experiments, especially in chemistry. He early recognized the importance of weighing substances with the greatest accuracy, provided himself with the most delicate balances obtainable, and carried out his weighing with the greatest care. In 1775, the year after Priestley had prepared his dephlogisticated air, Lavoisier published his epochal paper, "On the nature of the principle which combines with metals during their calcination." He had prepared the same air which Priestley called "dephlogisticated air" by heating mercuric oxide but found that, when the oxide became a metal, it gave up something to the air. The metal when burnt into the oxide increased in weight, having taken something from the air. Two years later, he showed conclusively that the substance called by Priestley "dephlogisticated air," which combines with metals when calcined, is the characteristic constituent of acids.

Lavoisier proposed the name, "oxygen," or generator of acid, the name by which it has since been known.

The question has been hotly debated whether Lavoisier can be called "the discoverer of oxygen." He has been accused of appropriating Priestley's discovery as his own. However, this is surely unjust, for Lavoisier himself wrote in his *Mémoires,* "This air which Mr. Priestley discovered at about the same time as I; indeed, I believe before me." Also, at the beginning of his celebrated memoir, *Sur les fluides aériformes,* he remarks, "The experiments which I am going to report belong almost all to Dr. Priestley; I have no further merit than to have repeated them with care and especially to have arranged in the proper order to present the conclusions." On one point there is universal agreement: that Lavoisier and not Priestley understood the true meaning of the discovery. The former proved by it the fallacy of the phlogiston theory; the latter continued a faithful adherent of the phlogiston doctrine until his death. Foster states bluntly in speaking of Lavoisier, "He and he alone really discovered oxygen."

Lavoisier, upon the discovery of oxygen and of the true nature of oxidation, saw at once that respiration was oxidation, that air which had been respired resembled air in which metal had been calcined, that it had lost a certain amount of oxygen. And, he also found that expired air contained carbon dioxide. Two factors were

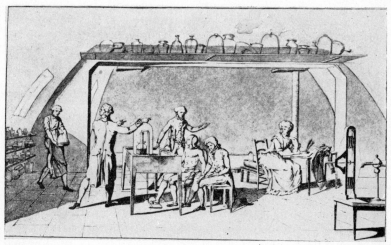

Grimaux, *Lavoisier,* Paris, 1888

LAVOISIER IN HIS LABORATORY

obviously important in respiration—the disappearance of oxygen and the appearance of carbon dioxide. These results were described in his paper, *Expériences sur la respiration des animaux,* 1777. Three years later, Lavoisier, in collaboration with the mathematician Laplace, published their memoir on heat, in which they concluded, "Respiration is therefore a combustion, slow it is true, but otherwise perfectly similar to the combustion of charcoal." Later, Lavoisier found that respiration was not a combustion of carbon alone. In 1793, he and Seguin published a paper, *Premier memoire sur la respiration des animaux,* which remains an excellent summary of the chemistry of the body although it contained one gross error, that the oxidation of the carbon and hydrogen supplied by the food takes place within the lungs.

Lavoisier's last paper on respiration was read before the *Académie des Sciences* in 1790. The French Revolution was now beginning. In 1792, the Academy was purged of the "enemies of the people"; in 1793, it was suppressed. On May 8, 1794, Lavoisier was tried on the charge that he was an enemy of France "in mixing tobacco with water and ingredients harmful to the health of its citizens." He was found guilty and executed the following day by the guillotine. As his friend Lagrange commented the next day, "A moment was sufficient to sever his head, but a hundred years will not be enough perhaps to produce another like it." Lavoisier's discoveries in the field of respiration are comparable to those of Harvey on the circulation. In the history of chemistry, Lavoisier will always be remembered as the destroyer of the phlogiston theory and as the father of modern chemistry.

The eighteenth century witnessed not only important discoveries in the physiology of respiration but also in the physiology of digestion. The work of Reaumur gave a great impetus to subsequent students of digestion.

Réné Antoine Ferchauld de Reaumur (1683-1757) stands out as one of the great men in science of this century. Born in 1683 at Rochelle, he was educated for the profession of law, but, possessed of an ample fortune, he went to Paris at the beginning of the century and devoted himself to scientific investigations. Elected to the Academy of Sciences in 1708, he read before that body a large number of papers dealing with nearly all branches of science. He invented the thermometer bearing his name, wrote papers on rivers, mines, forests and fossils. He devised the methods of tinning that are still employed and investigated the chemical differences between

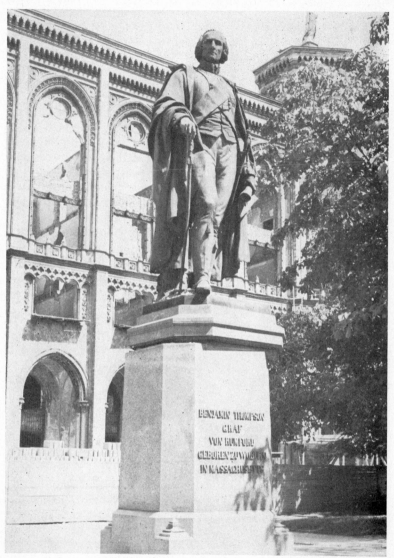

STATUE OF COUNT RUMFORD IN MUNICH

The life and labors of this remarkable American are described in the
Bibiographical Addenda. This photograph was taken in 1950 and shows
the bombed building in the background.

steel and iron. His great work, *Mémoires pour servir à l'histoire naturelle des insectes,* in six large quarto volumes, published during the years 1734-1742, remains one of the most monumental writings in the field of insect biology. His treatise on the digestion of birds, *Sur la digestion des oiseaux,* which appeared in 1752, is an important landmark in the history of digestion.

Reaumur began his experiments with a kite, a bird which has the well-known habit of rejecting from its stomach things that it has swallowed but cannot digest. He employed small tubes of metal with a fine mesh of wire at each end, into which he introduced small bits of meat or bone. The kite swallowed these tubes but subsequently rejected them, and Reaumur found that the bits of meat or bone were partially dissolved but showed no signs of putrefaction. Subsequently, he obtained the same results with dogs. These experiments employed an entirely new method and proved that gastric digestion was not simply a process of trituration or of putrefaction, as some had assumed, but that the gastric juice had the power of dissolving food. Next, he filled his tubes with small pieces of sponge and, squeezing out the sponge, obtained gastric juice, which he found had some digestive power *in vitro.*

These investigations were further extended by Spallanzani, who used the methods Reaumur had introduced. Lazzaro Spallanzani, was born at Scandiano in 1729, and, intended for the profession of law, received an excellent education. He showed, however, a great interest in natural science, studying physics at Bologna under his kinswoman, Laura Bassi. In 1754, he was appointed professor of logic, mathematics and Greek at Reggio but, in 1760, went to Modena as professor of natural history. After 11 years, he was called to Pavia as professor of natural history and remained there until his death in 1799. Before his appointment to a chair at Reggio, he had taken orders in the Church and is often referred to as the Abbé Spallanzani. His life was spent mainly in the study of natural history.

Employing tubes similar to those used by Reaumur, Spallanzani used birds and various other animals in his experiments and even made tests upon himself, swallowing perforated wooden tubes and regurgitating them. He also swallowed small linen bags containing meat, bread, and other substances, studying the contents of the bags after they had been passed *per anum.* He obtained samples of gastric juice, found that it dissolved meat *in vitro,* that this action was hastened by heat, and that gastric juice prevented putrefaction. Gastric digestion was obviously neither fermentation nor putrefaction. He concluded erroneously that gastric juice was not acid.

John Hunter, who was studying digestion, attacked both Reaumur and Spallanzani. He accused Spallanzani as being deficient in anatomical knowledge and added, "Like all mere experiment-makers, he is not satisfied even with those which are clear and decisive, but multiples them most unnecessarily." Hunter's hostility probably stemmed from the fact "that he distinctly belonged to the school of Stahl though he replaced the phrase 'sensitive soul' by that of 'vital

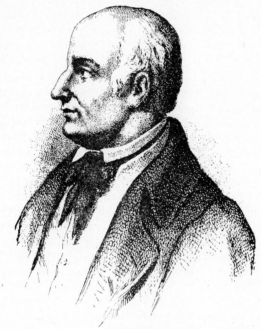

University of Kansas Collection

LAZZARO SPALLANZANI

principle' " (Foster). However Spallanzani was quite free from all vitalistic tendencies. Yet, Hunter was correct in stating there was an acid in the gastric juice although he later said, "It is only formed occasionally."

In investigating problems of respiration, Spallanzani corrected the error of Lavoisier that oxidation takes place in the lungs. The Abbé showed that the tissues, like the body as a whole, respire; that is, they consume oxygen and give off carbon dioxide; also that animals (snails) in an atmosphere of hydrogen or nitrogen give off carbon dioxide just as they do in air.

Spallanzani, early in his career, became an expert with the microscope, which he used in his work on infusoria. He demolished the doctrine of spontaneous generation by demonstrating that water after being boiled and sealed in a flask, developed no signs of life unless the seal was broken and air permitted to enter (1767). His experiments on fertilization were very important. He fertilized frog eggs by adding sperm from male frogs and injected dog sperm into the vagina of a female dog, who, "sixty-two days after the injection of the sperm, became mother of three little vivacious children, two males and the third female."

OBSERVATIONS ON ELECTRICITY

The subject of electricity had attracted the attention of philosophers since the days of Thales (600 B.C.), who observed that yellow amber, when rubbed, had the power of attracting light objects, such as feathers. The word, "electricity," itself is derived from the Greek ἤλεχτρον, the word for amber. William Gilbert (1544-1603), physician to Queen Elizabeth, author of De magnete, explained the phenomena of attraction as vis electrica and described a great variety of electrical experiments. Robert Boyle, Sir Isaac Newton, and Otto Guericke of Magdeburg, the inventor of the air-pump, made many experiments with electricity in the seventeenth century. In the eighteenth century, Hauksbee produced light by electricity, Stephen Gray showed that electrical attraction could be transferred by contact from one body to another, von Kleist of Kammin and Musschenbroeck of Leyden discovered the Leyden jar, and Benjamin Franklin introduced the concept of positive and negative electricity and demonstrated in his famous kite experiment that lightning is electricity. These discoveries were followed by the observation of Galvani that weak electrical currents caused muscular contractions, and, by his demonstration of animal electricity. Galvani also showed that dissimilar metals, when brought into contact with each other, generated electricity, an observation which led Volta to the discovery of the battery and of the voltaic pile.

These discoveries led quickly to the application of electricity in the treatment of disease. Joseph Priestley, in his History and Present State of Electricity, devotes a chapter to medical electricity. Benjamin Franklin treated paralysis with electrical currents. De Haen in Vienna employed "gentle shocks" and cured St. Vitus dance. The Rev. John Wesley, who found time from his arduous evangelistic labors to write Primitive Physick, which had a phenomenal circulation, made use of electricity in treating his patients. Electricity was soon extensively used by physicians and laymen in the treatment of disease, and some of its enthusiastic advocates claimed cures not only in paralysis, hysterical affections and toothache but even in lockjaw, blindness and deafness.

FRANZ ANTON MESMER AND MESMERISM

The eighteenth century, which began as a century of theorists and system makers, witnessed at its close the appearance of a new system which swept through Europe like a crusade, enrolling innumerable zealots from all walks of life in its ranks. This new system, which came to be known as mesmerism, was the creation not of an illiterate or untrained quack, but of a graduate of the Old Vienna School—Franz Anton Mesmer.

Franz Anton Mesmer was born at Iznang on the Lake of Constance in 1734 and studied first theology and philosophy. Later he went to Vienna, where he studied medicine under van Swieten, Störck and de Haen, graduating in 1766. His doctor's thesis, *De planetarum influxu* (On the influence of planets), outlined his doctrines of disease and healing which he subsequently followed throughout his remarkable career. He stated that, just as the planets exercise a well-known attraction for each other, so they exercise a direct effect upon all the tissues of the human body. This influence is produced by a mysterious fluid which penetrates all substances both living and inanimate, the *Gravitas Animalis* (animal gravity), which he later called "Animal Magnetism." He referred to the views of older physicians on the influence of the heavenly bodies upon disease, citing Galen's belief in the influence of the moon on epileptics and hysterical patients and Tulp's opinion that renal colic was related to the cycles of the moon.

After graduation, Mesmer settled in Vienna, began to practice medicine, and married Frau van Bosch, the wealthy young widow of an imperial councillor. They entertained lavishly, and Mesmer, who was musical, became a good friend of young Wolfgang Mozart, who wrote an operetta for him entitled, "Bastien and Bastienne," which was performed in Vienna. In 1774, Mesmer became much interested in the success of Maximilian Hell, an English astronomer, who was visiting in Vienna and claimed to have had successfully treated several cases of stomach cramps with a magnet. Mesmer experimented with magnets for a time but concluded that the cures were the result of animal magnetism. These views were published in his first book, *Schreiben über die Magnetkur,* Vienna, 1775. The same year, when he was in Munich, the Elector asked his opinion regarding the remarkable cures accomplished by Father Gassner,

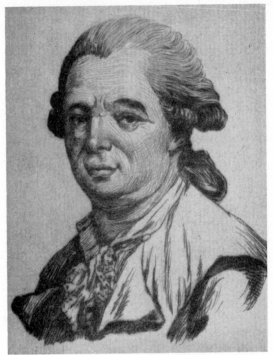

University of Kansas Collection

FRANZ ANTON MESMER

which were creating a great sensation at the time. Johann Joseph Gassner (1727-1779), after much reflection, had concluded that all diseases could be divided into two classes, those due to natural causes and those due to the Devil. He treated patients by exorcising the Devil according to the rites of the Church and drew large crowds of sufferers, whom he cured by the laying on of hands and commanding the Devil to leave the body of the afflicted. Mesmer gave as his opinion that Gassner was sincere and that his cures were not miraculous but were produced by animal magnetism.

In the winter of 1777-1778, Mesmer attracted the attention of all Vienna by his supposed cure of Maria Paradies, who had been blind since the age of three and a half years. Mesmer claimed that she was able to see after treatment for 14 days. Many prominent physicians, including Störck, denied his claims and attacked him violently. Vienna became an unpleasant place for Mesmer, and, in 1778, he went to Paris.

In Paris, Mesmer began to see patients and invited the *Académie des Sciences* to visit him and witness his cures, but the Academy did not answer the invitation. Likewise, his attempts to establish relations with the *Société de Médecine* were unsuccessful. He threatened to leave Paris, but Queen Marie Antoinette offered him a yearly lifelong pension of 20,000 livres and a house if he would remain there. Because of difficulties in arranging terms, the negotiations were broken off, and Mesmer departed for Spa, followed by many patients and admirers. Meanwhile, a group of friends and patients began a campaign to hold Mesmer in Paris, where he could heal the sick, instruct pupils, and spread his teachings. A sum of 340,000 livres was subscribed, each pupil paying 100 livres. These pupils later formed a society called "Société de l'harmonie," which had a ritual something like that of Masonic orders and presently had branches in several provincial towns.

Mesmer returned to Paris, and his name was soon on every tongue and his consulting rooms were crowded with patients from all walks of life, neurotic women of the upper classes predominating. The crowds became so great that patients had to reserve places in his treatment rooms days or weeks in advance. When the patient was finally fortunate enough to be admitted to the salon, he saw in the darkened room a group of people seated in a circle with joined hands around a large tub, or *Baquet,* from which at various points iron bars protruded. These iron bars were charged by the touch of Mesmer with animal magnetism, which flowed over into the circle of people when the bars were touched. Soon Mesmer appeared, clad in a lilac silk robe and carrying a wand. Moving slowly, he touched one of the group with his wand. Immediately the person touched began to twitch and writhe, and all in the circle became agitated. These were the crises it was necessary to produce before treatment could be attempted. The crises were then resolved by the animal magnetism which flowed from Mesmer.

In 1784, King Louis XVI appointed a committee, consisting of four members of the *Société de Médecine* and five members of the *Académie des Sciences,* to investigate Mesmer's claims. Among the members of the academy were Benjamin Franklin and Antoine Lavoisier. The report of the commission stated that examination of the *Baquet* with an electrometer and a compass showed no evidence of electrical activity and that the patients when blindfolded could not tell whether they were magnetised or not. The conclusion was that the effects produced were entirely the result of imagination. The committee added that "imagination without magnetism produces convulsions and that magnetism without imagi-

nation produces nothing" and also that "nothing proves the existence of the animal magnetic fluid; that this non-existent fluid is
therefore useless."

This adverse report, however, had no effect upon Mesmer's
popularity. His salon continued to be filled with patients, and the
number of his adherents continued to increase. Lafayette became

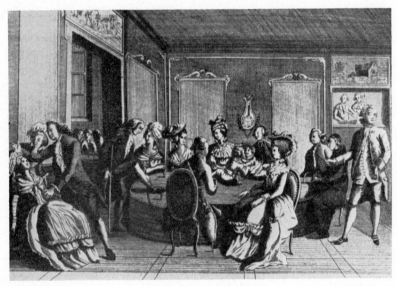

THE *BAQUET* OF MESMER

A group of patients are seated around the *baquet,* or tub, holding to bars
or ropes immersed in the magnetised water. On the left sits a lady who is
apparently recovering from a "crisis." On the right stands Mesmer with a
wand in the right hand, directing the action of the *baquet,* and, as an
admirer described him, "is serious, speaks little, his head always seems
loaded with great thoughts." (From a contemporary print.)

one of his enthusiastic disciples and wrote his friend, George Washington, that he was bringing to the new Republic something more
valuable than cannons or soldiers, he was bringing "the secret of
Mesmer, which is a great philosophical discovery." However, the
revolutionary mob crushed what the scientists had been unable to
check. Mesmer fled from Paris as Robespierre was rising to power.
He went to London, then to Vienna, and finally settled down in
Meersburg on Lake Constance, where he died in 1815 at the age of
81, unnoticed by the world. Mesmer was not, as his enemies charged,

a swindler but believed sincerely in animal magnetism with his last breath.

As Tischner has pointed out, we see in Mesmer "a second-rate intellect exercising a profound influence upon philosophy, science, and practical life, all the more remarkable since he himself misunderstood the essentials of what he had discovered." Tischner compares him to Columbus, who believed he had discovered a new trade route to India, and, like Columbus, "he never understood the true importance of his discovery."

One of Mesmer's disciples, Puységur, while working with mesmerism, rediscovered "artificial somnambulism," or, as it was later called, hypnotism. We say "rediscovered" since hypnotism in one form or another has been known from earliest times. In 1784, Puységur developed a technique for producing hypnosis; Recamier in 1821 applied a cautery under hypnosis; and, in 1829, Cloquet operated for cancer of the breast under hypnosis. Mesmerism and hypnotism became almost synonymous terms, and the practice of mesmerism spread far beyond the confines of France. John Elliotson, one of the leading physicians of London, unrivaled in his day as a teacher, took up mesmerism and spent the rest of his life quarrelling with his professional brethren. In America, Phineas Quimby, the founder of New Thought, after healing the sick with mesmerism or hypnotism, came to the conclusion that it was the faith of the patient that healed him. Among his patients was Mrs. Mary Baker Eddy. Mrs. Eddy later became the founder of Christian Science and scoffed at the suggestion that she had borrowed Quimby's teachings or methods, although a careful study of Quimby's writings and of the early editions of Mrs. Eddy's *Science and Health* shows an obvious similarity.

Mesmer was the forbear or spiritual ancestor of a number of later prophets of new religions closely allied with healing. Mesmerism was the catalyst that produced by a series of chain reactions, Christian Science, New Thought, Unity, Cueism, and a score of lesser cults. Hypnotism has been of great value to psychology in exploring new avenues of the mind, and it has been extensively employed as a diagnostic and therapeutic procedure in functional neuroses. Psychoanalysis, the latest technique in the study of neuroses, has an obvious close kinship with hypnosis or, as it was originally called, artificial somnambulism or mesmerism. The healing cults, which are the spiritual descendants of Mesmer, however vehemently they may deny the fact, have achieved their therapeutic successes through psychotherapy, a method of treatment that has gained fresh statue and attracted anew the attention of the medical profession.

Biographical Addenda

The EIGHTEENTH CENTURY

1660-1734—Georg Ernst Stahl.

1660-1742—Friedrich Hoffmann.

1660-1753—Sir Hans Sloane was born at Killeleagh, Ireland, studied at Paris and Montpellier, and graduated in medicine at the University of Orange. Returning to England, he became Fellow of the Royal Society and of the Royal College of Physicians. He went to Jamaica as physician to the Duke of Albemarle, where he collected a large number of specimens of animals and plants, which he brought back to London and described in *A Voyage to the Islands of Madeira, Barbados, Nieves, St. Christopher's and Jamaica*, the first volume of which appeared in 1707, the second volume in 1725. He was very successful in practice, was appointed first physician to King George II in 1727, and, the same year, succeeded Sir Isaac Newton as president of the Royal Society. On his death in 1753, he left his large collection of books, manuscripts, prints, medals, coins, drawings and pictures to the nation, and they formed the nucleus of the British Museum.

1661-1708—François Poupart, French naturalist and physician, achieved fame as an entomologist and anatomist. He described the ligament, since known as Poupart's ligament, in 1705 although it was clearly described by Falloppio in 1561.

1661-1719—Sir Samuel Garth, physician and poet, was author of the famous poem, *The Dispensary*, a satirical account of the opposition of certain physicians and apothecaries to the establishment by the Royal College of Physicians of a free dispensary where drugs were supplied to the indigent. He was a member of the Kitkat Club, was knighted by King George I, and appointed physician to the king and physician-general to the army.

1664-1726—Antonio Pacchioni, Italian anatomist, pupil of Malpighi, and colleague of Lancisi. He investigated especially the anatomy of the brain and its membranes and, in 1705, described the Pacchionian bodies.

1664-1742—Thomas Dover, physician and buccaneer, graduated B.A. Oxford in 1684 and M.B. Cambridge in 1687. He was a resident pupil of Thomas Sydenham and practiced in Bristol for a time. In 1708, he went with a vessel belonging to the Merchant Adventurers of Bristol to the Pacific, where they found and brought back Alexander Selkirk, the original of Robinson Crusoe. He originated the well-known Dover's powder and was the author of *The Ancient Physician's Legacy to His Country*, London, 1732, which went through eight editions.

1666-1709—William Cowper began the study of medicine as an apprentice to a surgeon of London and, in 1691, was admitted to the Barber

Surgeons' Company. He practiced as a surgeon in London and devoted much time to the study of anatomy. In 1694, he published *Myotomia Reformata,* a description of the muscular system and, in 1698, *Anatomy of Humane Bodies,* the latter a piece of scientific piracy at the expense of Godfrey Bidloo. In 1702, he described the glands which bear his name although Méry had described them in 1684. In 1705, Cowper, in a paper contributed to the Philosophical Transactions of the Royal Society, described and illustrated the valvular lesions of aortic insufficiency.

1666-1723—Antonio Maria Valsalva was born in Imola, studied at Bologna under Malpighi, and received his doctor's degree in 1687. In 1697, he was appointed professor of anatomy at Bologna and held this position until his death. His *De aure humana tractatus,* Bologna, 1704, is a remarkable book containing anatomical, physiological and pathological observations concerning the ear. He devised the method of inflating the Eustachian tube by closing the nose and mouth and employing a forcible expiration—Valsalva's experiment. He was deeply interested in pathology, and Morgagni's great work, *De sedibus,* contains much material collected by Valsalva, who was Morgagni's revered teacher.

1668-1707—Giorgio Baglivi.

1668-1738—Hermann Boerhaave.

1669-1760—Jacques Benigne Winslow, born in Odense, Denmark, studied in Holland and France and received his doctor's degree at Paris in 1705. In 1707, he became professor of anatomy at Paris and, from 1743 to 1750, he was professor in the Jardin du Roi. He was an excellent anatomist, made many advances in topographical anatomy, and became famous as a teacher, numbering Albrecht von Haller among his pupils. His chief work was his *Exposition anatomique de la structure du corps humain,* Paris, 1732. Winslow's foramen and Winslow's ligament commemorate his name.

1671-1743—George Cheyne, a native of Aberdeen, Scotland, studied in Edinburgh as a pupil of Pitcairn and, in 1702, settled in London after writing a tract, *The New Theory of Fevers,* which attracted much attention. As his practice grew, he both ate and drank too much. He became quite obese, weighing 445 pounds, was short of breath, and moved with great difficulty. He sought a cure from the waters of Bath, where he spent a part of each year. He described his own experiences in his best known works, *An Essay on the True Nature and Due Method of Treating the Gout,* London, 1720; *An Essay of Health and Long Life,* London, 1724; and *The English Malady,* London, 1733, which ran through six editions and is, in mainly, a discourse on neurasthenia and hypochondriasis.

1673-1754—Richard Mead was one of the most celebrated and successful British physicians of the eighteenth century. He was born in Stepney, studied at Utrecht, Leyden and Padua, receiving his degree at Padua in 1695. On his return to England, he published his first work, *Mechanical Account of Poisons,*

1702, and, the following year, was elected Fellow of the Royal Society. The University of Oxford conferred upon him the degree of doctor of medicine in 1707. He succeeded to Radcliffe's practice on the latter's death and earned for years between 6 and 7,000 pounds annually, an enormous sum for that period. He was a great collector of books, statues, gems, prints, drawings and medals, which he housed in his spacious mansion. A printed catalogue of his library contained 6,592 separate numbers. He kept constantly in his pay several scholars and artists. His writings deal with the plague, measles and smallpox, the diseases described in the Bible, and medical precepts. He was known as the "princely Mead."

1674-1760—John Louis Petit, of Paris, was one of the greatest surgeons of his time. "Since Ambroise Paré, no one has contributed as much to the progress of this branch of the healing art." (Biograph. méd., 1824.) He devised many new operations and was the first to perform a cholecystotomy and to open the mastoid.

1675-1721—Martin Naboth, professor of medicine at Leipzig, described in 1704 the ovules or follicles which have since borne his name.

1675-1728—John Freind, physician, classical scholar, and the first English medical historian, was educated at Oxford, receiving his A.B. in 1698 and his M.B. in 1703. While an undergraduate student at Oxford, he edited a Greek and Latin edition of Aeschines and Demosthenes and revised a new edition of Ovid's *Metamorphoses.* After serving for

two years in the army in Spain, he settled in London, was created doctor of medicine at Oxford, and was elected Fellow of the Royal College of Physicians and of the Royal Society.

In 1722, Freind was elected a member of parliament and, the same year, was confined to the Tower for suspected participation in the so-called "bishop's plot." While a prisoner, he wrote *The History of Physick,* the first work of its kind in English, which was published in two volumes in 1725 and 1726 and remains a valuable work.

1679-1759—Gaspar Casál, a Spanish physician, practiced medicine at Oviedo in the Asturias from 1720 to 1751, when he moved to Madrid, where he was appointed physician to King Ferdinand. Three years after his death, his *Historia natural y medica de el principado de Asturias* was published in Madrid. This remarkable work, the fruit of 30 years' observation, describes the topography, climate, winds, waters, flora, fauna, minerals, metals, epidemics and diseases of the Asturias. In this book, the author describes in great detail the "Mal de la Rosa," now known as pellagra.

1697-1763—William Smellie, "one of the most important obstetricians of all times and countries," was born in Lanark, Scotland, studied medicine at Glasgow, began practice at Lanark in 1720, and, in 1738, moved to London. There he taught midwifery by demonstrations upon a "machine" and by attending the poor in their own homes. He invented several obstetrical instruments, including forceps with a simple lock, perforation, and blunt hooks. He made fundamental observations on the mechanism of labor and was the first to measure the diagonal conjugate diameter. William Hunter was his pupil.

1681-1737—Giovanni Domenico Santorini was born in Venice, studied at Bologna, Padua and Pisa, receiving his doctor's degree from Pisa in 1701. He was appointed professor of medicine at Venice the same year and, in 1706, became demonstrator of anatomy.

He was one of the most exact and careful dissectors of his day. His name and influence would have been far greater if death had not called him away before the completion of his chief work which was not published until 38 years after his demise, and then only in part (Choulant).

His chief works were *Observationes anatomicae*, Venice, 1724, of which Haller remarked, "In this unique book, the most subtle of dissectors sets forth many new discoveries"; and his *Septemdecim tabulae*, Parma, 1775. Santorini's anatomical works are characterized by their lucid descriptions and excellent artistic illustrations. "Even today a facial muscle (risorius), a pair of cartilages (cornicula) of the larynx, the emissary veins of the skull, and a part of the superior and inferior turbinates of the ethmoid are named after Santorini" (Choulant).

1682-1772—Giovanni Battista Morgagni.

1683-1758—Lorenz Heister was born at Frankfurt am Main, received his doctor's degree at Harderwyk, and served for a time as surgeon in the Dutch Army. In 1710, he was appointed professor of surgery at Altdorf and, in 1720, became professor of surgery at the University of Helmstedt, where he remained until his death. Heister was an extraordinarily industrious man, an indefatigable student, an excellent botanist, an accomplished linguist, and one of the outstanding surgeons of his time. His best known works were his *Institutiones chirurgicae*, Leyden, 1739; and his *Medizinische. Chirurgische und Anatomische Wahrnehmungen*, Rostock, 1753. In the latter work, he described a case of acute appendicitis observed while "dissecting the body of a malefactor."

1684-1751—Abraham Vater, graduate of the University of Wittenberg, professor later of anatomy and botany in his alma mater. In 1710, he described the papilla named after him.

1684-1766—Jean Astruc graduated at Montpellier in 1703, became professor of anatomy at Toulouse in 1711 but returned to Montpellier, and, in 1716, was appointed professor of medicine. He remained at Montpellier for 10 years, resigning to accept the position of professor of medicine at the *Collège Royal de France* in Paris.

Astruc is best known for his *De morbis venereis*, Paris, an invaluable history of syphilis and venereal diseases; and his *Memoires pour servir à l'historie de la faculté de médecine de Montpellier*, Paris, 1767, an indispensable source book on the history of Montpellier. He was also the author of *Traité des maladies des femmes*, Paris, 1761. Astruc's historical sketch of syphilis contains references to some 600 authors and defends with great skill the theory of the American origin of syphilis.

1686-1732—Adrian Christian Thebesius was educated at Leipzig, Halle and Leyden. He graduated at Leyden in 1708, and his doctor's dissertation, *De circulo sanguinis in corde,* described the Thebesian veins *(venarum minimarum)* and the Thebesian valve *(valvula sinus coronarii).* In 1709, he began practice in Hirschberg in Silesia, became town physician in 1714, and lived there until his death.

1688-1752—William Cheselden was one of the most famous English surgeons and anatomists of the eighteenth century. He was born in Leicestershire, received a sound classical education, and, at the age of 15, became a pupil of William Cowper, the anatomist, and was subsequently apprenticed to Mr. Ferne, surgeon and lithotomist to St. Thomas' Hospital. He was admitted to the Barber Surgeons' Company in 1710 and, the following year, gave lectures on anatomy. In 1719, he became surgeon to St. Thomas' Hospital, was appointed surgeon to Queen Caroline in 1727; and, when the French *Académie royale de chirurgie* was founded in 1729, he was the first foreign member elected. Cheselden was very successful as a surgeon, enjoyed a large practice, and was held in high esteem by the public, as expressed in the well-known verse of Pope:

I'll do what Mead and Cheselden advise
To keep these limbs, and to preserve these eyes.

Cheselden's *Anatomy of the Human Body* was first published in 1713 and went through 13 editions. His greatest work, *Osteography, or anatomy of the bones,* published in 1733, contains numerous beautiful plates, very accurate and of the highest artistic merit.

1688-1756—John Freke was one of the most prominent London surgeons of his time, a man of broad culture, well versed in natural science, a connoisseur in art, and a judge of music. He was surgeon to St. Bartholomew's Hospital and first curator of its museum. A Fellow of the Royal Society, he read before that body in 1736 one of the earliest accounts of *myositis ossificans.*

1693-1769—Antoine Ferrein, born in Frespech, France, studied first theology; but, fascinated by Borelli's *De motu animalium,* he studied medicine at Montpellier, where he received his doctor's degree. He served as an army surgeon from 1732 to 1735 and, in 1742, was chosen professor of medicine and surgery at the *Collège Royal* of Paris. He was the author of a handbook of practical surgery and published an anatomical study of the lachrymal glands.

1693-1770—Jean Baptiste Senac was born in Gascony and was intended by his parents for the Protestant ministry. Instead, he embraced Catholicism, became a Jesuit, and later studied medicine at Rheims, where he received his degree. In 1752, he was appointed physician to Louis XV, councillor of state, and later member of the *Académie royale des Sciences.* His *Traité de la structure du coeur de son action et de ses maladies,* Paris, 1749, in two volumes, was the first comprehensive systematic book on the anatomy, physiology and pathology of the heart and on heart disease. He noted exaggerated pulsation of the cervical arteries in enlargement of the left ventricle and marked pulsation of the cervical veins in enlargement of the right ventricle. He described ossification of the coronary vessels and insufficiency of the cardiac valves, and he even mentioned an endocardial murmur that could be heard at a distance. He also wrote books on chemistry, anatomy, lithiasis, and the plague, but these works were overshadowed by his *Traité*.

1694-1768—John Huxham was a native of Devon, studied medicine for three years at Leyden under Boerhaave, and then went to Rheims, where he received his doctor's degree. He returned to England, settled in Plymouth, and eventually obtained a high reputation and a considerable fortune. His *Essay on Fevers*, 1739, brought him great fame. His dissertation, *On the malignant, ulcerous sore throat,* 1750, contains an excellent description of diphtheria, but the author confuses it with the angina of scarlet fever. His *Method of preserving the Health of Seamen in Long Cruises and Voyages* advises the use of fresh vegetables and fruit juices to prevent scurvy. His *Dissertation on the Devonshire Colic,* 1758, ascribed this disease to the presence of crude tartar in the cider. He introduced the term "influenza" to describe the "vernal catarrh" of 1743.

1697-1767—Alexander Monro Senior *(primus).*

1697-1770—Bernhard Siegfried Albinus was born at Frankfort-on-the-Oder and studied at Leyden, where he took his doctor's degree in 1719. Two years later at the age of 24, he was appointed, on the recommendation of Boerhaave, professor of anatomy, a position he held for 50 years. His anatomical works contain what are probably the most artistic and accurate representations of the human body that have ever been published. His chief books were *Historia musculorum hominis,* Leyden, 1734; *Tabulae sceleti et musculorum humani,* Leyden, 1747; and *Tabulae ossium humanorum,* Leyden, 1753. Choulant describes Albinus as "the pioneer of a new epoch in human anatomy."

1698-1775—John Rutty, a native of Wiltshire, England, graduated in medicine at Leyden in 1723 and then settled in Dublin, where he practiced until his death. A very devout Quaker, he lived sparely, sometimes dined on nettles, and frequently fasted. His *Spiritual Diary,* in which he accused himself of irritability and of too much love for materia medica, meteorology, and good food, excited the mirth of Samuel Johnson. His *Chronological History of the Weather and Seasons and of the prevailing Diseases in Dublin,* London, 1770, contains the first clear description of relapsing fever.

1699-1767—Paul Gottlieb Werlhof was born at Helmstedt, began his medical studies at the University of Helmstedt at the early age of 17, graduating in 1723. In 1760, he became physician to the court of Hanover and achieved an European reputation as a physician and scholar, his clientele extending from Moscow to Rome. He also composed poetry and wrote hymns. In 1735, he described purpura haemorrhagica, since known as *morbus maculosus Werlhofi*. His *Opera omnia* was published at Hanover in 1775.

1700-1772—Gerhard van Swieten.

-1784—Matthew Dobson, a native of Yorkshire, graduated at Edinburgh in 1756 and practiced in Liverpool. He was a Fellow of the Royal Society and a member of the Medical Society in London. In 1776 he described sugar in the urine of a diabetic—the first demonstration of this fact. Dobson also wrote *A Medical Commentary on Fixed Air*, London, 1779, describing experiments with carbon dioxide.

1704-1776—Anton de Haen.

-1775—François Thiéry was a native of Nancy and took his medical degree at Paris in 1740. While physician to the French ambassador to Spain, he met Gasper Casál and, hearing from him an account of the new and strange malady, "Mal de la Rosa" (pellagra), sent a report of it to Paris, where it was published in the *Journal de médecine, chirurgie et pharmacie* in 1755.

1708-1777—Albrecht von Haller.

1708-1779—Thomas Cadwalader.

1710-1786—Jacques Gautier d'Agoty was a physician, an anatomist and an artist. He claimed the discovery of the four-color process of printing and employed color plates in the illustration of his numerous works on anatomy. Choulant observed, "His anatomic illustrations, while they may be perhaps fascinating to the layman, on account of their size and vivid execution . . . do not recommend themselves to the student of anatomy."

1710-1790—William Cullen.

1710-1801—William Heberden.

1711-1746—Johann Nathanael Lieberkühn, born in Berlin, studied at Halle, Jena and Leyden, receiving his doctor's degree at Leyden in 1739. He settled in Berlin in 1740 and practiced there until his death. He was an excellent anatomist and described the glands since called by his name in a treatise, *De fabrica et actione villorum et intestinorum tenium*, published at Leyden in 1745.

1712-1780—John Fothergill was born in Yorkshire and, after an apprenticeship to an apothecary, entered the University of Edinburgh with the plan of qualifying as an apothecary. He attracted the attention of Monro *primus*, who urged him to study medicine. He followed this advice and graduated in medicine in 1736. After graduation, he went to London, studied for two years at St. Thomas', and began practice among the poor. He soon attained a large practice and such a reputation as a skilled practitioner that, as he said later, "I climbed on the backs of the poor to the pockets of the rich."

Soon his practice became one of the largest and most lucrative in London. He purchased a large estate, where he laid out a very extensive botanical garden, which in a short time acquired a European reputation. He was a Quaker, a great humanitarian and philanthropist. He was very active in prison reform, in the improvement of medical education, and in the abolition of slavery.

Fothergill was the first graduate of Edinburgh to be admitted to the Royal College of Physicians (1744) and, in 1763, was elected a Fellow of the Royal Society. In 1774, he was offered the post of Royal physician but declined the appointment. His *Account of the Putrid Sore Throat attended with Ulcers,* London, 1748, was an early classic account of diphtheria; his account of *tic douloureaux* is an early clear description of this affection; and his paper on angina pectoris contains the first record of sclerosis of the coronary arteries in this disease—an observation confirmed later by Jenner and by Parry.

1713-1788—Percivall Pott was born in London and, at the age of 16, was apprenticed to Edward Nourse, surgeon to St. Bartholomew's Hospital. In 1745, Pott was appointed assistant surgeon to St. Bartholomew's and full surgeon in 1749, retiring in 1778 at the age of 75.

Pott has been often described as a surgical genius. He wrote treatises on wounds, fractures, dislocations, hydrocele, fistulae and cataracts. His *Some few general remarks on fractures and dislocations,* London, 1769, depicts the fracture since called Pott's fracture—a fracture Pott himself received when thrown from a horse. His *Remarks on that kind of palsy of the lower limbs, which is frequently found to accompany curvature of the spine,* London, 1779, describes the condition now known as Pott's disease. His *Chirurgical Works* appeared in London in 1771.

1716-1794—James Lind.

1717-1783—Linnaeus, or Carl von Linné, botanist, professor of physic and botany at Uppsala and physician to the King of Sweden. He is called "the father of systematic botany."

1718-1783—William Hunter.

1719-1813—Francis Home, a native of Scotland, served as a regimental surgeon from 1742 to 1748 in Flanders and, during lulls in the campaign, studied medicine at Leyden. After the war, he entered the University of Edinburgh, where he received the degree of doctor of medicine in 1750. He taught materia medica, the institutes of medicine and agriculture at his alma mater. His *An Enquiry into the Nature, Cause and Cure of the Croup,* Edinburgh, 1765, according to some authorities, contains the first, clear, systematic study of diphtheria. He also, "in the same way as the Turks have taught us to mitigate the smallpox," vaccinated children with material from measles and apparently produced some degree of immunity. Home was also the first observer to point out that yeast fermented the sugar in diabetic urine.

1721-1770—Mark Akenside was born in Newcastle, England, studied medicine first at Edinburgh and later at Leyden, where he received his M.D. degree in 1744. He practiced medicine in London and achieved some reputation as a poet, his best known poem being *The Pleasures of Imagination,* published in 1744.

1721-1809—Sir George Baker.

1722-1763—William Hillary, an English physician, was a pupil of Boerhaave and received his M.D. degree from Leyden in 1722. He practiced first at Ripon and Bath, then went to the Barbados, where he remained six years. On his return to England, he settled in London, where he remained until his death. Hillary's *Observations on the changes of the air and the concomitant epidemical diseases of the island of Barbados*, London, 1759, contains the first account of sprue in the English language.

1722-1776—Théophile de Bordeu, a native of Iseste, France, graduated in medicine at Montpellier and was for many years director of the baths in the Pyrenees. He was one of the founders of the school of vitalism and taught that health was a co-ordination of the individual life of each organ in the body. The most important organs of the body are the stomach, heart and brain, and the glands are very important in the economy of the body. Bordeu maintained that every disease was cured by a crisis and in his therapy aimed to produce a crisis, which, in chronic diseases, he produced by stimulants.

1722-1789—Pieter Camper, physician, anatomist and naturalist, was born in Leyden and studied medicine at the University of Leyden, where he graduated in 1746. He was successively professor at Franeker, Amsterdam and Gröningen. A skilled artist as well as an anatomist, he made, while in London, several plates for Smellie's *Set of anatomical tables* dealing with obstetrics, and he illustrated his own works on anatomy, pathology and anthropology. His *Demonstrationum anatomico-pathologicum*, Amsterdam, 1760, treats of anatomic, pathologic and surgical observations, with ex-cellent illustrations by the author. His *Verhandeling over het naturlijk verschil der wezenstrekken in Menschen*, etc., Utrecht, 1791, contains investigations on the mathematical structures of the human body and describes the "facial angle" as a criterion of race. Camper discovered the processus vaginalis of the peritoneum and the fibrous structure of the lens and made excellent topographic studies of the arm, pelvis, inguinal canal, and proposed symphysiotomy in labor.

fl.1771—Francesco Frapolli graduated at Pavia in 1757 and practiced medicine in Milan, where he was physician to the Ospedale Maggiore. In 1771, he wrote an account of pellagra and gave this name to the disease. He died in 1773.

1725-1813—Leopoldo Marco Antonio Caldani was born in Bologna, where he obtained his medical degree. He later studied at Padua with Morgagni, became professor of anatomy at Bologna in 1760 and professor at Padua in 1771. He was the author of *Icones anatomicae*, Venice, 1801, and *Iconum anatomicarum explicatio*, Venice, 1802, which, according to Choulant, "comprised the best anatomic representations of past periods."

1728-1793—John Hunter.

1728-1799—Joseph Black.

1731-1802—Erasmus Darwin, physician, philosopher, physiologist and poet, was born in Elton, England, and was educated at Cambridge and Edinburgh. He practiced at Nottingham, Lichfield and Derby. His poem, *Botanic Garden*, 1792, contains much botanical information but is lacking in poetic quality. His

Zoonomia, 1794, emphasized the gradual evolution of complex organisms, the struggle for existence, sexual selection, and the influence of environment, thus anticipating the work of his famous grandson, Charles Darwin.

1731-1810—Henry Cavendish.

1733-1804—Joseph Priestley.

1733-1817—Alexander Monro *secundus.*

1735-1788—John Brown.

1735-1789—John Morgan.

1734-1815—Friedrich Anton Mesmer.

1733-1794—Caspar Friedrich Wolff was born in Berlin, received his medical degree at Halle in 1759 and lived for several years in Berlin, teaching logic, physiology, pathology and therapy. In 1767, he went to St. Petersburg as a member of the Academy of Sciences and worked there until his death. Wolff is regarded as "the father of modern embryology" and described the Wolffian duct and Wolffian body in his doctor's thesis of 1759.

1736-1808—William Shippen.

1736-1822—Domenico Cotugno was born at Ruvo in the province of Bari, Italy, studied medicine at the University of Naples, where he later became professor of anatomy. His best known work was his *De ischiade nervosa commentarius,* Naples, 1765, in which he demonstrated, by heating, albumin in the urine. He also discovered the aqueduct of Cotugno, described the intestinal lesions of typhoid and the skin lesions of smallpox.

1737-1798—Luigi Galvani was born and spent his life in Bologna. He graduated at Bologna in 1759, became professor of operative surgery and, in 1766, professor of anatomy. In his *De viribus electricitatis in motu musculari commentarius,* 1791, he showed that two dissimilar metals, when brought into contact with each other, produced an electrical current which caused contraction of a frog's muscle and that electricity could be generated in animal tissues—animal electricity.

1739-1774—William Hewson was born at Hexham, Northumberland, England, studied anatomy with William Hunter in London, and later attended lectures at Guy's Hospital and at Edinburgh. In 1762, he entered into partnership with the Hunters. He became celebrated as a teacher of anatomy and was elected Fellow of the Royal Society. He demonstrated the presence of lymphatics in birds, reptiles and fishes, and, in his *Experimental Inquiry into the Properties of the Blood,* Phil. Trans., 1770, he demonstrated the role of "coagulable lymph," now called fibrinogen, in coagulation. "A man of genius, he died of a dissection wound" (Garrison).

1740-1827—John Haygarth, a native of Yorkshire, England, graduated at Cambridge in 1766 and settled in Chester. In 1798, he moved to Bath, where he analyzed his clinical records accumulated while physician to the Chester Infirmary and published them in his *A Clinical History of Acute Rheumatism,* London, 1805.

1740-1819—Eduard Sandifort, born in Dortrecht, Holland, studied at Leyden, where he received his doctor's degree in 1763. In 1772, he was called to Leyden as professor of anatomy and surgery and remained there until his death. He was an outstanding anatomist, and, while he followed the methods of Albinus and was much interested in accurate and artistic illustrations, yet he treated anatomy in its relationship to disease and pictured diseased as well as healthy states. Cruveilhier called him "the father of pathological iconography." He wrote many books, among them *Observationes anatomico-pathologicae,* Leyden, 1777-1781, which contains the first known illustration of vegetative endocarditis in a patient with pulmonary stenosis and interventrical septal defect (Fallot's tetralogy).

1741-1799—William Withering.

1742-1786—Carl Wilhelm Scheele.

1742-1821—Samuel Bard.

1742-1787—Maximilian Stoll.

1743-1794—Antoine Laurent Lavoisier.

1744-1815—John Coakley Lettsom was born on the island of Little Vandyke in the West Indies and, at the age of six years, was sent to England for his education. He attended the lectures of Dr. Cullen in Edinburgh and subsequently studied at Paris and at Leyden, receiving his medical degree at Leyden in 1769. He settled in London under the patronage of Dr. Fothergill and was very successful. "For many years he enjoyed the largest medical business in the city" (Munk). A Quaker and a great philanthropist, he was on intimate terms with the most eminent men of the period. His chief works were *Reflections on the General Treatment and Cure of Fevers,* London, 1772; and *The Natural History of the Tea Tree,* etc., London, 1772.

1744-1829—Jean Baptiste Lamarck, French naturalist, was born in Bazantin, Picardy, and, after serving in the army, began the study of medicine. Later, however, his interest shifted to botany, and his *Flora française,* published in 1778, gained him admission to the *Académie des Sciences.* In 1793, at the age of 50, he was appointed professor of zoology at the Jardin du Roi. He now began work actively in his new field, and, in 1815, his *Histoire naturelle des animaux sans vertèbres* appeared which established his fame as a naturalist. He was the father of the modern doctrine of evolution that new organs develop in animals as the result of a new want continuing to be felt and that such changes are preserved and transmitted to new generations.

1745-1813—Benjamin Rush.

1745-1821—Johann Peter Frank.

1756-1810—Jean Louis Baudelocque, a great name in the history of obstetrics, was born in Heilly, Picardy, France, studied in Paris and worked for many years at the Hôpital de la Charité. In 1776, he was elected to the *Collège de Chirurgie* and, in 1798, was appointed professor of obstetrics at the École de Santé and was soon the leading obstetrician in Paris. Napoleon appointed him accoucheur to the Empress Maria Louise, but he did not live to officiate. His *Principes des accouchements,* Paris, 1775, went through five editions.

1747-1832—Antonio Scarpa, surgeon and anatomist, was born in Motta, Italy, and studied anatomy under Morgagni at Padua and surgery under Rivera at Bologna. In 1783, he became professor of anatomy at

Pavia and later of surgery also. He wrote the first accurate description of the anatomy of clubfoot. He was an excellent artist and engraved most of the plates for his anatomical works. "His anatomic prints are therefore models of anatomic representation as regards faithful differentiation of the tissues, correctness of form, and the utmost perfection of engraving". (Choulant). Noteworthy were his *Anatomicarum annotationum,* Ticini and Milan, 1779 and 1785; and his masterpiece, *Tabulae nevralogicae,* Ticini, 1794. His *Saggio di osservationi e d'esperienze sulle principali malattie degli occhi,* 1801, was the first Italian text on ophthalmology.

1748-1794—Félix Vicq d'Azyr, famous French anatomist and scholar, was born in Valognes, studied medicine at Paris, and, while still a student, gave lectures on anatomy. He became secretary of the *Societé Royale de Médecine* and read many papers before this organization. In 1789, he was appointed first physician to Queen Marie Antoinette and, although pursued by the revolutionaires, died a natural death. He was an excellent anatomist as well as physiologist. His chief work was his *Traité d'anatomie et physiologie,* Paris, 1786.

1749-1823—Edward Jenner.

1752-1815—Paolo Mascagni was born in Castelleto (Siena), became professor of anatomy at Siena in 1774 and professor of anatomy at Pisa in 1800. One year later, he was appointed instructor in anatomy and physiology in the hospital of Santa Maria Nuova in Florence. Mascagni's great work, *Vasorum lymphaticorum corporis humani historia et ichnographia,* Siena, 1787, is a faithful and masterful representation of the lymphatics and remains unsurpassed in its field for accuracy and artistic beauty.

1753-1814—Benjamin Thompson, Count Rumford, scientist, soldier, administrator and philanthropist, was born in Woburn, Massachusetts, but, sympathizing with the British during the Revolution, went to London, where he was appointed Under-Secretary of State and also pursued investigations on gunpowder, firearms, and signaling at sea. He was elected a Fellow of the Royal Society, was knighted by the king, and, in 1784, went to Munich at the invitation of Prince Maximilian. He remained in Munich, where he reorganized the army, introduced measures to improve the condition of the people, and carried out experiments on heat, devising a thermoscope and calorimeter to aid in his tests. In addition, he studied many practical problems relating to the heating and ventilation of houses. He was created Count Rumford by the grateful Elector. Rumford returned to London, where, in 1800, he founded the Royal Institution of Great Britain for the study of science, securing as professors Humphry Davy, Thomas Young, and Michael Faraday. Rumford moved to Auteuil near Paris in 1804 and continued his scientific investigations until his death.

1754-1846—Benjamin Waterhouse.

The Nineteenth Century— The First Half

NAPOLEONIC WARS AND THE INDUSTRIAL REVOLUTION

THE NINETEENTH CENTURY witnessed the emergence of modern medicine. The century began in the turmoil of war and revolution, in kaleidoscopic changes in the political, economic and social structure of Europe, the effects of which spread far beyond the boundaries of that continent. The towering figure of the Corsican, Napoleon, spread its shadow over the Continent for both good and evil; the ferment of the French Revolution and the profound influence of the growing Industrial Revolution, which changed the social structure of nations, exerted deep and lasting changes on the evolution of medicine.

The Napoleonic wars carried social reforms into Italy and the Rhineland, but new diseases followed in the wake of French arms, and the general level of health declined. Napoleon's dream of European domination was shattered at Waterloo in 1815 but had received a mortal wound three years previously in the ill-fated campaign against Russia. In June, 1812, Napoleon led an army of 363,000 men into Russia, an army later reinforced by reserves. When this army, after incredible sufferings, retreated from Russia and crossed into East Prussia in December of the same year, Larrey described it as follows: "Three thousand men of the best soldiers of the guard, part infantry, part cavalry, almost all from the central provinces of France, were the only ones who had really resisted the cruel vicissitudes of the retreat." He adds that this small army was "the remnant of an army of more than 400,000 men, which the inhabitants of the country had seen march six months before in all their strength and in all their splendor."

Disease played a decisive role in the defeat of Napoleon's army. The French troops crossing into Poland were immediately attacked by typhus and typhoid, which decimated the soldiers by the thousands. Kerckhoffs, a Dutch army surgeon who served in Napoleon's army and has left us a vivid account of the sufferings of the soldiers, remarked that, if Napoleon had contented himself with occupying Poland and reorganizing sanitation there, the campaign would have been a success and the whole course of history would have been changed. Larrey, who accompanied Napoleon on all his major campaigns, also described in vivid terms the losses from battle, privation and disease. The soldiers returning from Russia brought back the same diseases that had decimated their comrades. Central Europe, during the next three years, was a hot bed of typhus fever, typhoid fever and dysentery.

The Industrial Revolution, while not so spectacular as either the French Revolution or the Napoleonic Wars, produced an equally profound change in creating a new kind of society. The great inventions of the eighteenth and nineteenth centuries—the steam engine patented by James Watt in 1769, the discovery of methods for using coal in blast furnaces, the invention of new machines for the manufacture of textiles—led to an unprecedented development of the iron and textile industries and to the conversion of the rural peasant society into an urban industrial one. This revolution was further accelerated by the invention of railways, the rise of engineering, and the discovery and utilization of electricity. The Industrial Revolution began in England and spread to the continent of Europe and to America.

The rapid increase in the population of the towns in England, caused by this industrial expansion, found that country without any effective system of local government. The new towns, which sprang up so rapidly as the textile and metal industries expanded, were unable to handle the new problems. Overcrowding, unsanitary housing conditions, the lack of proper supervision of water supply and food, all emphasized that life in these congested centers was becoming increasingly hazardous to the inhabitants. As William Farr, the best known statistician of this period, observed, "It is proven beyond doubt that, if the population be the same in other respects, an increase in density implies an increase in mortality; and that the ratio of increase . . . is as certain roots of density."

This increase in mortality brought into sharp relief that the medical profession was quite as unable under the existing conditions to combat the rising tide of disease as the country squires, acting as local magistrates, were unable to deal with the complex problems presented by the mushroom-like growth of the industrial towns and cities. There was a growing realization that health was a concern of the public and that public health was a responsibility of the state as well as of the individual. This thought, with all its implications, had as its powerful and influential champion Johann Peter Frank, often called "the Father of Public Health."

JOHANN PETER FRANK AND HIS
MEDICINISCHE POLIZEY

Johann Peter Frank was born in the town of Rodalben near Lake Constance in 1745 of mixed German and French ancestry, a "rare and happy mixture of German thoroughness and French intelligence" (Garrison). Against the opposition of his parents, he decided to study medicine and went first to Heidelberg, then to Strassburg, and back to Heidelberg, where he received his doctor's degree in 1766. At the time of his examination, he had a noteworthy conversation with Dr. Oberkamp, dean of the medical faculty at Heidelberg, who asked him what he intended to do. Young Frank, age 21, answered that he thought many diseases were of such a nature that some kind of public control was necessary and that, since there was no work describing the principles of this sort of control, he proposed to write such a book. When Dr. Oberkamp asked him what he was going to call a work like this, the student answered promptly, *"Medicinische Polizey,"* for it would be medicine administered by the state.

Frank began practice in Rodalben and, in 1768, had completed the first volume of his *Medicinische Polizey*. This, however, was refused by the publisher. The young author, discouraged by the rebuff, says, "I took my despised manuscript with both hands, tore it furiously in a thousand pieces, and delivered these to the flames." During the next 10 years, Frank was active in practice, had charge of the garrison hospital at Rastadt, saw severe epidemics of typhoid fever, dysentery and smallpox, practiced obstetrics, and established a school for midwives. Meanwhile, he began work anew on his *Medicinische Polizey,* and the first volume of his *System einer vollständigen medicinischen Polizey* appeared in 1779, a second volume in 1780, and the third volume in 1783. From these, Frank achieved a great reputation. He was appointed professor at Göttingen in 1784 but remained there only one year, leaving to accept a similar post in Pavia. Here he remained for 10 years and was presently *Protophysicus,* or medical director, of Austrian Lombardy. In Pavia, in addition to teaching, he revised the medical curriculum, established courses for midwives and apothecaries, founded a medical library, a pathological museum, and a chemical laboratory, published numerous articles, and completed volume four of his *Medicinische Polizey*. In 1795, he went to Vienna as director of the *Allgemeines Krankenhaus* and as professor of clinical medicine in the university. Here he revised the curriculum, established the pathological museum, and soon directed a medical clinic, recognized as one of the most outstanding in Europe. Students from all over the Continent flocked to Vienna to hear his lectures, always delivered in Latin, and to follow his ward rounds and clinical demonstrations.

After nine years in Vienna, Frank went to Russia as physician to the Czar and as director of the Medical-Surgical Academy in St.

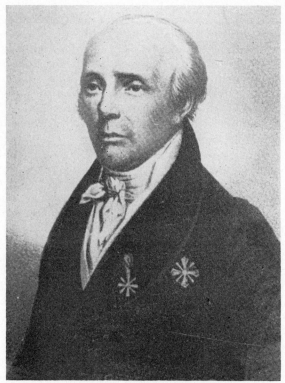

Sigerist, *Grosse Ärzte*, München, 1932

JOHANN PETER FRANK

Petersburg. The climate disagreed with him, and, in 1817, he returned to Vienna, where he enjoyed a very large practice, numbering among his patients Beethoven and the young King of Rome, the son of Napoleon by Marie Louise. Richard Bright, who was in Vienna in 1814, wrote:

Of all I have mentioned, Dr. Frank is best known to the world by his numerous and learned writings. . . . His wish was to avoid practice and to devote himself to his literary pursuits; but, notwithstanding this, he has much practice forced upon him as a consulting physician. .... He is a man of the most instructive and pleasing conversation, with great knowledge both of books and men, and most universally respected.

Volume five of Frank's *Medicinische Polizey* was published in 1813. Volume six appeared in 1817-1818. He died in 1821.

The *Medicinische Polizey* is the first comprehensive treatise on public health. In the preface to this great work, the author states his *credo:* "to prevent evils through wise ordinances." He discusses in great detail vital statistics, marital hygiene, infant and maternal welfare, child welfare, infectious diseases, food inspection and sanitation. His views aroused much discussion as well as hostility. His contention that all physically and mentally healthy persons should marry and that most men and women were unsuited to celibacy aroused clerical circles. His statement that unmarried mothers and their children were entitled to the same care and protection as married women and legitimate children seemed radical at that time. His naïve enthusiasm for the regulations he proposed and his belief that laws could transform theories into facts, betray a deep ignorance of human nature and a disregard for the instinct of personal independence. "It never seems to have occurred to him that health education might be necessary before the public could be expected to respect and observe his laws" (Baumgartner and Ramsey).

Frank's public health measures, excellent though most of them were in theory, breathed the spirit of absolutism, which was characteristic of Austrian political thinking at that period. They had little influence upon contemporary thought. Even Frank himself, who had devoted his entire life to writing his *Medicinische Polizey,* won his European reputation, not as a reformer and the pioneer in public health, but as a skilled physician and as an outstanding medical teacher. Several decades later, after the din and confusion caused by the Napoleonic wars had subsided and a more stable and peaceful atmosphere had appeared on the Continent, his ideas of public health reform took firm root and spread.

THE PARIS SCHOOL

The early years of the nineteenth century saw in France a constant succession of brilliant physicians and great surgeons. Paris, at this period, had almost an excess or plethora of brilliant minds. As soon, it seemed, as one comet came across the horizon, another appeared to dim its lustre. There can be no doubt that the god of medicine, which had once had his habitation in Greece, then wandered to Alexandria, from there to Baghdad, thence to Italy during the Renaissance, and from there to the Netherlands, had now taken up his abode in Paris.

The political and economic ferment unloosed by the French Revolution and the Napoleonic Wars produced some of the greatest military leaders and statemen in history. It coincided also with the appearance in France of a large number of outstanding scientists and physicians, whose achievements, though less spectacular than those of Napoleon, Marshal Ney and Talleyrand, were of more enduring value. Whether this resurgence of French science was produced by the political and military upheavals of this period, or whether the great scientists and physicians developed in spite of these upheavals, is a moot point. Some of these men were closely connected, both politically and personally, with the affairs of Napoleon; others were as far removed as possible, considering the powerful impact of Napoleon on every phase of French life.

One of the great surgeons during this time was Dominique Jean Larrey (1766-1842), devoted friend and follower of Napoleon, who accompanied his master in his campaigns in Italy, Germany, Egypt and Russia, and was by his side at the fateful Battle of Waterloo. Faithful until the last, Larrey received on Napoleon's death a legacy of 100,000 francs with the notation, *"C'est l'homme le plus vertueux que j'aie connu."*

Larrey was born in the village of Beaudéan and received his first training under his uncle, Alexis Larrey of Toulouse. After studying in Paris under Louis and Desault, he entered the navy and, after a brief service, returned to Paris and entered the *Collège de Chirurgie*. In 1792, he joined the Army of the Rhine and henceforth spent most of his active days as an army surgeon. He rose by sheer force of character and ability; was named, with Desgenettes, chief of the medical service in the Army of the Orient, which invaded Egypt; was created a baron after the Battle of Wagram; and was named surgeon-in-chief of the *Grande Armée,* which had such a disastrous campaign in Russia. After the banishment of Napoleon to Alba, Larrey went into retirement but joined his master on his return. He served at the Battle of Waterloo. The Duke of Wellington, following the fighting from the heights of Mount St. Jean during the battle, saw Larrey working directly under the fire of the English cannon. When told it was Larrey, the Duke said, "Go tell them not to fire on that side, give this brave fellow time to collect

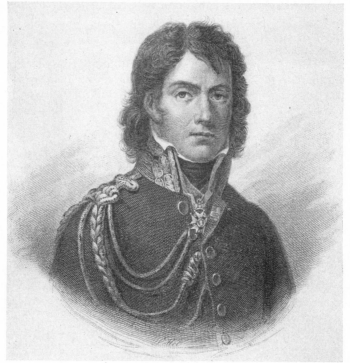

University of Kansas Collection

DOMINIQUE JEAN LARREY

his wounded." Larrey was captured at the end of the battle and sentenced to death. Led out for execution, he was recognized and released through the intervention of Blücher, whose son's life he had saved in a previous campaign. Larrey, who always shared the dangers and privations of the troops, took part in 60 battles, 400 engagements, and was wounded three times.

His *Relation historique et chirurgicale de l'expedition de l'armée d'Orient,* Paris, 1803, and his *Clinique chirurgicale,* Paris, 1829, are vivid accounts of his surgical experiences with the armies of Napoleon in Italy, Germany, Egypt and Russia. At Borodino, he performed 200 amputations in 24 hours. He was probably the first to describe "trench foot" (1812), to point out the contagious nature of Egyptian ophthalmia, and he described vividly the ravages of scurvy in the French army in Egypt. He employed a flexible rubber catheter passed into the stomach to feed a soldier who had received a severe

wound of the glottis at the Battle of Aboukir. He invented the celebrated "flying ambulances," with which he picked up wounded
soldiers as soon as the battle began and not at its end, which had
been the custom up to this time. Thus originated the rule of "first
aid to the wounded" in the modern sense. His professional life ends
with the fall of Napoleon. Upon the return of the Bourbons, Larrey,
as a follower of Napoleon, was deprived of his honors and his pension. He suffered no bodily harm, as did many of Napoleon's followers, because his hold on the affections of the people was too
strong.

Pierre François Percy (1754-1825), Larrey's colleague and life-
long friend, also spent most of his active professional life in Napoleon's armies. He was for a long time surgeon-in-chief of the
army, was succeeded by Larrey as chief during the invasion of Russia, but again became chief at the Battle of Waterloo. He was created a baron by Napoleon and, during his long service as an army
surgeon, introduced many improvements in the treatment of the
wounded, in ambulance service, and in the organization of the
medical department of the army. He was the author of *Manuel du
chirurgien d'armée,* Paris, 1792, a highly prized and notable book
on military surgery.

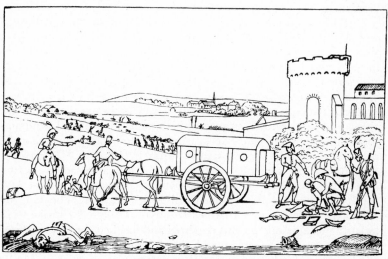

Cabanès, *Chirurgiens et Blessés à travers l'Histoire,* Paris, 1918
LARREY'S "FLYING AMBULANCE"

A very different type of person was Guillaume Dupuytren, whom Percy described as the "first of surgeons and the last of men." He rose to eminence not through long service on the battle field but by long and careful training in anatomy, pathology and surgery. Born at Pierre-Buffière in 1777, the son of a poor advocate, he was a boy of unusual charm and intelligence and attracted the attention of a cavalry officer stationed in the town. This officer took him to Paris, where he was sent to the *Collège de la Marche*. After finishing college, he returned home with the idea, it is said, of becoming a soldier, but this was overruled by his father, who told him he must become a surgeon. He went back to Paris, where he entered the medical school but where he suffered great hardships because of his poverty. A year later at the age of 18 he obtained a position as prosector at the *École de Santé* and presently was placed in charge of all autopsies at the medical school, an unrivaled opportunity of which he made the most. In 1801, he was appointed *chef des travaux anatomiques* and began his anatomical studies with his characteristic energy. Soon, however, he turned his attention to pathology and announced that he was writing a treatise on pathological anatomy based on findings in 1,000 autopsies. He gave a course in pathology with Bayle and Laennec as assistants but lost interest in that field. Meanwhile he had a violent quarrel with Laennec, who resented his attempts to belittle Bichat and to appropriate Bichat's work as his own.

In 1802, Dupuytren obtained the position of surgeon of the second class at the Hôtel Dieu, where he worked until his death, being elected, after a bitter contest, to the chair of operative surgery in 1812 and becoming surgeon-in-chief in 1815. He reigned alone and supreme, disliked by his colleagues, but performing an incredible amount of work, and soon was recognized, even by his enemies, as the outstanding surgeon of his day. Garrison calls him, "the ablest and best trained surgeon of his time . . . cold, hard, contemptuous, unscrupulous and overbearing, and more respected than beloved." Dupuytren was created a baron by Louis XVIII and was appointed first surgeon to Charles X. He amassed a fortune and, after the dethronement of Charles, offered the exiled king a gift of 1,000,000 francs—one-third of his fortune. The king declined the generous gift. In 1833, Dupuytren suffered a stroke while lecturing to his students, but persisted and finished the lecture. From that time on, he was an invalid, dying some 15 months later.

The surgical achievements of Dupuytren were numerous. He devised an enterotome to be used in the making of an artificial anus,

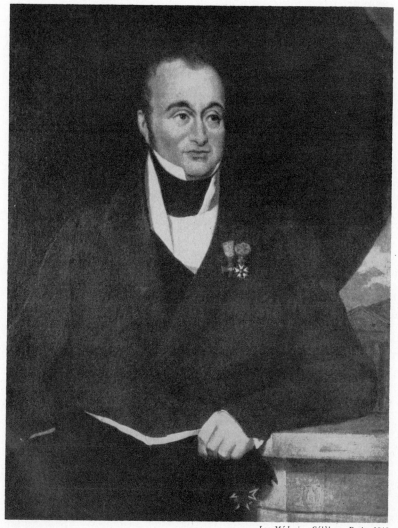

GUILLAUME DUPUYTREN
Artist unknown. Hôtel Dieu, Paris.

first removed successfully the lower jaw, sectioned the sterno-cleido-mastoid muscle for wry-neck, first successfully ligated the external iliac, described the condition now known as Dupuytren's contracture, and cured it by operation. He was a clear, forceful and logical lecturer. He never operated if an operation could be avoided, but, once the decision to operate was made, he studied the patient with great care, made all necessary preparations, and operated with an unshakable cold bloodedness. His *Leçons orales,* his clinics at the Hôtel Dieu, were published by his pupils, de Boismont and Mark, in four volumes, Paris, 1830-1834, and were translated into German, English, Italian and Danish. Dupuytren lived and died true to his maxim, "Nothing should be feared so much for a man as mediocrity" *(Rien n'est pas tant à redouter pour un homme que la médiocrité).*

Marie François Xavier Bichat (1771-1802), who began his professional career as a surgeon and assistant to the well-known surgeon, Pierre Joseph Desault, later turned his attention to anatomy and physiology and has been described as "the father of descriptive anatomy." Bichat was born at Thoirette in the Department of Jura, studied first at Montpellier, then at Lyons, and later at Paris, where he became the favorite pupil of Desault. In 1797, he gave lectures on anatomy, physiology, surgery and pathology and, four years later, was appointed physician to the Hôtel Dieu. Deeply interested in the problems of life and death, he threw himself passionately into the study of pathology, even sleeping at times in the morgue, and performed more than 600 autopsies during one winter. Worn out by excessive work, which had undermined his already frail constitution, he died in 1802 at the early age of 31, following a fall down the staircase of the Hôtel Dieu.

Bichat was deeply influenced by Bordeu's vitalistic doctrines and by Haller's demonstration of the irritability of muscular tissue. While Haller had demonstrated that irritability was a property of muscular tissue, Bichat extended this concept to cover all living tissue. While John Brown saw life as the result of the stimulation of external forces, Bichat considered it as something primordial, original and independent. Like John Hunter, he believed that disease was primarily an alteration of the vital principle. These views were expounded in his *Recherches physiologiques sur la vie et la mort,* 1818, containing a large number of physiological and pathological observations. This work begins with his oft-quoted definition, *"La vie est l'ensemble des fonctions qui résistent à la mort,"*

(Life is the sum of forces which resist death), a definition which, as has been often pointed out, is merely a question-begging truism. Bichat also assigned to each tissue a specific vital property, a view since shown to be untenable.

His most important work was his *Anatomie générale,* Paris, 1801, a detailed description of the tissues of the body in health and in disease. While previous anatomists and pathologists had confined their attention to the study of individual organs, Bichat stressed the importance of the systems of the body, the cellular tissues, the arteries, veins, lymphatics, bones, muscles and glands in diseased state. This book had a profound influence upon pathology and, particularly, upon clinical medicine. Its influence is apparent in the writings of Broussais, Corvisart and Laennec.

A physician whose interests lay in a different field was Philippe Pinel, who is remembered by posterity as a great psychiatrist, one of the first to treat insane patients in a humane manner. Pinel was born in 1755 near Lavour in southern France, was destined for the Church, but decided to study medicine, and entered the medical school of Toulouse, where he received

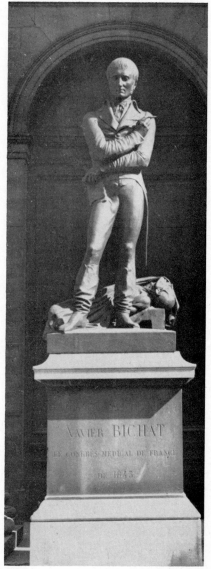

XAVIER BICHAT

Statue in the court of the École de médecine, Paris.

his doctor's degree in 1772. After further study at Montpellier, he went to Paris in 1778, where he supported himself by teaching mathematics. During this period, he published papers on the mechanics of bones and joints, which attracted so much attention that he was appointed to a position at the Jardin des Plantes.

Deeply moved by the death of a friend who became insane, ran away to the forest, and was devoured by wolves, Pinel resolved to devote himeslf to the study of mental diseases and soon attained such proficiency that he became in 1792 physician to the Bicêtre, a hospital for the insane. He found many patients chained and treated like wild beasts, being often shown to the curious, who paid an admission to see the spectacle. He removed the chains from the poor unfortunates and introduced humane treatment of the patients. His experiences with the insane were described in his *Traité medico-philosophique sur l'aliénation mentale ou la manie,* Paris, 1801, a landmark in the history of mental disorders.

Even though Pinel is remembered by posterity chiefly for his introduction of humane methods of treatment in psychiatry and as a great humanitarian, he was more eminent in his day as a system-atizer. His chief work was considered to be his *Nosographie philo-sophique, ou la méthode de l'analyse appliqué à la médecine,* Paris, 1789. According to him, medicine is only a branch of natural science and should be studied such as one studies botany, zoology and min-eralogy. Diseases are entities and can be classified, just as the dif-ferent plants and animals. He distinguished 2,700 diseases and di-vided them into classes, orders, genera and species.

The idea was not original. Carl von Linné (1707-1778), who was both a botanist and a physician, had published in 1737 his *Genera plantarum,* which is considered the starting point of modern botany. Becoming through his later writings a European celebrity, he turned his attention to medicine and published in 1763 *Genera morborum,* wherein he attempted to classify diseases as specifically as he had classified plants. Cullen's *Nosographia,* published in 1772, attempted a somewhat similar feat. Pinel's more ambitious work, along simi-lar lines, was a great success. It went through six editions and made its author famous. In 1794, he became physician to the Salpêtrière and, 1802, published *La médecine clinique,* based, as he writes, on his observations at the Salpêtrière and in which he extended and amplified the *Nosographie.* Pinel was later professor of hygiene and of internal pathology in the medical faculty. He died in 1826.

The artificiality of Pinel's system is apparent. His classifications are often based upon the symptoms and signs which patients present. If a patient with fever had marked cerebral and gastric symptoms, the disease was diagnosed as *fièvre meningo-gastrique;* if he had headache with glandular enlargement, *fièvre adeno-meningée.* Under the class of internal hemorrhages, we find grouped together such diverse conditions as menorrhagia, hemoptysis, hematuria,

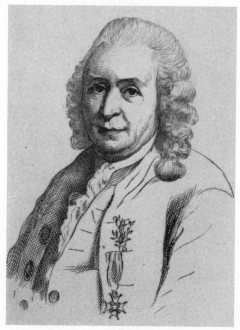

University of Kansas Collection

C. LINNÉ

hemorrhoids and aneurysm. There is no consideration of the etiology, and the autopsy reports are extremely sketchy.

A very different method of investigating disease was pursued by Corvisart. He was not obsessed with the idea that medicine was an exact science and could answer all questions definitely and positively. It was an attractive idea and very comforting for those who could believe. For Corvisart, medicine was an *ars conjecturalis* (the art of conjecture). The physician's task was to study the interrelation of cause and effect, to determine the cause of disease by a careful in-

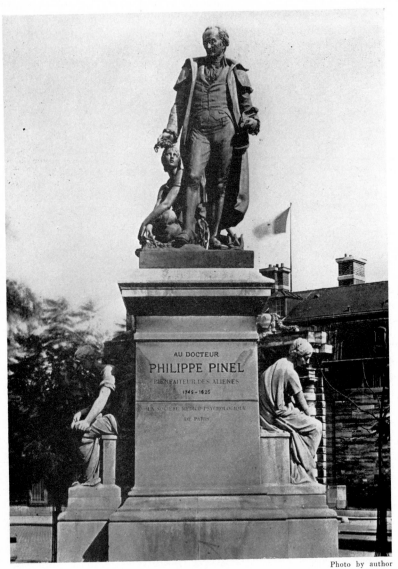

PHILIPPE PINEL

Statue in front of the Salpêtrière Hospital, Paris.

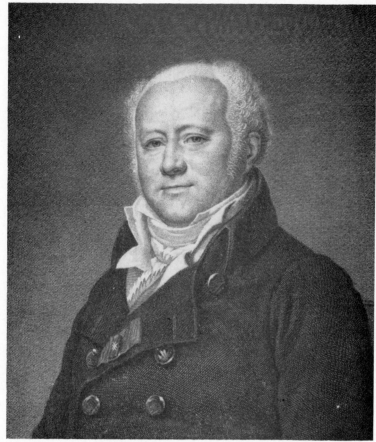

JEAN NICOLAS CORVISART
Engraving by Blot from painting by Gérard.

vestigation of the effects it produced, that is, the symptoms and signs
the patient presented and the pathological changes found at postmortem examination.

Jean Nicholas Corvisart, the premier and outstanding physician
of this period, was born in the small village of Dricourt in Cham-
pagne in 1755. He was intended for the bar and entered the College of St. Barbe at the age of 12, but he was an indifferent student
and showed no signs of future greatness. He began the study of
law but, finding it dull, wandered off to Paris, where he heard

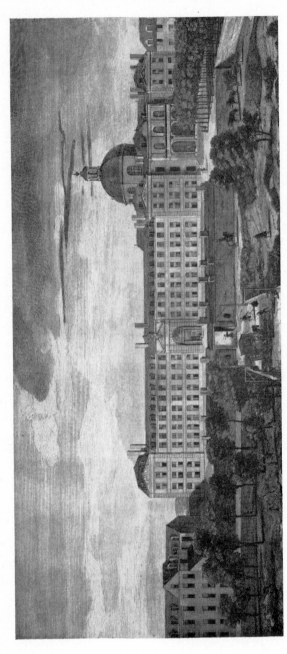

THE SALPÊTRIÈRE AT THE BEGINNING OF THE NINETEENTH CENTURY

The Salpêtrière was erected during the reign of Louis XIII as an arsenal—the name signifying "salt-peter works." In 1656 through the efforts of St. Vincent de Paul, it was transformed into an asylum for old women, abandoned prostitutes, and the insane. After serving for more than a century as a poorhouse, hospital, and insane asylum, it gradually became a hospital for mental and nervous diseases. (From an old print.)

Desault lecture and was so much impressed that he decided to study medicine. Being without funds, he obtained a clerical position at the Hôtel Dieu, prepared anatomical specimens for Desault, and received his doctor's degree in 1785. He was offered a position by Mme. Necker in the hospital she founded but refused when he learned he must wear a wig. In 1788, he was appointed physician to the Charité Hospital and immediately threw himself into the work of clinical instruction in the wards. Having asked a student one day what he wished to do and receiving the reply, "To study," he turned to his patients and said, "These are your books. Read them, but you will find them more difficult than those printed" (Brown). In 1797, he was appointed professor of practical medicine in the Collège de France, the highest teaching honor in France.

Corvisart examined his patients with great care, noted their physiognomy, their complexion, the color of their eyes and lips, their voice, their facial muscles, the rate and character of their respiration, the rate and quality of their pulse. On one occasion while examining a portrait, he remarked, "If the painter has been exact, the original of this portrait died of a disease of the heart." An investigation revealed that Corvisart's diagnosis was correct. Reading in the works of Stoll an account of the new method of percussion discovered by Auenbrugger, he employed this new method of examination and was soon convinced of its great value. Called to see Napoleon, he examined him with such care that the emperor was delighted, named him his personal physician, and, later, created him a baron. Corvisart suffered a cerebral hemorrhage in 1815, retired from his practice, and died from a second stroke in 1821.

Two notable books, which exercised a great influence on medicine, were written by Corvisart. His first was *Essai sur les maladies et les lésions organiques du coeur et des gros vaisseaux,* Paris, 1806, the outstanding book on cardiac disease of its time. He classified heart disease on the basis of the anatomical structures involved—pericardium, heart muscle, endocardium and valves. He employed the term, "organic lesion," made a distinction between hypertrophy and dilatation of the heart, and differentiated between right and left heart failure. He described with great accuracy mitral and aortic valvular lesions, and tricuspid stenosis. He made no mention of angina pectoris, however, and referred only casually to the coronary arteries. He stressed unduly the importance of what he called "aneurysm" of the heart, which we today should call hypertrophy and dilatation. He referred to "carditis" as a conception of inflam-

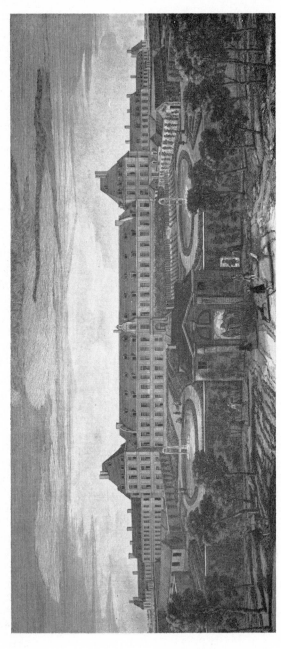

THE BICÊTRE AT THE CLOSE OF THE EIGHTEENTH CENTURY

The name Bicêtre is derived from Jean de Pointoise, Bishop of Winchester, who built a château here in 1285. The name Winchester went through the successive corruptions of Bichester, Bicestre, and finally emerged as Bicêtre. Louis XIII commenced the present building in 1632 as a hospital for military invalids. Early in the nineteenth century, the Bicêtre became a general asylum for the indigent, a lunatic asylum, and a prison. In 1792, it housed more than 100 psychiatric patients. Pinel was appointed physician-in-charge in 1793. (From an old print.)

mation of the heart as a whole, a conception later revived by other authors.

The *Nouvelle Methode pour reconnaître les maladies internes,* Paris, 1808, was Corvisart's second great book. It was a translation of Auenbrugger's *Inventum novum,* to which Corvisart added his own observations based on "a long experience" with percussion. This work rescued Auenbrugger's study from an ill-merited oblivion, and percussion, backed by the European reputation of Corvisart, was soon used in medical clinics everywhere.

Corvisart's fame as a teacher drew brilliant pupils who were attracted by his skill as a diagnostician, by his clarity as a lecturer, and by his frankness, fairness, independence, and generosity as a man. Among his pupils were Bayle, Laennec and Bouillaud.

Gaspard Laurent Bayle (1774-1816), whose death at the age of 42 was a great loss to medical science, was one of those restless spirits, like Bichat and Laennec, whose flagging body was never quite equal to the strain and stress he placed upon it. Born in Vernet in Provence, he studied first theology, then law, and finally medicine, pursuing his studies at the École de Médecine in Paris and receiving his degree in 1801.

Bayle worked regularly until midnight, met his students at dawn when he made ward rounds, and then held a clinic in the amphitheatre, where the most interesting cases were shown and discussed. The class then adjourned to the morgue, where the postmortems of the day were performed, each preceded by a résumé of the history and followed by a discussion, in which an attempt was made to correlate the history and the clinical course with the autopsy findings.

The results of Bayle's investigations were summarized in his *Recherches sur la phthisie pulmonaire,* published in 1810, a work that had a profound influence upon his own generation, particularly upon his friend and colleague, Laennec. Bayle pointed out that tubercles may be present in patients before symptoms appear; correlated tubercles and cavity formation; described acute miliary tuberculosis, tubercular laryngitis, lymphadenitis and enteritis; and insisted that tuberculosis was a specific disease, a disease *sui generis* and not a degenerative condition following other diseases. Bayle's reputation and practice grew rapidly following publication of this work. He was finally unequal to the strain and died in 1816 of tuberculosis.

RENÉ THÉOPHILE HYACINTHE LAENNEC

The most famous pupil of Corvisart was René Théophile Hyacinthe Laennec, to whom one can justly apply that often banal word —immortal. He was born at Quimper in 1781. His father, Théophile-Marie Laennec, was a rather futile but entertaining person, a lawyer by profession, a writer of mediocre verse, and an inveterate office seeker. His mother died when he was six, and, at the age of eight,

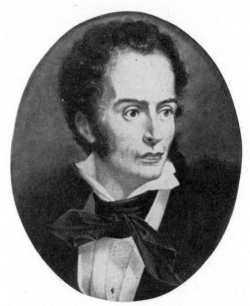

Les Médecins Célèbres, Paris, 1917

RÉNÉ THÉOPHILE HYACINTHE LAENNEC
Artist unknown. Faculté de médecine, Paris.

he went to live with his uncle, Guillaume, a physician of Nantes. At the age of 14, he began his medical studies with his uncle. These studies were interrupted by the civil wars, in which he served as a surgeon in 1799 and 1800. In 1801, he went to Paris, where he enrolled at the Charité as a pupil of Corvisart and received his doctor's degree in 1804. He became a close friend of Bayle in Paris, and, as mentioned previously, the two young men were for a time assistants to Dupuytren, then busy with his projected work on pathological anatomy. The study of pathological anatomy, which had been given such a powerful stimulus by the brilliant work of Bichat, had a great fascination for Laennec, with the result that his first pub-

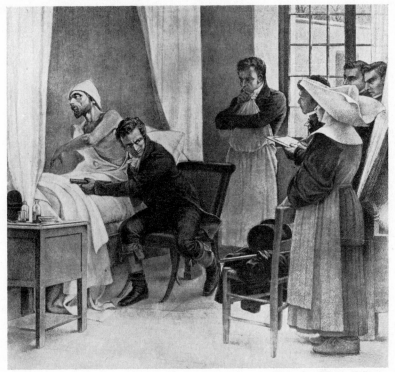

University of Kansas Collection

LAENNEC EXAMINING A PATIENT AT THE NECKER HOSPITAL

lished papers were on pathological anatomy. He was deeply influenced by the work of Bayle, whose *Recherches sur la phthisie pulmonaire* was the point of departure for Laennec's subsequent work on tuberculosis. Laennec, slight of figure, unprepossessing in appearance, modest, if not timid, in bearing, presently achieved through hard work, the reputation of an expert pathologist, an excellent teacher, and a skillful physician. He was appointed in 1814 physician to the Necker Hospital.

In 1816, Laennec invented the stethoscope. The story of this invention has been told so many times that it has almost taken on the character of a legend. However, his friend, Lejumeau de Kergaradec, wrote,

The author told me himself, the great discovery which has immortalized his name was due to chance. . . . One day walking in the court of the Louvre, he saw some children, who, with their ears glued to the two ends of some long pieces of wood which transmitted the sound of the little blows of the pins, struck at the opposite end. . . . He conceived instantly the thought of applying this to the study of diseases of the heart. On the morrow, at his clinic at the Necker Hospital, he took a sheet of paper, rolled it up, tied it with a string, making a central canal which he then placed on a diseased heart. This was the first stethoscope.

This story is confirmed in its essential details by Laennec in the Introduction to his *De l'auscultation médiate,* which was published in 1819.

At first, Laennec gave no name to the new instrument but finally chose the name, "stethoscope," from the Greek words, στηθος (the chest) and σκοπεῖυ (to look at). After numerous experiments, for he was an expert woodturner, he produced a cylinder of wood either cedar or ebony, 30 centimeters (12 inches) long and three centimeters (one and one-fourth inches) in diameter with a central canal five millimeters (c. one-fourth inch) in diameter. The cylinder was also divided in the middle, so the two parts could be separated and more easily carried.

Laennec's *De l'auscultation médiate* was the product of three years of the most intensive work with his new stethoscope and, also, of more than 18 years of close study of problems in pathology and clinical medicine. It is far more than a manual for the stethoscope. It is, also, a treatise on diseases of the lung and of the heart, a mine of information on the clinical aspects of pulmonary and cardiac disease, with an accurate description of the pathological anatomy of these conditions. Laennec heard with his stethoscope sounds never before heard or described and for which no terms existed in medical literature. He was the creator of a large number of words now currently employed in physical diagnosis, such as râles, bronchophony, pectoriloquy and egophony. His book, unlike Auenbrugger's *Inventum novum,* did not wait 47 years for recognition. It was immediately accepted as an epoch-making work, and auscultation was soon used in medical clinics throughout the world.

The first part of the book is devoted to diseases of the lungs. The author describes the symptomatology, the clinical course, the physical findings, and the pathological anatomy of pneumonia, "apoplexy" of the lungs, gangrene, emphysema, cysts of the lung, tuberculosis, pleurisy, pleural effusion, pneumo-thorax, and edema of the lungs. Many case histories are included as well as autopsy findings. He described and christened cirrhosis of the liver, "because of its color." While he devotes much attention to auscultation in his description of physical findings, he stresses the importance of percussion, which he learned from his master Corvisart, and the value of inspection and palpation.

The section devoted to diseases of the heart suffers perhaps by comparison with the section on pulmonary diseases. The physiology of the heart was poorly understood at the time. "Starting with the false hypothesis (that) the second sound was auricular in origin, he never found his way out of the jungle" (Thayer). He overlooked the embolic nature of some of his cases of pulmonary "apoplexy"; he did not appreciate the significance of the *frémissement cataire* (presystolic thrill), which he described; and he overestimated the importance of blowing murmurs.

Following the appearance of his work, Laennec, exhausted by his labors and showing unmistakable symptoms of pulmonary tuberculosis himself, retired to his country place, Kerlouarnec, in Brittany. His health improved gradually, and, after two years, he returned to Paris. Here he was appointed physician to Her Royal Highness, the Duchess of Berry, and was made professor at the Collège de France and professor of the medical clinic of the Charité. The next four years were spent in the preparation of the second edition of his book, which was published in 1826 with a slightly altered title, *Traité de l'auscultation médiate et des maladies des poumons et du coeur*. Much of the time while he worked on this second edition, Laennec was ill, suffering from a constant cough, pains in his right side, fever, shortness of breath and diarrhoea. "In taking the last year in order to finish my book," he wrote, "I knew that I risked my life, but the book that I am going to publish will be, I hope, of more value than the life of a man, and in consequence my duty was to finish it, whatever might happen to me." The same year the book was published, he retired once more to his home in Brittany, where he died on August 13, 1826.

This second edition was largely re-written. The admirable sections on pulmonary disease were re-cast, and many new observations were recorded. He differentiated pulmonary tuberculosis, pulmonary abscess and gangrene, bronchiectasis, emphysema, infarction and pneumothorax. He described in detail râles and their varieties, vesicular and bronchial breathing, bronchophony, pectoriloquy, egophony, amphoric and cracked-pot resonance, and metallic tinkling. "He found phthisis pulmonalis a conglomeration of disease, pulmonary and general, and left it a clear-cut entity" (Brown).

The section on heart disease in this second edition was again the least satisfactory part of the book. Apparently, Laennec had not found his way out of the jungle. In the first edition, he devoted much attention to blowing murmurs *(bruit de soufflet)* and stated, "The time and the place where one hears them indicates obviously which orifice is affected." In the second edition, he observed that some patients having this murmur showed no cardiac lesions at autopsy, and "he denied to them from that time any diagnostic value, falling thus, in condemning himself, into a new error worse than the first" (Potain). Even with its defects and at times its vagueness, Laennec's contribution to cardiology was impressive. He introduced a new method of studying the heart, and he gave a certain precision to many pathologic concepts, previously in a state of confusion. Laennec was without question one of the greatest physicians of all time. His *Traité* is one of the outstanding medical books of history; and, with it, clinical medicine entered into a new and modern era.

One of Laennec's most determined adversaries, with whom he had a long series of verbal clashes, was François Broussais (1772-1838). In many respects the antithesis of Laennec, Broussais was a man of powerful physique, of impressive bearing, dogmatic in his views, and, in his prime, an excellent lecturer, whose oratory often convinced his skeptics. Born near St. Malo in Brittany, where his father was a doctor, he began his medical studies with his father, for whom he delivered prescriptions. In 1799, he went to Paris to continue his studies, working particularly under Halle, Corvisart and Bichat. He received his degree four years later, but, as practice came slowly, he joined the army, serving five years in Belgium, Holland, Germany, Austria and Italy. In 1808, he returned to Paris and brought out his first work, *Histoire des phlegmasies ou inflammations chroniques,* Paris, 1808, which attracted little attention. The following year, he joined the army in Spain and served five years as the chief medical officer. With the fall of Napoleon, he returned to Paris after 10 years' service in the army, was appointed second medical officer at the Val-de-Grâce Military Hospital, and subsequently was made first medical officer.

In 1816 he published his *Examen des doctrines médicales et des systèmes de nosologie,* a work expounding his medical theories, particularly his "physiological medicine," which were further developed in later publications. Broussais called his system "physiological medicine" since he attached more importance to disorders of function than to anatomical changes. All diseases were due to irritability of tissues, a statement that calls attention to the similarity between "physiological medicine" and the theories of John Brown. However, Brown maintained that 97 percent of patients owed their

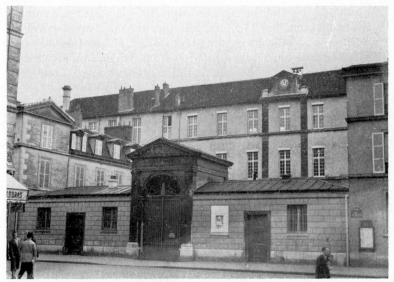

Photo by author

NECKER HOSPITAL

The tablet to Laennec is seen to the right of the entrance. The Necker Hospital was founded in 1778 on the initiative of Mme. Necker, wife of the powerful finance minister of Louis XVI. Originally it was called L'Hospice de Charité, during the Revolution it was known as L'Hospice de l'Ouest, in 1802 the name was changed to Hôspital Necker in honor of Mme. Necker.

illness to asthenia and required stimulation, whereas Broussais declared that 97 percent of his patients were sthenic and required sedation, a difference which led to the remark that the "physiologism" of Broussais was "Brownism" turned inside out. Disease entities, or specific diseases, do not exist; disease results from inflammation. The seat of these inflammations is the stomach and intestines; cancer, syphilis, tuberculosis and malaria are simply the end result of chronic inflammation of the alimentary tract.

Laennec, whose careful pathological studies revealed to him the absurdity of Broussais's pathology, and Bretonneau, who had already proved the specificity of certain diseases, were prominent among the opponents of "physiologic medicine." Broussais greeted Laennec's *Traité* with a certain disdain and called it a "sublime romance, a fastidious collection of undigested facts or of useless discoveries," but he himself employed the stethoscope at the Val-de-Grâce Hospital.

Broussais's "physiologism," like Brownism, gained a large number of adherents and, for 15 years, was the predominant doctrine in Paris. Broussais believed in the great efficacy of bleeding and had himself bled six times when suffering from indigestion and had 15 applications of 50 to 60 leeches. As the result of Broussais's teaching,

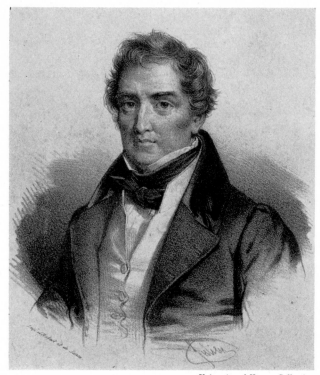

University of Kansas Collection

FRANÇOIS BROUSSAIS

bleeding and the application of leeches grew so popular that the supply of leeches in France became exhausted and enormous numbers had to be imported from abroad.

About 1828, Broussais became interested in phrenology, was elected president of the *Société de Phrénologie,* and began to lecture on the subject. On one occasion, the police suspended the lectures because of excitement caused by the rumor that he was going to deny the existence of God and of the soul. The lectures were con-

tinued after Broussais, well known as a free-thinker, said that he believed in God, not from the bottom of his heart like the ordinary
man, but as a phrenologist should from the anterior part of his
brain. As for the soul, he could not attempt to defend it as a phrenologist.

The doctrines of Broussais declined, not so much because of the
attack of greater minds upon them, as because of his methods of
treatment. Copious bleedings and a starvation diet produced few
cures. Oliver Wendell Holmes, writing of Paris in the 1830's, noted,

> Broussais was in those days like an old volcano, which has pretty nearly
> used up its fire and brimstone, but is still boiling and bubbling in its in-
> terior, and now and then sends up a spurt of lava and volley of pebbles. His
> theories of gastro-enteritis, of irritation and inflammation as the cause of
> disease, and the practice which sprang from them ran over the fields of
> medicine for a time like flame over the grass of the prairies.

Broussais developed an intestinal affection, which proved to be a
carcinoma of the rectum, from which he died in 1838.

The doctrines held by Broussais that most ills arose from gastro-
enteritis and that diseases were not specific entities were discredited
even before his death. A powerful opponent, whose heavy blows
assisted in demolishing these two foundations of Broussais's creed,
was Pierre Fidèle Bretonneau, who was born at St. Georges-sur-Cher
in the province of Touraine in 1778. At the age of 17, he was sent
to Paris to study medicine and entered the École de Santé, where he
had as fellow students Dupuytren, Bayle and Recamier. His studies
were interrupted by ill health, but, in 1799, he returned and followed the courses of the faculty of medicine, especially the clinics
of Corvisart, whom he admired greatly and whose methods he afterwards followed. He failed to obtain his doctorate, was forced to content himself with the title, *officier de santé,* and returned to Chenonceaux, where he began to practice.

At Chenonceaux, he acquired such a reputation that he was invited to go to Tours as chief physician to the hospital there. Since
it was necessary to have the title of doctor to fill this position, he
returned to Paris and, having passed the examinations, received his
degree in 1814.

Bretonneau was chief physician to the hospital at Tours for 23
years. He was very active during these years, dividing his time between his clinical rounds, which began at six in the morning, and
the autopsy room, where he correlated his clinical findings with the

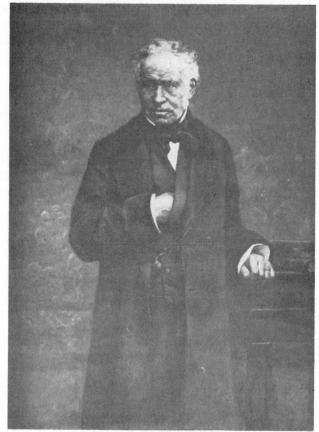

Photo by author

PIERRE BRETONNEAU

Portrait by Moreau in the Hospice Général, Tours.

revelations of the necropsy. He was a great favorite with his students, two of whom, Velpeau and Trousseau, achieved great fame in Paris and spread Bretonneau's reputation as an investigator and teacher.

Epidemic forms of sore throat and of continued fever, both taking a heavy toll of life, were two diseases which especially interested Bretonneau. "If called to a patient, he would tell his servant to ask if it was a case of sore throat or fever, and, if it was neither, to say that his master was not at home" (Trousseau). In 1819, he studied a severe epidemic of sore throat in Tours, performed 60 autopsies on the victims, and read before the Paris *Académie de Médecine* in 1821 a paper in which he asserted that "croup," "malignant angina," and "scorbutic gangrene of the gums" were all the same malady, a specific disease, for which he proposed the name, "diphtheritis." This paper was the basis for his work, *Des inflammations spéciales du tissu, muqueux, et en particulier de la diphthérite, ou inflammation pelliculaire,* Paris, 1826.

Between the years 1821 and 1827, Bretonneau studied a great many cases of typhoid fever in the wards and the autopsy findings in 120 persons. In all of them, he demonstrated the characteristic ulcers on Peyer's patches, pointed out the difference between typhoid ulcers and tuberculous ulcers, and described both intestinal hemorrhage and perforation. He maintained that the lesions on the intestinal mucosa were specific and went through various stages, as does the eruption of smallpox. For some reason, he declined to publish this work, but it was published by his pupil Trousseau in 1826.

Bretonneau insisted on the specificity of infectious disease. "The specificity of diseases," he said, "is proved by such a mass of facts, and there is probably no truth better demonstrated and more fruitful." He died in 1864 before the birth of bacteriology, which proved so clearly the correctness of his views regarding infectious diseases. His funeral services were held at Tours in the presence of a large part of the population, and an eulogy was pronounced by the president of the *Académie de Médecine,* Bouillaud.

Jean Baptiste Bouillaud was born in 1796 and died in 1881 at the age of 89. During his long life span, beginning with the French Revolution, he lived through the Napoleonic era, the restoration of the Bourbons, the European revolutions of 1848, the reign of Napoleon III, the defeat at Sedan, the Paris Commune of 1871, and the German occupation of Paris. He saw the invention of the stethoscope, the era of physical diagnosis, the creation of cellular pathology, the birth of bacteriology, and the rise of experimental medicine.

Bouillaud, the son of a tile maker, was born in the small hamlet of Bragette near Angoulême. His medical studies were begun at the Cochin Hospital in Paris but were interrupted by the return of Napoleon from Elba, at which time the young man joined the army of the emperor. After Waterloo, he returned to Paris, studied under Corvisart, Laennec, Dupuytren and Magendie, and received his doctor's degree in 1823. He was quite active in carrying out investigations and wrote papers on dropsy, aneurysm of the aorta, asthma and cholera. In 1825, he wrote a paper based on experiments, controlled by clinical and autopsy findings, which confirmed the view

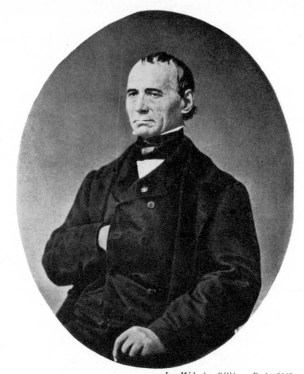

Les Médecins Célèbres, Paris, 1947

JEAN BAPTISTE BOUILLAUD

Academy of Medicine, Paris. Photograph by Trinquart.

of Gall, that the center for articulate speech is located in the anterior lobes of the brain. He went further and pointed out the difference between the ability to create words and the ability to articulate them—internal and external language.

The rise of Bouillaud was rapid. In 1826, he became professor agrégé and, in 1831, professor of clinical medicine, to the great delight of his students, who carried him about in triumph on their shoulders. He became a follower of Broussais and a partisan of venesection but, in spite of these vagaries, was an excellent physician and is remembered today chiefly for his contributions to cardiology, especially for his *Traité clinique des maladies du coeur,* Paris, 1835; and his *Nouvelles recherches sur le rhumatisme articulaire aigu,* Paris, 1836.

In the preface to his *Traité,* Bouillaud writes, "I have given the name of endocardium to the inner lining of this organ and that of endocarditis to its inflammation," thus introducing these terms into medicine. He was the first to describe accurately the endocardium and endocarditis, noting the changes in endocarditis, beginning with exudation and terminating with cicatrization and deformity of the valves. In the *Nouvelles recherches,* he pointed out the association between endocarditis and acute articular rheumatism. He also made other important contributions to the subject of cardiology and corrected some of the errors of Laennec. He elucidated the mechanism and significance of the normal heart sounds, described the positive venous pulse in the neck, stressed its value in the diagnosis of tricuspid insufficiency, and described the *bruit du diable,* gallop rhythm, the double sound at the apex in mitral stenosis, the friction in pericarditis, extrasystoles, and auricular fibrillation.

The year after Bouillaud's death, Oliver Wendell Holmes said in an address, "Where now is the fame of Bouillaud, Professor and Deputy, the Sangrado of his time?"—a comparison of Bouillaud with the blood-letting physician of Lesage's novel, *Gil Blas,* and intimating that Bouillaud's fame had evaporated. But Holmes's impression of Bouillaud has proved to be quite wrong. Bouillaud's work has placed his name among the immortals of cardiology.

Another physician of that period, however, drew unstinted praise from the lips of young Oliver Wendell Holmes, then a post graduate medical student in Paris. Pierre Charles Alexandre Louis was, according to Holmes, "the object of our reverence, I might almost say idolatry." Louis seems to have been a particular favorite of the American students. Osler has listed the names of 37 Americans who studied under Louis, most of whom later became well-known physicians and leaders in American medicine.

Pierre Charles Alexandre Louis was born in 1787 at Aï and studied medicine at Rheims and at Paris, taking his degree at Paris in 1813. Shortly after graduation, he went to Russia with a friend of his family, M. le Comte de Saint-Priest, who was the governor of one of the provinces there. He wandered about Russia for three years with his friend and then settled in Odessa, where he practiced with great success for four years. During his last year there, he saw a severe epidemic of diphtheria attended by a high mortality, which impressed him so deeply that he resolved to give up the practice of medicine for a few years and devote himself to further study.

He returned to Paris, and an old friend Chomel, physician to Charité, allowed him to work in its wards. Later he was made *chef de clinique.* He remained there for nearly seven years, and, from the age of 33 until 40, he refused all private practice, lived in a room at the hospital, and devoted his entire time to rigorous impartial observation—carefully collecting facts and carefully analysing them. He called this method the "Numerical Method," and, in his hands, it proved an invaluable instrument of research. He be-

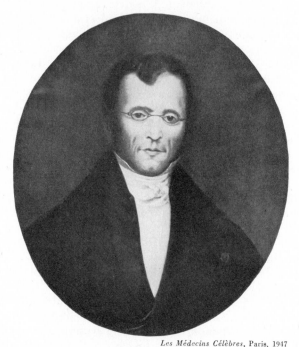

Les Médecins Célèbres, Paris, 1947

PIERRE CHARLES ALEXANDRE LOUIS
Artist unknown. Academy of Medicine, Paris.

lieved that the edifice of medicine rests entirely upon facts and that the truth can be elicited only from those facts which have been well and completely observed.

Louis's first publication was *Recherches anatomico-pathologiques sur la phthisie,* Paris, 1825, based on the study of 123 cases observed in Chomel's clinic. The lesions in the various organs are described with meticulous care and great accuracy, and the symptoms and clinical course of each patient is written with clarity and exactness. More than 80 years later, Osler said, "I do not know of any single work on pulmonary tuberculosis which can be studied with greater profit today by the young physician."

The second great work of Louis was his *Recherches anatomiques pathologiques et therapeutiques sur la maladie connue sous les noms de fièvre putride, adynamique, ataxique, typhoïde,* etc., Paris, 1829. It was a notable contribution to medical literature, in which he studied 138 patients suffering from typhoid, analysing the lesions that 50 showed at autopsy and comparing them with the intestinal lesions of patients dying from other diseases. It has been described as dealing the death blow to Broussais's "physiologism" and his doctrine that all diseases originate in the gastro-intestinal tract. Louis's *Recherches sur les effets de la saignée,* 1835, gave further offense to the followers of Broussais by showing through his "numerical"—we should say statistical—methed that blood-letting never arrested an attack of pneumonia and that its beneficial effect upon the course of the disease was difficult to prove.

Louis impressed all by his sincerity, his honesty, and his total lack of ostentation. He died in 1872.

We may recall that Dupuytren, in the course of his spectacular rise to the highest pinnacle in French surgery of his time, was deeply interested in pathological anatomy and had, as an assistant, a young man named Cruveilhier, who assisted him in his work of preparing specimens for his projected book. This work was abandoned, but Cruveilhier, 30 years later, published an atlas of pathological anatomy that probably gives us some idea of what Dupuytren had in mind.

Jean Cruveilhier was born at Limoges in 1791, the son of an army surgeon. In early life, he wished to be a priest, but, at the command of his father, he went to Paris in 1810 to study medicine. The first autopsies he witnessed produced in him such an aversion to medicine that he fled from the medical school and entered the Seminary of St. Sulpice as a candidate for holy orders. His father hastened from Limoges and compelled his disobedient son to recommence his medical studies. Dupuytren, a friend of the elder Cruveilhier, took the young student under his protection and awakened in him an interest in pathological anatomy.

After receiving his doctor's degree in 1816, Cruveilhier practiced for a time in Limoges but, in 1823, went to Montpellier as professor of surgery. Two years later, he went to Paris as professor of anatomy and, in 1836, became the first professor of pathological anatomy. This was a new chair created by a legacy from his old

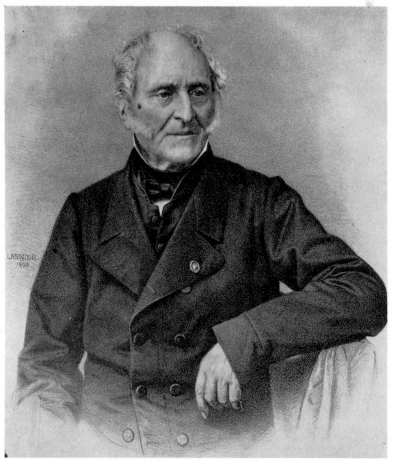

University of Kansas Collection

JEAN CRUVEILHIER
From an engraving by Lasnier.

patron Dupuytren. He held that position for 30 years and, in addition, was physician to the Salpêtrière and the Charité. He died in
1874.

Cruveilhier was the author of several works on anatomy and
pathology, the best known of which is his *Anatomie pathologique
du corps humain*, Paris, 1830-1842. This work is one of the most
sumptuous pathological atlases ever published, and the illustrations,
mostly in color, have never been surpassed or even equaled artisti-

cally. In this atlas, the author described and illustrated for the first time disseminated sclerosis, gave an early description of progressive muscular atrophy, and pictured several cases of gastric ulcer—still called by the French "la maladie de Cruveilhier." Having not used the microscope, he made the erroneous deduction that pyemia is the result of phlebitis and stated, "Phlebitis, in a way, dominates all pathology."

The early years of the nineteenth century, which saw in Paris the rise of such a group of eminent clinicians, also witnessed the beginnings of experimental medicine. Physicians in the past had, of course, experimented, two notable examples being Galen and Harvey. Never before, however, had medical experiments been pursued so systematically and so perseveringly as the physician's chief interest and occupation. The initiator of this movement was unquestionably François Magendie.

François Magendie was born in Bordeaux in 1783, the son of a surgeon, who was an intense republican and who, when François was eight years of age, moved his family to Paris in order to take part in the stirring political events of the day. The father was a devoted follower of Rousseau and took so seriously his advice on education, "The first education ought to be purely negative. . . . Leave your pupil to himself in perfect liberty, and observe what he does without saying anything to him," that Magendie received no schooling until he was over 10 years of age.

Later, Magendie's father persuaded "Citizen" Boyer, who later became Napoleon's personal surgeon and a baron, to take his son as a pupil. François soon became an excellent anatomist and presently gave courses in anatomy. In 1801, Napoleon, then first consul, had a statute passed reforming medical education, at that time in a chaotic state, and providing that no one should practice medicine who did not have a diploma certifying that he was a doctor of medicine. Bichat had died without possessing one, Dupuytren had to write a thesis and defend it, and even the great Boyer himself, although nearly 50, had to submit to an examination. Magendie took his examination, wrote a thesis on the uses of the soft palate, and received his degree in 1808.

His first notice was achieved in 1809 by an article in which he attacked Bichat's conception of vitalism. He criticized the distinction between vital and physical phenomena and laid down "the two principles which guided him throughout his whole scientific life, distrust of theory and firm faith in experiment" (Olmsted).

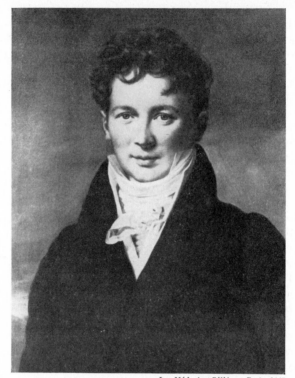

Les Médecins Célèbres, Paris, 1947

FRANÇOIS MAGENDIE
Portrait by Guérin. Collège de France, Paris.

In 1809, Magendie made his initial appearance before the Paris
Académie des Sciences and described the effects upon animals produced by the absorption of a poison obtained from Java. This work
marks the beginning of experimental pharmacology. In 1813, Magendie, who had been trained by Boyer and who, from his work in
anatomy, was apparently destined for a surgical career, resigned his
post as prosector in the anatomical laboratory, gave up all previous
ideas of practicing medicine and surgery, and resolved to devote his
life to the pursuit of experimental physiology. His subsequent work
forms a large chapter in the history of physiology. He founded in
1821 the first periodical devoted exclusively to that field, the *Journal
de physiologie expérimentale*. His fame rose steadily. In 1836, he
was appointed professor of medicine at the Collège de France and,
during the next decade, was quite active in the Paris *Académie des*

Sciences, reading many papers before that body. He died in 1855.

Magendie once described himself as a rag-picker *(chiffonier)* who wanders through the field of science, picking up stray facts. In his eulogy of Magendie, Claude Bernard regrets that his empiricism, his love of experimentation led to a lack of plan in his work. Magendie discovered many important isolated facts, but, as he failed to associate them with each other, he arrived at no important generalizations.

He carried out important work on deglutition and on the mechanics of the digestive tract, studied the effects of excision and section of the cerebellum, the properties of the cerebrospinal fluid, the mechanics of circulation, and the physiology of the heart beat, advancing the erroneous explanation that the heart sounds were caused by the heart striking the chest wall. His experiments on the circulation convinced him of the absurdity of "points of election" in bleeding, and further observation and experiments convinced him of the uselessness, and even harm, resulting from this universal and hallowed method of treatment. Called once in consultation, where the question of bleeding the patient simultaneously from the right arm and the left foot was hotly debated, Magendie said it reminded him of some of the best scenes on the comic stage. His investigations in pharmacology included observations on the effects of bromine, iodine, strychnine, morphine, veratrine, brucine and emetine. In 1839, he showed that rabbits who tolerated a single injection of egg albumin often died following a second injection— the first observation of anaphylaxis.

In one of his early papers read before the *Académie des Sciences* in 1822, Magendie described what was probably his greatest contribution, the proof that the anterior spinal nerves are motor and the posterior, sensory in function. This led to an acrimonious dispute with Charles Bell, who maintained his priority in this discovery, a dispute renewed as recently as 1938. Olmsted has reviewed the whole controversy and concludes, "The physiologist is therefore inclined to give all the credit for this discovery to Magendie." "The term, 'Bell-Magendie rule,' " he adds, "represents a compromise between the points of view of the older type of anatomist who arrived at function by way of inference and the physiologically-minded investigator who insists upon experimental verification."

A comparatively late comer to the medical life of Paris was Franz Joseph Gall, who was born near Tiefenbrunn in Baden in 1758. He studied first at Strassburg, then proceeded to Vienna, where he studied under van Swieten, received his doctor's degree in 1785, and

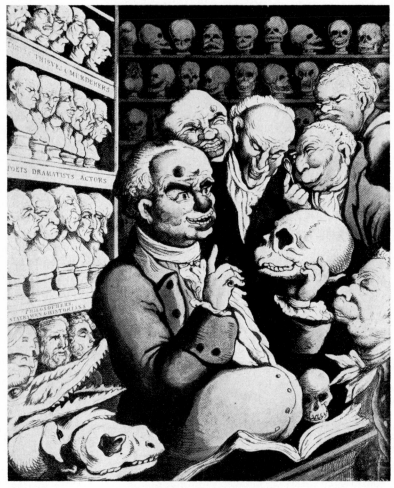

A LECTURE BY DR. GALL
Caricature by J. Rowlandson.

began to practice. He had long been impressed by an apparent association between the features of his fellow students and their mental
capacity, those showing prominent eyes usually having excellent
memories. He was at first interested in physiognomy, but, becoming
dissatisfied with it, as well as with craniology, he turned to the
subject of cerebral physiology—"The cranium is only a faithful cast
of the external surface of the brain." Gall made a large collection

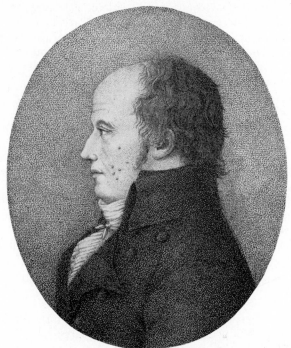

University of Kansas Collection

FRANZ JOSEPH GALL

of skulls and casts of skulls and gradually reached the conclusion
that the talents and mental characteristics of men depend upon the
functions of the brain, that these characteristics cause variation in
the development of certain areas on the surface of the brain, and
that this can be determined by a careful study of the external appearance of the skull.

Gall began to expound these views in his lectures, which attracted
a great deal of attention and made many converts, one of whom,
Johann Caspar Spurzheim (1776-1832), was closely associated with
him for several years. The Emperor Francis II, alarmed by the stir
these lectures were creating, wrote in his own hand a letter to the
chancellor complaining,

Many are losing their heads (*Kopf*) over this phrenology (*Kopflehre*),
which leads them into materialism and also seems to contradict the first
principles of morals and religion.

The chancellor forbade further lectures. Gall left Vienna in 1805 and, accompanied by Spurzheim, went for a lecture tour through Germany and adjacent countries, reaching Paris two years later and remaining there until his death in 1828. In Paris, he found a supporter in Broussais, in the philosopher Comte, and in Bouillaud, who had postulated in 1825 the existence of a motor speech center in the anterior portion of the brain. Gall's chief work, *Anatomie et physiologie du système nerveux,* appeared in four volumes in 1810-1819.

In general, the physiologists opposed Gall, but many philosophers became his partisans, and the general public applauded the novel theory. Later anatomical studies pointed out that the skull was commonly not a faithful cast of the external surface of the brain and that there were normally great variations in the thickness of the skull, in the size of the frontal sinus, and in the prominence of the centers of ossification. Gall's work did stimulate investigation of the physiology of the brain, investigations which presently localized certain activities in definite areas of the brain and demolished completely the fanciful system of Gall.

THE IRISH SCHOOL

Although Paris, in the early decades of the nineteenth century, was the unquestioned center of medical progress and discovery, the *Civitas Hippocratica,* yet this spirit of inquiry appeared elsewhere, partly as an overflow from the French capital, partly as an indigenous plant developing on its own soil. In Ireland, there appeared at Dublin a small group of men whose achievements in medicine were noteworthy and who formed what has been called the "Irish School." This group had a profound influence upon its time and has left a notable record in the annals of medical history.

The first of this group, Abraham Colles, who was born near Kilkenny in 1773, was not a physician but a surgeon. Colles matriculated at Trinity College, Dublin, where he received his bachelor's degree in arts in 1795, and, the same year, obtained a diploma from the College of Surgeons. The same year also, he entered the University of Edinburgh, where he received his M.D. in 1797. From Edinburgh, he went to London, walking the entire distance of 400 miles in eight days. Spending only a short time there, he returned the same year to Dublin and began practice.

The first year in practice was not financially very successful for Colles as his receipts for the year totalled only £8, 16s, 7½d. The following year, he was elected Resident Surgeon at the Steevens' Hospital. In 1804, he was appointed professor of anatomy and surgery at the College of Surgeons, a position he held 32 years, during which time his contributions to surgery played an important role in establishing the reputation of the Irish school. He was soon recognized as a master surgeon and an outstanding teacher.

Colles's *Treatise on Surgical Anatomy, Part the First* appeared in Dublin in 1811 and was favorably received and reprinted in Philadelphia. No further parts ever appeared, however. His paper, *On Fracture of the Carpal Extremity of the Radius,* published in the *Edinburgh Medical and Surgical Journal* in 1814, was such a masterful treatise on the subject that this fracture is still known as Colles's fracture. In 1837, he published *Practical Observations on the Venereal Disease, and on the Use of Mercury,* in which he noted, "A child born of a mother who is without any obvious venereal symptoms . . . and shows this disease when it is a few weeks old . . . will infect the most healthy nurse . . . and yet this child is never known to infect its mother"—an observation since known as Colles' law. Although the observation was original with Colles, it had been made much earlier, in 1565, by Simon de Vallambert.

Colles resigned from his position at Steevens' Hospital in 1842 because of ill health. He died the following year.

Another notable physician of this group was John Cheyne, born at Leith, Scotland, in 1777. He graduated in medicine at Edinburgh and saw service with the British Army in Ireland, being present at the Battle of Vinegar Hill, where the Irish rebels were defeated by the British under the command of Sir John Moore. Returning to Scotland, Cheyne spent the next nine years assisting his father in his practice, also studying pathology and dissecting with Charles Bell. During this period, he was especially interested in diseases of children, and his first book, *Essays on the Diseases of Children,* was published in 1801 at Edinburgh. This work contained chapters on croup, on the pathology of the larynx and bronchi, on bowel complaints, and on acute hydrocephalus.

Cheyne settled in Dublin in 1809, was appointed physician to Meath Hospital, and was elected two years later professor of medicine in the College of Surgeons. He was very successful in practice, an enthusiastic student of pathology, an excellent teacher, and much interested in the problems of medical education. He has been generally known as the "founder of the Irish school of medicine." During his professional activity in Dublin, he wrote books on apoplexy,

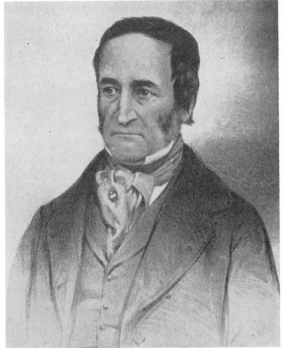

Ormsby, *Medical History of the Meath Hospital*, Dublin, 1888

ROBERT JAMES GRAVES

on hydrocephalus, and an important monograph on typhus fever which raged in Dublin from 1817 to 1818. His name is best remembered for his account of Cheyne-Stokes respiration, published in 1818.

Robert James Graves, whose family was descended from a colonel in Cromwell's army, was born at Dublin in 1797, the son of a distinguished clergyman. He was a brilliant student and graduated M.B. at Dublin in 1818. The next three years, he studied in London, Edinburgh, and on the Continent, working in Göttingen and Berlin. He had a great talent for languages and, on one occasion, was imprisoned for 10 days in Austria as a German spy, the authorities disregarding his statement that he was English "insisting that no Englishman could possibly speak German as he did." (Bettany) It is also related that, while Graves was in Italy, he lived and traveled with the celebrated painter Turner for months without either of them inquiring the name of his companion.

In 1821, Graves returned to Dublin and, the same year, was elected physician to Meath Hospital, a position he held for 22 years. He was a handsome man, endowed by nature with unusual charm and tact, an excellent speaker, and an interesting and thought-provoking teacher. He reorganized medical teaching, insisting that advanced medical students take charge of the patients and report the diagnosis, treatment and progress to the physicians during ward rounds. His *Clinical Lectures on the Practice of Medicine,* Dublin, 1848, was received most enthusiastically and was translated into French. Trousseau wrote a communication which appeared in the French translation, stating, among other things, "Graves is, in my acceptation of the term, a perfect clinical teacher."

Graves was very much interested in fevers and greatly opposed to the restricted diets then in vogue. He taught that fever patients should be placed on liberal feedings, and, one day while passing through the hospital wards, he was struck by the healthy appearance of the patients who were convalescing from typhoid fever. "This is all the effect of our good feeding," he exclaimed, "and lest, when I am gone, you may be at loss for an epitaph for me, let me give you one in three words: HE FED FEVERS." In 1835, he described in a paper published in the *London Medical and Surgical Journal* "a newly observed affection of the thyroid gland in females," since known as Graves' disease, although, as we know today, this condition was first described by Parry. Graves died in 1853.

William Stokes, colleague of Graves, had a reputation during his lifetime of being quite as great a clinician and teacher as Graves himself. The two men were, however, not rivals but colleagues, close friends who worked together in complete harmony and comradeship for nearly 30 years. Stokes, eight years younger, was born at Dublin in 1804, the son of Whitley Stokes, Regius Professor of Medicine, a brilliant man and a devoted Irish patriot. William studied chemistry at Glasgow and then went to Edinburgh for his medical education, receiving his degree in 1823. Before he left Edinburgh, he published in 1825 a little book on *The Use of the Stethoscope,* which was the first treatise on this new instrument in the English language.

In 1825, Stokes returned to Dublin and, the same year, was appointed physician to Meath Hospital. Although only 22, he was soon lecturing and giving clinical instruction to large classes of students, always pointing out the importance of the stethoscope and emphasizing that auscultation has "added more to the facility, certainty and utility of diagnosis than anything that has been done for centuries."

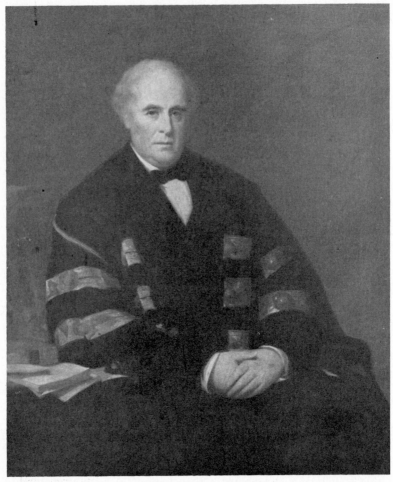

DOMINIC JOHN CORRIGAN
Portrait by W. Catterson Smith. Royal College of Physicians, Dublin.

Stokes's first book, *Diseases of the Chest,* Dublin, 1847, brought him great fame. It was immediately hailed as the first modern treatise on the subject in the English language and the best book since Laennec. His *Diseases of the Heart and the Aorta,* Dublin, 1854, based on the added experience of 20 years, was not immediately so popular as his first work but has been of more permanent value. It is a comprehensive treatise, showing great clinical acumen, mature judgment, and an intimate familiarity with the literature of cardiology. It contains an early, if not the earliest, account of paroxysmal tachycardia and the description of Cheyne-Stokes respiration. Stokes's description of heart block, since known as Stokes-Adams disease, was published in 1846 in an article in the *Dublin Quarterly Journal.* The first description of this condition in the English language was, however, published by Robert Adams in 1827. This is mentioned in Stokes's article. In *Lectures on Fever,* London, 1874, Stokes maintained the view that typhoid and typhus were but varieties of the same fever. "His fame would have been greater if he had not written his monograph on Fever" (Riesman). The prevention of disease was a subject in which Stokes was deeply interested and about which he constantly talked and wrote "before," as Bettany says, "sanitary science had come into fashion."

"My father," remarked Stokes, "left me but one legacy, the blessed gift of rising early." He often arose at four or five, studied or wrote until eight, when he began the day's work, which lasted often until far into the night. Many honors came to him, honorary degrees from Edinburgh, Oxford and Cambridge, physician to the Queen, Fellow of the Royal Society, and the coveted Prussian order Pour le Mérite.

In 1875, Stokes resigned as physician to Meath Hospital, after holding the position for nearly 50 years. He died in 1878 after a long life "with honour, love, obedience, troops of friends."

Dominic John Corrigan, another eminent member of the Irish school, colleague and friend of Graves and Stokes, was, unlike them, of pure Irish ancestry. He was born in Dublin in 1802 and, after pursuing medical studies there, went to Edinburgh, where he took his medical degree in 1825. On his return to Dublin, he devoted himself particularly to the study of pathological anatomy and obtained a position in the Meath Hospital out-patient department. Later, he was appointed physician to the Jervis Street Hospital, where his service consisted of only six beds. Nevertheless, by carefully choosing his patients and studying them with great care, he made here his great reputation as a physician, pathologist and teacher.

In 1832, Corrigan published in the *Edinburgh Medical and Surgical Journal* a paper on the "Permanent Patency of the Mouth of the Aorta or Inadequacy of the Aortic Vales," in which he described the typical pulse of aortic insufficiency, since commonly called the "Corrigan pulse." The article was accompanied by three excellent illustrations showing the morbid appearance of the aortic valves.

Corrigan was very popular as a teacher and extremely successful as a physician, developing a large practice which netted him for many years 9,000 pounds per annum, an enormous sum for those days. In 1866, he was created a baronet and, four years later, was elected as the representative of Dublin in Parliament. While chiefly remembered for his studies on the heart, he published a notable series of lectures on fevers in 1853, in which he stated that typhoid and typhus fevers were distinct diseases. He died in 1880.

After Corrigan, the preeminence of Dublin and the Irish school waned. It had made important contributions to the progress of medical science, some of the most important of which are constantly recalled by the eponyms, "Colles' fracture," "Colles' law," "Graves' disease," "Stokes-Adams syndrome," "Cheyne-Stokes respiration," and "Corrigan pulse."

THE GREAT MEN OF GUY'S

Guy's Hospital was founded by Thomas Guy, a citizen of London, who made a fortune in the publishing business and in speculation on the stock market. The hospital was built during the last year

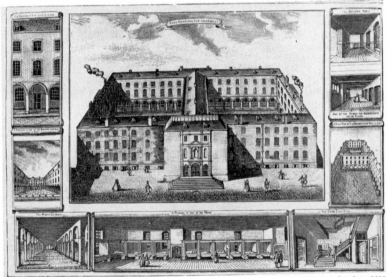

Wilks and Bettany, *Biographical History of Guy's Hospital*, London, 1892

GUY'S HOSPITAL IN 1725

Engraving by John Bowler.

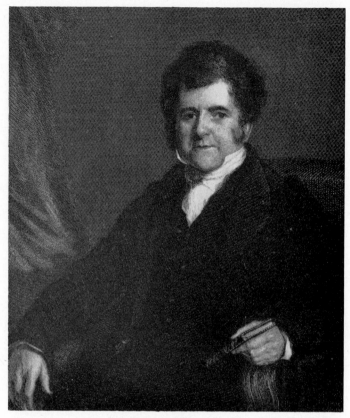

RICHARD BRIGHT
Portrait by T. R. Say.

of his life and was opened on January 6, 1725, ten days after his death. During the century, it had on its staff a succession of excellent physicians and surgeons but no outstanding figures. At the beginning of the nineteenth century, however, four remarkable men joined the staff—Bright, Addison, Hodgkin and Cooper, whose contributions to medical science raised Guy's Hospital to an eminence equal to that attained by Meath Hospital through the work of Graves and Stokes. These men of Guy's, like their counterparts at Meath, were investigators and teachers and active in establishing and directing a medical school in the hospital to which they had dedicated their professional lives.

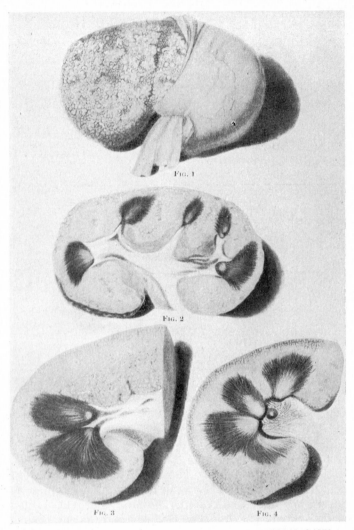

ILLUSTRATION FROM BRIGHT'S *REPORTS OF MEDICAL CASES*

"Showing a hard contracted and granulated state of the kidney, which was connected with the secretion of albuminous urine, and was accompanied by repeated and obstinate anasarca, and by effusion into the cavities."

The first of these men was Richard Bright (1789-1858), the son of a wealthy banker of Bristol, who had spared nothing in giving his son an excellent education and opportunity to travel. Bright entered Edinburgh University in 1808, and, after studying mathematics, botany and zoology, entered the medical school, then presided over by Monro *tertius*. In 1810, after a trip to Iceland, where he studied the flora and fauna of the island, he came to London and served two years as a resident officer in Guy's Hospital, "a foretaste of the forty years' residence which he practically made within its walls" (Bettany). Returning to Edinburgh in 1812, he took his degree in 1813. The following year, he went to the Continent, became fluent in French and German, and, in 1815, traveled extensively in Hungary, then *terra incognita* to most Britishers. He wrote an interesting account of his trip, *Travels from Vienna through Lower Hungary,* which was published at Edinburgh in 1818. This book is an excellent account of the social and economic conditions in Hungary and is illustrated with numerous charming full page sketches by Bright himself, who was an accomplished artist. This artistic talent of Bright, his ability to see clearly and to draw accurately what he saw, was of inestimable value to him in his study of pathological anatomy.

In 1820, Bright took a house in Bloomsbury Square for the practice of medicine and was appointed assistant physician to Guy's Hospital. For many years, he spent six hours a day in the hospital, studying the patients in the wards and their pathology in the postmortem room. He was a handsome man, possessed of a remarkably even and cheerful disposition, and these qualities, combined with his industry and intelligence, presently attracted a large following. In later years, when his large practice absorbed most of his time, he looked back with nostalgia on the days when he could spend most of his time in the hospital.

Bright's *Reports of Medical Cases,* which was printed at London in 1827, established his fame among his contemporaries and for posterity. In this work, he pointed out the association between diseased kidneys, dropsy and albuminous urine and clearly defined the disease since known by his name. The work was illustrated by striking illustrations in color, and, as Bright states, "The drawings and engravings were executed under my own immediate superintendence." Others before him had noted that, in some cases of dropsy, the urine was scanty and contained albumen and that certain of these patients showed small hardened kidneys. Yet, no one before him had stressed the association of albuminous urine, sclerosis of the kidneys and dropsy, grouped them together as a clinical entity, or pointed out the frequency of this syndrome. He also pointed out the frequency of cardiac hypertrophy in this condition and in the increase of urea in the blood.

Besides his *Reports,* Bright wrote numerous articles—on pancreatic diabetes, acute yellow atrophy of the liver, unilateral convulsions, and "status lymphaticus." The second volume of the *Reports of Medical Cases,* published in 1831, contains accurate accounts of acute otitis, laryngeal phthisis, cerebral hemorrhage, paralysis and tetanus, with striking plates of the pathologic lesions in typhoid fever, nephritis, acute yellow atrophy, and cerebral lesions. "Bright could not theorize, but he could see, and we are struck with astonishment at his powers of observation, as he photographed pictures of disease for the study of posterity" (Wilks).

During his lifetime, Bright was better known abroad than any British physician of modern times. He died in 1858 at the age of 69, and the postmortem examination revealed an extreme aortic stenosis but normal kidneys. He did not die of "his own disease," as has often been said.

Thomas Addison, Bright's colleague at Guy's, was a man of very different background and temperament. Addison was born in less comfortable circumstances, had not enjoyed the advantage of extensive travel, and personally, unlike the sunny, genial, likeable Bright, was taciturn, unapproachable, and often gruff, hiding an innate shyness under the cloak of gruffness.

He was born near Newcastle in 1793 and first went to school there, becoming such an excellent Latin student that, when he went to Edinburgh to study medicine, he took his lecture notes in Latin. He received his degree in 1815, began practice in London, and went to Guy's in 1820 for further study. He soon attracted the attention of the authorities and, in 1824, was appointed assistant physician, later becoming physician and serving on the staff for 36 years. He died in 1860.

Addison's fame rests chiefly on his description of what he termed "melasma suprarenale," bronzed skin associated with disease of the suprarenal glands, a syndrome since known as Addison's disease. A brief report of this first appeared in the *Medical Gazette* of March 15, 1849. The report was later expanded in his monograph, *On the Constitutional and Local Effects of Diseases of the Suprarenal Capsules,* London, 1855, which contained some excellent plates of the condition. In the same report, he also described "idiopathic anemia," since known as pernicious anemia or Addisonian anemia. In 1850 Addison published a paper in *Guy's Hospital Reports,* in which he described for the first time xanthoma diabeticorum.

During his lifetime, Addison's reputation did not rest upon his discoveries, his description of suprarenal disease being regarded simply as a curiosity, but upon his skill as a physician and upon his remarkable ability as a teacher. His painstaking examinations and his uncanny diagnoses became a legend. He was described by a critic as "a fine dashing, big, burly, bustling man, proud and pompous as a parish beadle in his robes of office. . . . Every sentence is polished, is powerful; he prefers the grandiloquent. Slow and studied are his opening sentences, studied the regularity of his intonations." Students worshipped him, but feared him rather than loved him.

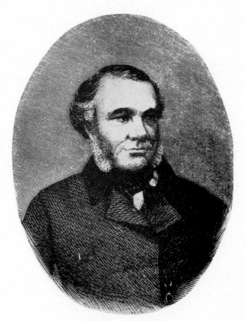

THOMAS ADDISON

Frontispiece of *A Collection of the Published Writings of Thomas Addison,* London, 1868.

The personal power which he possessed was the secret of his position, much superior to what Bright could ever claim, and equal, if not greater, than that of Sir Astley Cooper. For many years, he was the leading light of Guy's, so that every Guy's man, during the 30 or 40 years of his teaching, was a disciple of Addison, holding his name in the greatest reverence and regarding his authority as the best guide in the practice of the profession. (Wilks and Bettany.)

Thomas Hodgkin, another notable member of Guy's group, was a gentle Quaker, born in Tottenham in 1798, and, like Bright and Addison, a graduate of Edinburgh, where he took his medical degree in 1823. On his return to London, he became interested in the formation of a medical school at Guy's Hospital and was appointed curator of the museum and demonstrator of morbid anatomy. He did an enormous amount of work in his new position, collecting and assembling specimens as well as making an extensive catalogue, this experience forming the basis of his *Lectures on the Morbid Anatomy of the Serous and Mucous Membranes*, London, 1836. After serving for 10 years as lecturer on pathology, he resigned after his unsuccessful candidature for the post of assistant physician. He continued to practice in London, but, being very generous by nature and careless in collecting fees, he soon abandoned practice and devoted himself to philanthropy. While traveling in the Orient, he died at Jaffa in 1866.

Hodgkin's notable work was in the field of pathology. In his *Lectures,* he described clearly acute appendicitis and, in 1827, wrote an account of aortic insufficiency with an excellent pathological description, three years before the appearance of Corrigan's classic paper. In 1832, he published in the *Medical Chirurgical Transactions* an account of the disease since known as Hodgkin's disease, describing seven cases. However, a restudy of the tissue with the aid of the microscope, which Hodgkin did not employ, has shown that only three of these cases are what we today understand as Hodgkin's disease.

No account of Guy's Hospital at this period would be complete without the name of Astley Cooper, probably the best known surgeon of his time. He was already at the height of his fame when young Bright first joined the staff. Cooper was born in Brooke, near Norwick, in 1768, the son of a clergyman and grandson of a surgeon. He studied at Edinburgh, then returned to London, where he studied under John Hunter. In 1789, he was appointed demonstrator in anatomy at St. Thomas' and, in 1800, surgeon to Guy's, one of his pupils at that time, Benjamin Travers, describing him as the handsomest, most intelligent looking, and finely formed man he ever saw.

Cooper came into possession of a fortune by marriage and was able to devote himself to study and teaching. He went to the hospital even before breakfast to dissect, his passion for anatomy being so great that he is said to have dissected every day of his life, even when traveling. His dissecting passion threw him in close touch with body snatchers or resurrectionists so that he became one of their main supporters. He spent hundreds of pounds for bodies, and, when the resurrectionists were caught and imprisoned, he often advanced considerable amounts of money to defend them

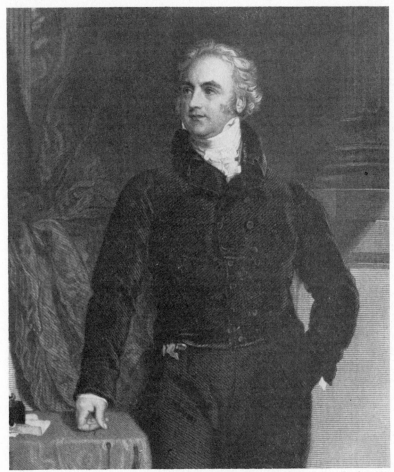

Cooper, *Life of Sir Astley Cooper*, London, 1843
SIR ASTLEY COOPER
Portrait by Sir Thomas Lawrence.

in court and, if they were convicted, to support them and their families during their imprisonment. This truly shocking state of affairs was primarily due to the laws which made it almost impossible legally to obtain a body for dissection.

Few men have worked so hard or so incessantly as Cooper. He rose at six, dissected until eight, breakfasted on two rolls and a cup of tea, saw poor patients until nine, saw private patients or operated until one, then drove to Guy's Hospital and made rounds, lectured at St. Thomas' Hospital at two, then worked in the dissection room for an hour or more, saw his private patients or operated until seven; then he bolted his dinner, and, after forty winks of sleep, he was off again to lecture or to visit patients until midnight. As he drove from place to place in his carriage, every spare moment was occupied in dictating to his assistants.

Cooper was one of the best operators of the day. "It is of no consequence what instrument Mr. Cooper uses," said his colleague Mr. Chandler, "They are all alike to him, and I varily believe he could operate as easily with an oyster-knife as the best bit of cutlery in Laundy's shop." In 1808, Cooper successfully ligated the common carotid and the external iliac arteries for aneurysms and, in 1817, the abdominal aorta. A successful operation for a small tumor on the head of George IV was rewarded with a baronetcy. Cooper's books on *Hernia,* 1804; *Injuries of the Joints,* 1822; *Diseases of the Breast,* 1829; *Diseases of the Testes,* 1830; and *The Anatomy of the Thymus Gland,* 1832 were widely read. Cooper's fascia (the fascia transversalis) and Cooper's hernia (retroperitoneal hernia) are terms still employed in surgical nomenclature. Sir Astley Cooper died in 1841. "No surgeon, before or since," says Bettany, "has filled so large a space in the public eye."

Thus did the men of Guy's make medical history, as did the men of Meath's. And like their contemporaries in Dublin, Bright, Addison, Hodgkin and Cooper also left their names on diseases, eponyms which recall their brilliant studies.

HOMEOPATHY AND SAMUEL HAHNEMANN

The early years of the nineteenth century, which witnessed such phenomenal advances in medical science, advances high-lighted by the schools of Paris, Dublin and London, also saw the growth of two strange phenomena which seemed a retrogression from the field of experimental science to the domain of pure, unchecked speculation. The first of these movements was homeopathy.

The founder of homeopathy was Samuel Friedrich Christian Hahnemann, who was born in Meissen, Germany, in 1755, the son of a porcelain painter at the well-known porcelain works. He entered the University of Leipzig as a medical student and then went to Vienna, where he studied under von Quarin, the first director of the *Allgemeines Krankenhaus,* physician to the emperor, and one of the most noted Viennese physicians of that period. Forced by

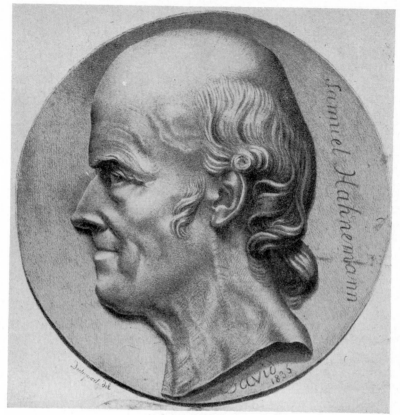

SAMUEL HAHNEMANN   University of Kansas Collection

pecuniary difficulties, Hahnemann left Vienna to become physician
to a nobleman in Hermannstadt and, in 1779, received his doctor's
degree at Erlangen.

After practicing in several places, he went to Leipzig, where he
worked on a translation of Cullen's *Materia medica*. While studying
the section on the action of quinine, he discovered, he said, the
principle upon which he founded his system of therapy. He saw, he
states, that quinine, which was widely used to treat fevers would also
produce fever—"the tincture of an ounce of cinchona-bark . . . will
certainly produce a cinchona fever of several days' duration." He
pondered long on this observation, which most pharmacologists
have been unable to verify, and concluded, "A disease can only

be destroyed and cured by a remedy which has a tendency to produce a similar disease." This conception that he later expressed in the well-known phrase, *Similia similibus curantur* (Likes are cured by likes), became the corner-stone of the medical system he later created.

In 1792, Hahnemann became interested in mental diseases, advocated humane treatment of the insane, and for a time directed an establishment near Gotha in a castle placed at his disposal by Duke Ernst II. He remained there some two years and, after practicing in six or seven localities, wrote his *Organon der Heilkunst*, the first part of which appeared in 1811. From 1811 to 1821, he practiced in Leipzig with great success, lectured on his new method of therapy, and, in 1821, became a *Privatdozent* in the University of Leipzig. He resigned from this position to become court physician to the Duke of Anhalt-Köthen and held this place until, at the age of 80, he married a second wife, a young French woman, and moved to Paris, where he practiced with success and found many disciples. He died in 1843 at the age of 88.

Hahnemann's system is outlined in his chief work, *Organon der Heilkunst*, Dresden, 1811-1833. He also wrote numerous articles from time to time. His biographer and champion, Wilhelm Ameke, has collected his bibliography, which totals 114 items. There are three cardinal tenets of his doctrine—that like cures like; that medicines increase in potency with their dilution; and that a large number of diseases are due to, or related to, a condition he called *Psora*.

The first tenet, *similia similibus curantur*, is the *leitmotif* which is clearly discernible in all his writings. In addition to the classic experiment on himself with cinchona, he experimented upon himself with a variety of drugs, noted the symptoms they produced, and then used them to treat diseases having symptoms like those produced by ingestion of the drug. In scarlet fever, which is associated with a sore throat, he employed belladonna, which, as well known, causes dryness of the throat. "A disease," he stated emphatically, "can only be destroyed and cured by a remedy which has a tendency to produce a similar disease, for the effects of drugs are in themselves no other than artificial diseases."

His second tenet that medicines increase in potency with their dilution is clearly formulated in the *Organon*. Eight drops of almost any medicinal tincture given in one dose have only a quarter of the effect of eight drops of the same tincture given in one drop doses every four or two hours. He further extends this doctrine and states, "A single drop of a tincture to a pound of water, if administered in doses of two ounces every two hours, will produce more effect than a single dose of eight drops of the tincture." Holmes observes that, in some of Hahnemann's prescriptions, he employed dilutions as high as one-sextillionth (one, followed by 21 zeroes) and observed powerful effects from their administration.

The third great doctrine of Hahnemann was the assertion that *Psora* (the itch) "is the sole true and fundamental cause that produces all the countless forms of disease, which go under the names of nervous debility." He continues, naming 31 diseases, including rickets, cancer, gout, jaundice, dropsy, asthma, cataract and amaurosis, that "appear in our pathology as so many peculiar distinct and independent diseases."

These doctrines had some supporters in Germany but more opponents. The same was true in France. The leading physicians, the professors in the medical faculties were not impressed by the new theories. Prof. Andral reported to the Paris *Académie de Médecine* that he had treated more than 100 patients with homeopathic remedies and had seen no effects whatever. Still, the movement spread. Five homeopathic medical journals appeared in France, homeopathic physicians in increasing numbers appeared in France, England, Germany, and the United States, where several homeopathic medical schools and hospitals were founded.

Today homeopathy is not merely on the wane; it has waned and practically disappeared. The foundation stone of homeopathy, the experiments of Hahnemann on himself and his friends have been shown by pharmacologists to be largely the results of self delusion. Every student of medicine, pharmacy and chemistry at the present time knows that the potency of a drug is diminished and not increased by dilution. And, as for Hahnemann's doctrine of the *Psora,* opposed even during his life time by some of his followers, any serious student of medicine would be highly amused at the suggestion that the 31 various diseases listed by him are all due to *Psora.*

However, homeopathy had certain beneficient effects upon the development of medicine. Hahnemann's protests against the employment of violent emetics, strong purgatives, the frequent bleeding, cupping and blistering, so commonly used, were not without their effects. His advocacy of few medicines in treatment was a welcome protest against the well-nigh universal and commonly irrational polypharmacy of the time. His prescriptions with their enormous dilutions, of course, had no medicinal effects, but they did no harm and impressed the physicians anew with the healing powers of nature, although Hahnemann himself had gone "so far as to say that no one had ever seen the simple efforts of nature effect the durable re- covery of a patient from a chronic disease" (Holmes). Since Hahne- mann's doses were so minute and usually prepared with pleasant flavors, many patients preferred homeopathic remedies, a lesson which was not lost on the regular medical profession.

NATURPHILOSOPHIE

The second movement which had a profound influence for a time, particularly on German medicine, was the creation of the German philosopher, Friedrich Wilhelm Joseph von Schelling (1775-1854). Schelling, the son of an esteemed theologian and Orientalist, first studied theology and, later turning to philosophy, was professor of philosophy successively at Jena, Würzburg and Berlin. His work, *Erster Entwurf eines Systems der Naturphilosophie,* 1797, marked the beginning of a new philosophical school that influenced deeply the philosophical thinking of his time and medicine as well. *Natur- philosophie* embraced not only what had been considered as the field of speculative philosophy but the entire field of natural science, of which medicine is a part.

Schelling taught, among other things, the identity of the subjec- tive and the objective; the unity of knowledge and what is known; that consciousness is the process of expansion and contraction, and sensation is the equilibrium resulting from the two forces; that the three principal phenomena of nature—electricity, chemistry and magnetism—appear in the organic world as the power of reproduc- tion, sensibility and irritability; and that the microcosm is the image of the macrocosm.

It is difficult to see what bearing all this speculation had upon the science of medicine, yet Hermann Horn, *Privatdozent* of the University of Munich, wrote the following statements indicative of the reasoning employed by the enthusiastic adherents of *Natur- philosophie* in his *Physiologisch-pathologische Darstellung des Schleimfiebers,* Augsburg, 1846:

Compare the blood cells with the earth and the similarity is striking. The earth is round and flattened at the poles. The blood cell of man is round and flattened at the sides. The earth has a nucleus (the earth itself) and a shell (the atmosphere). The blood cell has a nucleus and a shell. The earth turns on its axis, the blood cells turn on their axes. The earth is controlled by the sun, the blood cells by the nervous system. . . . All the properties of the blood cell we must also allow to the earth.

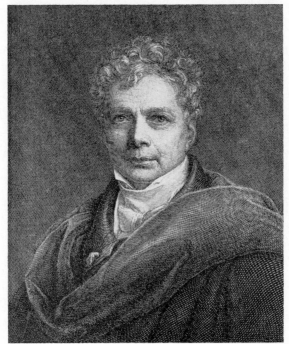

von Leixner, *Geschichte der deutschen Literatur*, Leipzig, 1903

FRIEDRICH VON SCHELLING

Engraving by Schultheis from painting by Stieler.

Leaving aside the fact that Horn's physiology is notoriously at fault, the student of today asks what progress in medicine the jargon of such "physiologic pathological" descriptions proclaims. The answer is simple—none, but a marked retrogression. Yet, appearing during the Romantic period, when the models of classic antiquity were being intensively studied as never before, this new movement swept many physicians, especially in Germany, off their feet, intoxicated by the fascinating new terms and the dialectic subteties of the leader and his enthusiastic disciples. However, as Hirschel remarks, "Whoever loves the light of day and the bright torches of truth and objective investigation, calls these *Naturphilosophers* neither naturalists nor philosophers, but rather poets and dreamers."

Naturphilosophie contributed nothing to the healing of disease, which is the *raison d'être* of the medical profession. It substituted speculation and phantasy for the scientific study of disease. However, some good features of the movement cannot be denied. The interest excited by the discussions regarding the nature of man led to a renewed study of many physiological problems, and the comparisons between the nature of man and that of the world at large led to important discoveries in comparative anatomy, in embryology, and in natural history. The broad generalizations of the *Naturphilosophers* regarding the progression of lower forms of organic life into higher forms, including man, according to some, led to the later generalizations of Lamarck and Darwin and the birth of the theory of evolution. Johannes Müller, the greatest German physiologist of his time and one of the greatest medical naturalists of all time, and Johann Lucas Schönlein, the founder of modern clinical teaching in Germany, were both in their younger years followers of the school of *Naturphilosophie*.

Biographical Addenda

THE NINETEENTH CENTURY—THE FIRST HALF

1753-1825—Jean Devèze was born at Rabartens and practiced many years in Santo Domingo. Returning to France, he published a noteworthy treatise on yellow fever, *Traité de la fièvre jaune,* Paris, 1820, in which he maintained that yellow fever was not contagious.

1754-1808—Thomas Beddoes was born at Shifnal, Shropshire, and was a student at Pembroke College, Oxford. He studied medicine under John Sheldon in London and then returned to Oxford, where he received his M.D. in 1786. After visiting Paris, where he became acquainted with Lavoisier, he went back to Oxford, and he was reader in chemistry until 1792. He established in 1798 the "Pneumatic Institute" at Clifton for the treatment of diseases by the inhalation of gases, the first superintendent being Humphry Davy, who carried out there his well-known investigations on nitrous oxide. His apparatus for the inhalation of gases was constructed by James Watt, the inventor of the gasometer. The Institute later became a hospital.

1754-1825—Pierre François, Baron Percy.

1755-1826—Philippe Pinel.

1755-1824—James Parkinson was the son of a physician and practiced in Hoxton, Middlesex, England. We have no details of his education or professional activities. He was the author of several political pamphlets, was interested in reform, and, in addition, was an excellent geologist and paleontologist. He wrote treatises on health, on chemistry, on the gout, and on insanity, and, in 1812, published in the *Medical Chirurgical Transactions* a paper on a *Case of Diseased Appendix Vermiformis,* describing a fatal case with necropsy findings. He is best remembered for his *Essay on the Shaking Palsy,* 1817, a disease since known as Parkinson's disease.

1755-1821—Jean Nicolas Corvisart.

1755-1830—Samuel Thomas von Soemmering was born at Thorn, Poland, the son of the city physician of Thorn, and, in 1774, entered the University of Göttingen as a medical student. In addition to studying medicine, he devoted much time to the study of languages and learned the art of engraving. He also engaged in anatomical research and, in 1778, received his degree, presenting as a doctor's thesis a remarkable paper on the cranial nerves, introducing a classification which eventually superseded that of Willis. Later, he visited England, Scotland and Holland, where he worked with John and William Hunter, Monro, and Pieter Camper. In 1784, he became professor of anatomy at Mainz, holding this position for 11 years, after which he practiced medicine in Frankfurt-am-Main. Later, he worked in Munich, becoming interested in astronomy, paleontology and physics. He studied sun-spots, meteors, fossils and invented an electric telegraph. His greatest achievement was his anatomical work, which drew unstinted praise from Choulant. He also described and pictured a case of achondroplasia, one of the earliest on record.

1755-1843—Samuel Christian Friedrich Hahnemann.

1757-1817—William Charles Wells was born in Charleston, South Carolina, and graduated in medicine at Edinburgh in 1780. In 1782, he returned to America and commenced publication of a weekly newspaper at St. Augustine, Florida. Two years later, he went to London, began the practice of medicine, and was physician to St. Thomas' Hospital from 1800 until his death.

Wells was a gifted and versatile investigator. In 1810, he published what is perhaps the earliest account of cardiac complications in rheumatic fever and described in 1811 albuminous urine in dropsy. In 1813, he proposed the theory of natural selection, later developed by Charles Darwin, and, in 1814, he explained in his *Essay on Dew* the manner in which dew is formed.

1758-1828—Franz Joseph Gall.

1760-1818—Caspar Wistar.

1761-1823—Matthew Baillie, the nephew of William and John Hunter, was born in Lanarkshire, Scotland, and educated at Oxford, where he took his M.B. in 1786. He began practice in London, was elected physician to St. George's Hospital, and, in 1789, became a Fellow of the Royal Society of Physi-

cians. Upon the retirement of Dr. Pitcairn, Baillie succeeded to his practice and soon had the largest and most lucrative practice in London. He was appointed physician to King George III and was offered a baronetcy, but declined the honor. He was the last to carry the gold-headed cane, the symbol of medical leadership in London, which had been successively carried by Radcliffe, Mead, Askew and Pitcairn. On Baillie's death, his widow presented it to the Royal College of Physicians.

Baillie's *Morbid Anatomy of some of the most important Parts of the Human Body,* London, 1793, is one of the landmarks in the history of pathology and the first great work on the subject written in English. It shows one of the earliest illustrations of a gastric ulcer and of cirrhosis of the liver.

1760-1839—Mathew Carey.

1761-1815—John Clarke, educated at St. George's Hospital, settled in London, lectured on obstetrics at William Hunter's school, and soon became one of the leading obstetricians of London. At the height of his success, he abruptly gave up the practice of obstetrics, moved to another part of the city, and devoted himself to diseases of women and children. His *Commentaries on Some of the Most Important Diseases of Children,* London, 1815, the completion of which was prevented by his death, contains what is probably the first account of infantile tetany.

1763-1820—John Bell, surgeon and anatomist, elder brother of Sir Charles Bell, graduated at Edinburgh in 1779 and, after extensive travels, returned to Edinburgh, where he taught anatomy, surgery and obstetrics. An accomplished artist, he drew some of the illustrations for *The Anatomy of the Human Body,* London, 1793, which he wrote in collaboration with his brother Charles. In addition to several anatomical works, he wrote *Principles of Surgery,* London, 1801-1808, a second edition of which was published by his brother in 1826-1828. John Bell was an accomplished classical scholar and one of the most skillful operators of his time.

1756-1832—Sir Everard Home was born in Hull and, in 1772, was elected to Trinity College, Cambridge, but chose instead to go to London to study with his brother-in-law, John Hunter. His first work, *A Dissertation on the Properties of Pus,* published in 1788, attracted much attention. He was closely associated with John Hunter for 20 years, interrupted by six years' service with the navy, assisted him in his experimental work, and soon achieved a reputation, which grew with the publication of his treatises on stricture of the urethra, ulcers of the leg, cancer and diseases of the prostate. On John Hunter's death, he was appointed by the terms of Hunter's will, custodian of Hunter's collections and unpublished after entific papers. He published after Hunter's death some 116 papers in the *Philosophical Transactions,* but it has never been determined how many of these were based on work done by Hunter or by Home. He burned a large number of Hunter's papers, an action severely criticized by posterity. Home's friends asserted that they were of little value

and added nothing to Hunter's reputation, whereas Home's enemies claimed that he destroyed them to hide the fact that many of his own alleged discoveries were the work of Hunter. Home himself explained his destruction of Hunter's papers in a communication to the Royal College of Surgeons--"I have not presumed to judge. He made me two requests; the one that his body should be opened, the other that his manuscripts should be destroyed. I have complied with both."

Home was surgeon to the King, professor at the Royal College of Surgeons, Fellow of the Royal Society, and, in 1813, was created a baronet. He was described by his pupils as an excellent teacher and surgeon, but was possessed of little originality. His interest in scientific surgery gradually faded after the death of Hunter, who had during his lifetime so completely dominated his brother-in-law.

1762-1836—Christoph Wilhelm Hufeland, one of the most widely known and respected physicians of his time, was born in Langensalza, in Thuringia. His father and grandfather had been court physicians at Weimar. Hufeland studied first at Jena and then at Göttingen, where he received his doctor's degree in 1783. After graduation, he returned to Weimar to assist his nearly blind father in his practice and had as patients Wieland, Herder, Goethe and Schiller, with all of whom he became intimately acquainted. In 1785, he wrote an article on mesmerism, expressing the view that its effects depended upon the imagination. In 1787, he wrote a treatise on smallpox, urging a strict quarantine as the only effective method of checking an epidemic of this disease. In 1793, he was called to Jena as professor. In 1796 after Jenner's discovery of vaccination, he took up the new method with great enthusiasm, and his championship played an important role in popularizing it in Germany.

Hufeland went to Berlin in 1800 as royal physician, director of the *Collegium medico-chirurgicum,* and chief physician at the Charité. He was eminently successful as a practitioner, teacher, and leader of the medical profession. He wrote many articles and two well-known books—*System der praktischen Heilkunde,* 1800-1805; and *Encheiridion medicum,* 1836. He was one of the pioneers of medical journalism in the nineteenth century, editing four journals, one of which the *Journal der praktischen Arzneikunde und Wundarzneikunst,* founded by him in 1795, continued publication until 1844 and, as *Hufeland's Journal,* had a deserved reputation as the most informative and respected medical journal of its time.

An opponent of medical "systems" in general, Hufeland was particularly outspoken in his hostility to Mesmerism and Brunonism. His *Makrobiotik,* 1796, a popular treatise on the prolongation of life, had a phenomenal success, went through numerous editions and translations, and was read literally throughout the world.

1764-1831—John Abernethy, a pupil of John Hunter, became assistant surgeon to St. Bartholomew's Hospital in 1787 and lecturer on anatomy, physiology, pathology and surgery. His lectures were so popular

that a building where he could teach was erected in 1790, and, on this account, he has been considered the founder of St. Bartholomew's Medical School. Deeply imbued with the spirit of Hunter, he carried out numerous anatomical and physiological investigations, established an anatomical and pathological laboratory, and achieved great popularity among medical students as a clear, forceful and dramatic lecturer. He wrote numerous surgical treatises and was appointed professor of anatomy and surgery in the Royal College of Physicians. A bold and skillful surgeon, he was the first to ligate the external iliac artery for aneurysm (1796) and ligated the common carotid for hemorrhage (1798). Although a kind and generous man, he often affected a brusque manner toward his patients on the ground that a masterful rudeness commands respect, while amiability might suggest weakness and a lack of self-confidence.

1766-1803—Kurt Sprengel, by general consent the greatest medical historian of his time and also an eminent botanist, was born in Boldekow, Pomerania, the son of a minister. He studied first theology at Griefswald but later changed to medicine, receiving his M.D. at Halle in 1787. The same year, he became a *Privatdozent* and, in 1797, became professor of medicine. He was an excellent classical scholar and, in addition, mastered Semitic languages. His *Versuch einer pragmatischen Geschichte der Arzneikunde,* in five volumes, was first published at Halle, 1792-1799, and later translated into French and Italian. In spite of the author's outspoken defense of the "vitalistic" standpoint in medicine and his severe criticism of its opponents, this work remains an exceedingly valuable source book, a mine of information, and "a marvel of solid learning" (Garrison).

1766-1842—Dominique Jean Larrey.

1766-1844—Sir Henry Halford, Bt., was born in Leicester, England, the son of James Vaughan, an eminent physician of that city. He was educated at Rugby and at Oxford, where he received his M.D. in 1791. He settled in London the following year and married the daughter of Lord St. John. He was elected physician to Middlesex Hospital but presently had such a large practice that he gave up his hospital connections. On the death of Lady Denbigh, widow of Sir Charles Halford, he inherited a large fortune, changed his name to Henry Halford, and was created a baronet. He was physician to four successive sovereigns and, in 1820, was elected president of the Royal College of Physicians. A successful and much sought-for physician, "his early success as a physician left him but little leisure for composition" (Munk). He wrote nothing of enduring worth.

1767-1828—René Joseph Hyacinthe Bertin was born near Rennes, studied medicine at Paris and at Montpellier, taking his degree at Montpellier in 1791. After serving as an army surgeon in the Napoleonic wars, he returned to Paris, was appointed chief physician to the Cochin Hospital, and was appointed in 1822 professor of hygiene in the medical faculty. His pathological studies on the heart were important, and the conception of "eccentric"

and "concentric" hypertrophy of the heart dates from his work. His chief publication was his *Traité des Maladies du coeur et des gros vaisseaux*, Paris, 1824.

1766-1859—Thomas Winterbottom was born in South Shields, England, and graduated in medicine at Glasgow in 1792. After graduation, he practiced medicine in Sierra Leone, Africa, for four years and then returned to his native town, where he practiced until his retirement some 20 years later. In 1803, he published *An Account of the Native Africans in the Neighborhood of Sierra Leone*, which contains probably the first account of trypanosomiasis, or "sleeping sickness," in the English language.

1768-1837—Philip Syng Physick.

1768-1841—Sir Astley Paston Cooper.

1769-1842—Thomas Spens was a native of Edinburgh, where he obtained his education and passed his professional life. In 1793, he published in *Medical Commentaries* the first description of heart block in English, 48 years before that of Adams and 53 years before that of Stokes, although the account of Morgagni anteceded Spens's 32 years.

1771-1802—Marie François Xavier Bichat.

1771-1860—John Blackall was born at Exeter, England, and educated at Oxford, taking his M.D. degree in 1797. He spent most of his professional career in Exeter and was generally regarded as the outstanding physician in that part of England. Blackall's *Observations on the Nature and Cure of Dropsies*, London, 1813, noted that dropsy is often associated with albuminuria and at times with diseased kidneys.

1771-1830—Ephraim McDowell.

1771-1843—Elisha North.

1772-1838—François Joseph Victor Broussais.

1773-1829—Thomas Young was born in Somersetshire, England, was a very precocious youth, and, at the age of 14, was familiar with Latin, Greek, French, Italian, Hebrew, Arabic and Persian. He studied medicine under John Hunter and Matthew Baillie, then proceeded to Göttingen, where he obtained his M.D. in 1796. While still a medical student, he read a paper on vision before the Royal Society and, in 1794 at the early age of 21, was elected a Fellow. In 1799, he began practice in London and, in 1801, was appointed professor of physics at the Royal Institution. He was physician to St. George's Hospital from 1811 until his death.

Young's contributions to medicine were slight; his contributions to physics and philology were most important. His experiments did much to establish the undulatory theory of light; he discovered the principle of the interference of light, explained the accommodation of the eye to distant objects, and first described astigmatism. As a philologist, he is remembered as the first to decipher partially the Rosetta Stone.

1773-1846—John Bostock was a native of Liverpool and graduated in medicine at Edinburgh in 1794. He began practice in Liverpool, removed to London in 1817, but soon afterwards gave up the practice of medicine to devote himself to science. He assisted Richard Bright in

his investigations of renal disease, translated Pliny's *Natural History*, wrote the first systematic treatise on physiology in English, his *Elements of Physiology*, and described "hay fever" in 1819.

1774-1816—Gaspard Laurent Bayle.

1774-1842—Sir Charles Bell was one of the six children of the Rev. William Bell, a clergyman of the Episcopal Church of Scotland. He began his medical studies under his elder brother John, already a well-known surgeon and anatomist in Edinburgh. Both brothers had unusual artistic ability, and Charles, while still a student, drew many of the illustrations for his brother's *The Anatomy of the Human Body*, 1793, and also contributed the sections on the nerves, sense organs and viscera. In 1799, he was admitted to the Royal College of Surgeons. Seven years later, he moved to London, where he taught anatomy at the Great Windmill Street School, founded by the Hunters, and, in 1812, was elected surgeon to Middlesex Hospital. In 1836, he was called to Edinburgh as professor of surgery, holding this position until his death.

Bell was by training an anatomist and disliked animal experimentation. He published several excellent anatomical treatises, with exquisite drawings by his own hand, particularly his *System of Dissections*, 1798; *Engravings of the Brain and Nervous System*, 1802; and *Bridgwater Treatise IV: The Hand*. He has been credited with the discovery that the posterior roots of the spinal cord have a sensory function while the anterior roots are concerned with motor function, but this claim has been disputed by many physiologists who hold that this fact was first demonstrated conclusively by François Magendie. Bell demonstrated that the fifth nerve is both sensory and motor, that the facial nerve is motor, and that a lesion of it produces paralysis of the face—"Bell's palsy."

In addition, Bell was an excellent surgeon and, after the Battle of Waterloo, went to Brussels, where he treated the wounded British soldiers. He published an *Essay on Gun-shot Wounds* as an appendix to the second edition of *A System of Operative Surgery, founded on the Basis of Anatomy*, 1814. In 1829, he was knighted for his services to science. Sir Charles Bell was an extraordinary man, equally distinguished as a surgeon, teacher, anatomist and physiologist. His drawings for their accuracy and artistic perfection have few equals in the history of anatomical illustration. "His various systems of anatomy, dissections, and surgery, still stand unrivaled for facility of expression, elegance of style, and accuracy of description" (Choulant-Frank).

1774-1844—John Conrad Otto.

1774-1856—Joseph Claude Anthelme Récamier, French physician and gynecologist, born at Rochefort, served in the army and navy during the Napoleonic wars. In 1801, he became physician to the Hôtel Dieu in Paris and held this position for 40 years, giving lectures and pathological demonstrations. He was appointed professor of medicine at the Collège de France, receiving the appointment although the *Académie des Sciences* preferred Magendie by a vote of 55 to five. Récamier was

dismissed from this chair in 1831 for refusing to take the oath of allegiance to Louis Philippe. He wrote several treatises on cancer.

1775-1843—Abraham Colles.

1777-1835—Guillaume, Baron Dupuytren.

1777-1836—John Cheyne.

1778-1856—John C. Warren.

1778-1851—Christian Friedrich Nasse was born in Bielefeld, Westphalia, graduated in medicine at Halle in 1800, and, after practicing in Göttingen, Leipzig, Dresden and Weimar, was called to Halle as professor of medicine in 1815. He went to Bonn in 1819 as professor and director of the medical clinic, where he remained until his death.

Nasse was an excellent teacher, a man of wide culture and learning and was very active in the new movement which stressed the physiological aspects of clinical medicine. He was the first German physician to introduce percussion and auscultation into his clinic and the first to employ the microscope in his clinical demonstrations. He wrote a large number of scientific articles and several very successful books, notably his *Handbuch der speciellen Therapie*, 1830-1838; and his *Handbuch der allgemeinen Therapie*, 1840. He was a pioneer in the scientific treatment of insanity and wrote a well-known text on the subject, *Die Behandlung der Gemüthskranken und Irren durch Nichtärzte*, 1844. He is also remembered as the formulator of "the law of Nasse" (1820)—that hemophilia occurs only in males and is transmitted by the unaffected females.

1778-1862—Pierre Bretonneau.

1781-1826—Réné Théophile Hyacinthe Laennec.

fl. 1823—V. Collin, assistant of Laennec, wrote a very popular manual of physical diagnosis, *Les diverses Méthodes d'Exploration de la Poitrine*, Paris, 1823, in which he described in great detail the pericardial friction sound.

1782-1855—François Magendie.

1785-1852—Daniel Drake.

1785—1853—William Beaumont.

1787-1872—Pierre Charles Alexandre Louis.

1787-1853 — Mathéo-José-Bonaventura Orfila, founder of experimental and legal toxicology, was a native of Minorca and, after studying at Valencia and Barcelona, graduated at Paris in 1811. In 1831, he became dean of the Paris faculty and held this post until 1848.

1787-1869—Jan Evangel Purkinje, born in Libochowitz, Bohemia, graduated in medicine at Prague in 1819 and, the same year, was appointed assistant in anatomy and pathology. In 1823, he went to Breslau, where he established a physiological institute, carried out important investigations, and stayed until 1849, when he returned to Prague as professor of physiology, remaining there until his death.

Purkinje's contributions were numerous and important. As a microscopist, he was the first to use a microtome, Canada balsam, glacial acetic acid, and potassium bichromate. He discovered the sweat glands of the skin, the ganglionic cells in the cerebellum, since called Purkinje's cells, and ciliary motion. In 1837, he pointed out the identity of plant and animal cells and the importance of finger prints in identification, long before Francis Galton. He made extensive studies on the physiology of sight, describing the visual images produced by poisoning with digitalis and belladonna. He studied extensively the pharmacologic effects of camphor, opium, belladonna, stramonium and turpentine.

1788-1858—August François Chomel, member of a family which produced several distinguished medical men, was born in Paris, where he received his medical degree and lived all his life. As a young man, he worked with great enthusiasm in anatomy and pathology, succeeded in 1827 to Laennec's position as professor of medicine at the Charité, and followed Récamier at the Hôtel Dieu in 1830. His reputation as a teacher grew rapidly, and students thronged to his lectures. He was elected member of the *Académie de Médecine* and appointed physician to King Louis Philippe. When the government of Napoleon III demanded in 1852 the oath of allegiance from the professors of the medical faculty, Chomel refused and gave up his position, retiring to his country home, where he died six years later.

Chomel wrote works on pathological anatomy and fevers, and his *Leçons de clinique médicale* enjoyed a great reputation. He was an excellent teacher, a genial person, and a man of high principles.

1789-1858—Richard Bright.

1790-1856—August Henschel, professor of medicine at the University of Breslau. In addition to lecturing on botany, physiology, pathology and medicine, he conducted courses in the history of medicine. He became well known as a medical historian and edited the original series of *Janus* (1846-1851), the first journal devoted to the history of medicine.

1791-1861—Johann Ludwig Choulant, a native of Dresden, received his M.D. at Leipzig in 1818. In 1821, he settled in Dresden as physician to the infirmary in Friedrichstadt, the following year began to lecture on medicine at the *Medicinisch-chirurgische Akademie;* and, in 1823, became professor of theoretic medicine and director of the clinic. He became in 1833 Medical Assessor and in 1844 Medical Referee, executive positions directing medical education and establishing procedures in medical jurisprudence; and, during this period, he made many contributions to legal medicine. He retired from the *Akademie* in 1860 after 38 years of great activity and died the following year.

Choulant wrote a textbook on medicine, *Lehrbuch der speciellen Pathologie und Therapie der Menschen,* which was published in 1831, passed through five editions, and was widely used. His lasting fame, however, rests upon his labors in the field of medical history. His medical chronology, *Tafeln zur Geschichte der Medicin,* 1822, a tabular arrangement, is an excellent introduction to the history of medicine. The *Handbuch der Bücherkunde für die ältere Medicin* (Bibliographical Handbook of Ancient Medicine), published in 1828, is a remarkable work, a monument to the author's industry, accuracy, and knowledge of languages. It remains indispensable to the student of Greek, Latin and Arabic medicine. His great

work, *Geschichte und Bibliographie der Anatomischen Abbildung* (History and Bibliography of Anatomic Illustration), published in 1852, is a comprehensive work with biographical details on the lives of the great anatomists, illustrations from their works, and a penetrating and judicious account of their achievements and their role in the development of anatomic illustration. An English translation of this work, translated and edited by Mortimer Frank, was published in 1920 and is itself a notable achievement.

1790-1857—Marshall Hall was born in Nottingham, England, and studied medicine at Edinburgh, where he received his degree in 1812. After practicing in Nottingham, he moved to London, where he practiced from 1826 until his death. Although busy with his professional duties, he found time to carry out physiological research, which brought him fame both at home and abroad. His most important discovery was the demonstration of reflex movements and that the spinal cord is a chain of segments whose functional units are separate reflex arcs. His memoir, *The Reflex Function of the Medulla Oblongata and Medulla Spinalis,* 1833, pointed out the differences between voluntary motion and unconscious reflexes. He was a very prolific writer, writing numerous memoirs on nervous diseases, on artificial respiration, on diseases of digestion, and on diseases of women.

1791-1875—Robert Adams was born in Dublin and received his M.D. degree from Dublin University in 1842. He served first on the staff of the Jervis Street Infirmary and later at the Richmond Hospital. He achieved a reputation as a teacher and surgeon, being appointed in 1861 Surgeon to the Queen and Regius Professor of Surgery in the University of Dublin. In 1827 before receiving his M.D. degree and while on the staff of the Jervis Street Infirmary, he published in the *Dublin Hospital Reports* an account of heart block, a condition later known as Adams-Stokes disease.

1791-1868—John Elliotson was born in London, entered the University of Edinburgh at the early age of 14, and remained there five years, receiving his M.D. in 1810. He returned to England and entered Jesus College, Cambridge, where he remained three years, receiving a Cambridge M.D. On his return to London, he was elected to the Royal College of Physicians, was appointed physician to St. Thomas' Hospital, and was made in 1823 professor of medicine at the University of London. As a clinical teacher, he was unrivaled. "His diagnosis of disease was accurate and minute, his teaching by the bedside impressive and effective. . . . He did not *lecture* but *taught*" (Munk).

At the height of his reputation, Elliotson became an advocate of mesmerism and phrenology and spent the rest of his life in conflict with his medical brethren. He lost most of his practice and died in poverty. Elliotson reported several surgical operations performed under hypnotism and, suspecting that pollen was the cause, proposed in 1831 the theory that hay fever was caused by the blossoms of graminaceous plants.

1791-1874—Jean Cruveilhier.

1792-1814—Johann Lucas Schönlein.

1793-1853—William Edmund Horner.

1793-1860—Martin Heinrich Rathke was born in Danzig, studied in Göttingen and in Berlin, where he received his doctor's degree in 1818. He practiced in Danzig for 10 years and was then appointed professor of physiology at the University of Dorpat, remaining there until he was called to Königsberg in 1835 as professor of zoology and anatomy. He was an outstanding anatomist and zoologist. "Rathke's pouch" commemorates his name in human embryology.

1793-1860—Thomas Addison.

1793-1876—Karl Ernst von Baer was a native of Esthonia, studied first at Dorpat, where he received his M.D. in 1814, and then proceeded to Würzburg, where he studied under Doellinger. He was subsequently professor of zoology at Königsberg and at St. Petersburg, Russia, where he lived for 30 years. He returned to Dorpat in 1867 and lived there until his death nine years later. While in Königsberg, he discovered the mammalian ova (*De ovi mammalium et hominis genesi*, Leipzig, 1827). Baer described also the formation of germ layers in the embryo and founded the science of modern comparative embryology. He was one of the founders of modern morphology, classifying animals as the result of his embryological studies into four groups—vertebrata, articulata, mollusca and radiata.

1794-1847—Robert Liston was born in Linlithgow, studied under John Barclay in Edinburgh, and was appointed in 1814 house-surgeon to the Royal Infirmary. After working for a time in the London Hospital and attending Abernethy's lectures, he returned to Edinburgh and began practice. In 1834, he was appointed professor of surgery in University College, London, and soon became noted as one of the most resourceful and skillful surgeons in the metropolis. A man of great physical prowess, he had arms and hands which were often likened to those of Hercules. "He would amputate the thigh single-handed, compress the artery with the left hand, using no tourniquet, and do all the cutting and sawing with the right" (Bettany). He wrote *Elements of Surgery*, London, 1830; and *A Treatise on Practical and Operative Surgery*, London, 1837, both works noteworthy for their clarity, simplicity and soundness. Liston was skillful not only in operations involving physical prowess but also in the most delicate operations, particularly plastic operations requiring both skill and dexterity. He was the first outstanding British surgeon to employ ether as an anaesthetic in a major operation—amputation of the thigh at University College Hospital, 1846.

1794-1879—Pierre Adolph Piorry, a native of Poitiers, France, began the study of medicine at 16 and received his M.D. in Paris in 1816. He practiced in Paris and is remembered as the discoverer of the pleximeter. His *Traité sur la percussion médiate*, Paris, 1828, was very successful and widely quoted. Piorry, however, over-refined percussion and described specific percussion tones for the various organs.

1795-1850—Justus Friedrich Karl Hecker was born in Erfurt and stud-ied at Berlin, where he received his M.D. degree in 1817. He became a *Privatdozent* in Berlin the same year, and in 1822 appeared the first volume of his *Geschichte der Heilkunde*, which made such an impression that a department of the history of medicine was created and Hecker appointed associate professor. In 1834, he was advanced to the rank of full professor and held this rank until his death. He wrote many noteworthy articles on medical history and, in addition to his history of medicine, is remembered particularly for his monographs on the Black Death, on the dancing mania, and on the English sweating sickness, all of which have been translated into English and published by the Sydenham Society in 1844 with the title, *The Epidemics of the Middle Ages*.

1795-1860—James Braid, born in Fifeshire, Scotland, practiced as a surgeon first in Edinburgh and later in Manchester. He became interested in hypnotism, and most of his works are on that subject.

1795-1873—Moritz Heinrich Romberg, a native of Meiningen, received his medical degree in Berlin in 1817 and practiced in that city until his death. He became professor in the University in 1838 and achieved a great reputation from his studies on the pathology of the nervous system. His classical *Lehrbuch der Nervenkrankheiten*, Berlin, 1840, was one of the best works on nervous diseases of its time. His name is remembered by "Romberg's sign."

1795-1878—Ernst Heinrich Weber was born in Wittenberg, where he received his degree in 1815. He became a *Privatdozent* at Leipzig in 1817 and professor of anatomy and physiology in 1821. He relinquished his chair of physiology in 1866 in favor of Ludwig and remained professor of anatomy until 1871, when he was succeeded by Wilhelm His. In 1845, he made the epochal discovery of the inhibitory action of the vagus nerve on the action of the heart. In this historic experiment, carried out in collaboration with his brother, Eduard Friedrich Weber, he showed that the heart could be brought to a standstill by passing a current from one pole placed in the nostril of a frog and the other on a cross section of the cord at the level of the fourth thoracic vertebra. Later studies showed that the vagi were the channels of communication. This memorable discovery was first read to the Congress of Italian Scientists at Naples and published in the *Annali universali di Medicina*.

The Webers collaborated in the famous *Wellenlehre*, 1825, in which they described their measurement of the velocity of the pulse wave, a discovery which disproved the contention of Bichat that the pulse is synchronous in all the arteries. Ernst Heinrich Weber was also the first to show that common sensation can be separated into visceral and muscular components and measured the sensations of pain, heat, pressure and smell.

1796-1883—James S. Combe was a native of Leith, Scotland, and practiced for many years in Edinburgh. In 1822, he published in the *Transactions of the Medical Chirurgical Society* a paper describing a case of pernicious anemia, more than 20 years before Addison's description.

1797-1853—Robert James Graves.

1797-1854—Gabriel Andral was born in Paris, where he received his medical degree in 1821. Three years later, he became *professeur agrégé* and, four years after that, professor of hygiene. In 1839, he succeeded Broussais as professor and taught with great success for 27 years. Andral had a clear, methodical, analytical mind, opposed all medical fads and dogmas, fought excessive bloodletting, and favored cold baths in the treatment of typhoid fever. His *Clinique médicale* is a valuable collection of medical cases with masterly descriptions of symptomatology of the patients and their clinical course. He urged the importance of studying the blood and believed in the existence of specific blood diseases.

1797-1866—Thomas Hodgkin.

1797-1891—Jean Baptiste Bouillaud.

1799-1854—Carl von Basedow was born in Dessau, Germany, studied medicine at Halle, and, after further study in Paris, settled in Merseburg, where he spent his life as a general practitioner. In 1840, he described a case of exophthalmic goitre, five years after Graves' description and 54 after Parry's. However, this disease is commonly known on the Continent as Basedow's disease and among English-speaking physicians as Graves' disease. In 1848, Basedow described a case of "exophthalmic cachexia" with an autopsy, probably the first protocol of an autopsy on a case of recognized exophthalmic goitre.

1799-1882—George Bodington, of Sutton Coldfield, England, was educated at Oxford, London, and Er-

langen, receiving his M.D. at Erlangen. He practiced medicine first
in Birmingham and then took over
the management of a private sanitarium for the insane, where he
worked until his retirement in 1868.
In 1840, he published his *Essay on
the Treatment of Pulmonary Consumption,* in which he attacked the
use of antimony, calomel and bleeding, urged a full nutritious diet, and
preferred cold, dry air to the moist
air of a sea voyage. He was severely
handled by the profession on account of his views and was so discouraged by these attacks that he
never pursued the subject further.

1800-1829—Henry Hill Hickman, a
forgotten pioneer in anesthesia, began practice in Ludlow, Shropshire,
England, about 1820. Impressed with
the pain produced by operations, he
began experiments on animals and
found that he could render them
insensible to pain by causing them
to inhale carbon dioxide. He could
not obtain a hearing from the physicians of England, so he wrote to
Charles X, King of France, asking
for permission to demonstrate his
method. The letter was referred to
the *Académie Royale de Médecine*
and was received with great deri-
sion, Larrey alone supporting Hickman's request and offering himself
as a subject for experiment. Hickman returned home and died a few
months later at the early age of 29.

1802-1880—Sir Dominic Corrigan.

1804-1878—Sir William Stokes.

1801-1841—James Hope was born in
Stockfort, Cheshire, and studied
medicine for five years at Edinburgh, after which he spent a year
in London at St. Bartholomew's Hospital and another year in Paris,
working under Chomel, who was delighted with his skill in sketching
pathological specimens. On his return to London, Hope, who did not
have a medical degree, passed his
examination as a licentiate of the
Royal College of Physicians and enrolled as a pupil at St. George's Hospital. At the latter place, he played
a leading role in proving the value
of auscultation, made many observations on the physical signs of cardiac
disease, and carried out experiments
on the production of the heart
sounds. In 1831 his *Diseases of the
Heart* appeared. "It outclassed all
other books on the subject that had
been published. . . . Hope struck a
new note in the literature of heart
disease. His volume has a modern
ring to it" (Herrick). This work had
a great and deserved success. In 1834
was published his *Principles and Illustrations of Morbid Anatomy,* a
book of high merit illustrated with
drawings made by Hope himself. He
was very successful in practice, became later physician to St. George's
Hospital, and died of phthisis at the
age of 40.

The Rise of American Medicine

EACH GROUP of early colonists coming to the New World brought to it the language, culture, religion and medicine of their homeland. Quebec looked back to France for its culture, New England to the British Isles; while, to the south, a large portion of the North American continent and all of the South American looked back to Spain and Portugal. The Spanish were the first to come and also were the first to organize medical schools and to build hospitals.

The first university in America was established in Santo Domingo (1538) and was followed by the University of Mexico, founded in 1551, more than a half a century before the English established their first settlement in the New World at Jamestown in 1607. The University of Mexico created the first chair of medicine in America in 1580. The Spanish had also established eight universities before Harvard was founded in 1636, three of which, Mexico (1551), Lima (1571), and Córdoba, Argentina (1614), have continued as seats of learning. Long before the early North American colonists established their first hospital on Long Island in 1663, Latin America had numerous hospitals for the sick and infirm. The first hospital was founded at Santo Domingo in about 1503, and, in 1523-1524, Cortés, the conqueror of Mexico, built there the "Hospital de la Purísima Concepción." The latter, now known as the Jesús Nazareno, still continues its service to the sick.

The Spanish *chronistas,* or chroniclers, who accompanied the conquerors and explorers to the New World, wrote vivid accounts of the topography, flora and fauna of the new lands as well as descriptions of the inhabitants, their diseases, and the remedies for them. Pietro Martire d'Anghiera (1457-1526), the first of the *chronistas,* an Italian like Columbus, mentions guaiac as a remedy for syphilis and describes many native therapeutic procedures. The first official *chronista,* Gonzalo Fernández de Oviedo, made no less than eight voyages to America and, in his *Historia general y natural de las Indias,* 1535, devoted four books with numerous illustrations to medicinal plants, describing copaiba, guaiac, cacao and tobacco. He also mentions in his *Sumaria,* 1526, bubas, or yaws, and notes, "The Spaniards coming to America in search of gold returned home gilded by jaundice instead and soon died" (Moll). José Acosta (1539-1600), a learned priest, went to Peru in 1571 and, on his return to Spain, wrote his celebrated *Historia natural y moral de las Indias,*

714

Seville, 1590, which was soon translated into Italian, French, Dutch, German, Latin and English. This work contains the first account of mountain sickness.

Bernardino de Sahagún (1499-1590), priest and missionary, called the "Pliny of the New World," came to Mexico at the age of 31 and remained there until his death. In his *Historia General de las Cosas de Nueva España,* he devoted one book to Mexican diseases

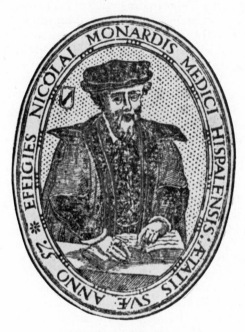

NICHOLÁS MONARDES
Portrait from the title-page of his
Dos Libros, Sevilla, 1569.

and drugs and described with illustrations the Mexican technique of treating wounds, of massage, and of administering enemata. Nicolás Monardes (1508-1588), a physician of Sevilla, became a deep student of American flora and established a botanical garden devoted exclusively to plants from the New World although he himself never crossed the ocean. He studied these plants for more than 40 years, tested their medicinal properties on his patients, and, after publishing two smaller works, published in 1574 his *Historia Medicinal,* which became well known to English readers under the arresting title of *Joyfull Newes Out of the Newe Founde Worlde,* London, 1577. This work was also translated into Latin, Italian, French, Flemish and German. Francisco Hernández (1517-1587), physician to Philip II, spent seven years in Mexico and wrote a monumental work, *Historia Natural de las Indias,* in 17 volumes, which, however, through a series of mishaps, remained unpublished for two centuries. Hernández described some 3,000 medicinal plants and wrote accounts of two devastating epidemics of typhus fever in 1570 and 1576 and of the autopsies performed on the victims.

The early colonists in North America were not accompanied by either official or semi-official *chronistas.* The first English colonists were not Spanish grandees in search of gold and glory, but people from the humbler walks of life seeking religious freedom. The terrain on which they landed was not a lush soil abounding in innumerable tropical plants and inhabited by a people who had developed a culture of their own, with a rich native materia medica and who had acquired much facility in the employment of native drugs as well as considerable surgical skill. The English landed on the bleak and inhospitable shores of New England, where the natives were a rough, savage race who devoted their talents to warfare rather than to the pursuits of peace.

The "Mayflower," which landed in 1620, had among its passengers, Deacon Dr. Samuel Fuller, who had lived with the Pilgrims in Leyden for 11 years before he came to America. He may have studied at the University of Leyden, although there is no record that he attended the University or that he ever received the degree of doctor of medicine. However, he served the colony as a physician faithfully and well until his death from smallpox in 1633. After his death, there was no outstanding physician in Massachusetts for a century. "Medicine was served by three classes: the governors, of whom John Winthrop the younger is the leading example; the ministers, typified by Thomas Thacher; and a host of minor physicians, ministers and schoolmasters, some with medical degrees and some without" (Viets). Thomas Thacher wrote the first medical paper published in North America, of which only one copy has survived, *A Brief RULE To guide the Common People of New England how to order themselves & theirs in the Small-Pocks, or Measels,* published in Boston in 1677, which, as Viets has pointed out, is an abbreviated extract from the writings of Thomas Sydenham. Thacher, the outstanding Puritan preacher-physician of his time, never attended a medical school but, while pastor of Old South Church in Boston, devoted much of his time to the practice of medicine.

Medical practice in the North American colonies followed closely the British pattern. Doctors in Boston, New York and Philadelphia followed Willis, then Sydenham, then Boerhaave, then Cullen, just as did their confrères in the old country. A few qualified physicians and surgeons emigrated to the colonies from time to time, but the number was too small to meet the needs of the steadily growing colonial population. To fill this need, young men were apprenticed to older physicians, and, in turn, became physicians themselves without ever attending a medical school. There were no prescribed courses and no examinations to determine the fitness of these young physicians to practice.

American medicine, as an independent growth, begins with the severance of the political ties that bound it to the Old World. This independence came first to North America, a circumstance explaining the earlier emergence of North American medicine.

The first medical school in the North American colonies was founded in Philadelphia only a short time before the outbreak of the Revolution. It was but natural that the founders of this school should be natives of Philadelphia, at that time the largest, the most influential, and the most cultured city in the colonies, and should

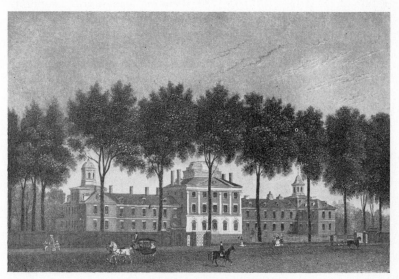

THE PENNSYLVANIA HOSPITAL
Drawn by McArthur.

have patterned their new school after those they had attended abroad. It was no mere chance that most of these young men had gone to Edinburgh. William Cullen reigned there, and his enthusiastic pupils placed his name alongside that of Sydenham as the two greatest names in British medicine.

Philadelphia, having been settled by Quakers, who laid great stress on charity and had no regular clergy to educate, had had the Pennsylvania Hospital since 1750. By contrast, the Puritans, who settled Boston, founded Harvard College in 1636, "dreading to leave an illiterate Ministry to the Churches when our present Ministers shall lie in the Dust," and did not establish a hospital until 1821.

Three men stand out in bold relief among the founders of the first medical school. They are Morgan, Shippen and Rush.

John Morgan was born in Philadelphia in 1735, the son of a wealthy and prominent citizen. He was educated at the Academy and College of Philadelphia and received his A.B. in 1757 in the first graduating class of that institution. His college work dovetailed with his early medical training, for he was an apprentice of Dr. John Redman, a graduate of Leyden and the leading physician of Philadelphia from 1751 to 1780, spending his last year as apothecary to the Pennsylvania Hospital. He served four years as an army surgeon in the French and Indian Wars and then proceeded to London, where he spent a year working with the Hunters and learning from them the method of making anatomical preparations by corrosion. From London, he went to Edinburgh, where he graduated in 1763 with the degree of doctor of medicine. His doctor's thesis, *De Puopoiesi* (Concerning the formation of pus), was a notable contribution, in which he maintained that pus was secreted from the blood vessels, a theory the correctness of which was first demonstrated by Cohnheim nearly a century later.

From Edinburgh, Morgan went to Paris, where he was elected to the *Académie Royale de Chirurgie,* and then traveled to Italy. Here he met Morgagni, who was deeply impressed by his ability, and presented him with a copy of his *De sedibus*. After five years abroad, young Morgan, now a licentiate of the Royal College of Physicians at Edinburgh and London, a member of the *Société des Belles Lettres* of Rome, an associate of the *Académie Royale de Chirurgie* of Paris, and a Fellow of the Royal Society, returned to Philadelphia with a great ambition—to establish a medical school equal to the best in Europe.

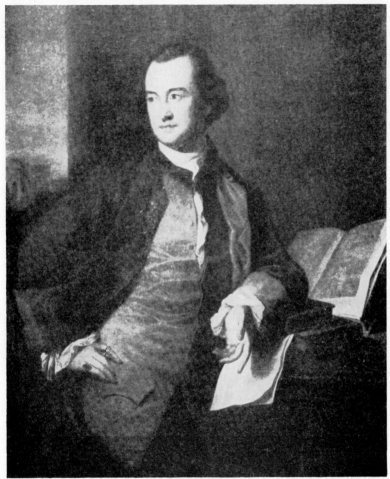

Packard, *History of Medicine in the United States*, New York, 1931

JOHN MORGAN

Immediately upon his arrival in Philadelphia, Morgan presented his plan to the trustees of the College, who received it favorably, established the medical school in 1765, and appointed him professor of the theory and practice of physic, the first medical professorship in North America. A few months later, William Shippen, Jr., was elected professor of anatomy and surgery. In 1768, the degree of M.B. was conferred on eight graduates. Adam Kuhn was added to

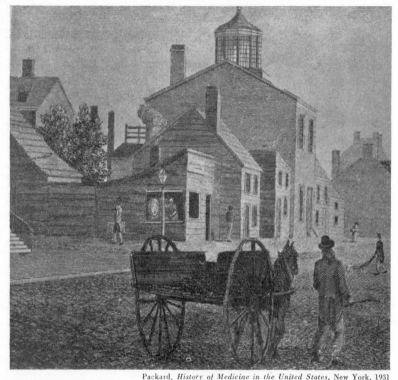

Packard, *History of Medicine in the United States*, New York, 1931

THE FIRST MEDICAL SCHOOL BUILDING IN THE UNITED STATES
The University of Pennsylvania, Philadelphia.

the faculty in 1768, and, the following year, Benjamin Rush, a
young protégé of Morgan, was elected professor of chemistry.

Morgan was thus a pioneer in American medical education. At
the foundation of the medical school, he delivered a memorable discourse upon the *Institution of Medical Schools* in America. In this,
he stressed the necessity for medical students of a good preliminary
education, including Latin, mathematics, natural science, and a
modern language, to be followed by a graduated course of medical
studies emphasizing anatomy, materia medica, botany and chemistry
as "the ladder by which we are to mount up to practice." Those
were revolutionary thoughts, for, in attacking the old apprentice
system, he was practically insulting most members of the medical
profession, since these had been trained under this system. When

he later announced that he was practicing only internal medicine but no surgery and that he employed a trained apothecary from England to fill his prescriptions, two other time-honored traditions were assailed. Most of the doctors in the Colonies practiced all branches of the healing art and compounded their own drugs, often earning more from their drugs than from their professional labors.

With the outbreak of the Revolutionary War in 1775, Morgan was appointed "Director General to the Military Hospitals and Physician-in-Chief to the American Army." His army experience was most unhappy. A violent quarrel broke out between him and his colleague Shippen, who was the head of the political faction seeking to oust Morgan from his position. He was charged with mismanagement and dismissed by Congress in 1777. Two years later, Congress exonerated Morgan, who, now vindicated, devoted most of his energies to attacking Shippen, whom he held responsible for his disgrace. After the war, work was resumed at the medical school, but Morgan refused to serve on the faculty with Shippen and did not teach although his position was held open until the year before his death. He became a recluse and dropped out of the medical life of Philadelphia.

Benjamin Rush in his *Commonplace Book,* a diary which he kept from 1789 until 1813, made the following entry for October 15, 1789:

> This afternoon I was called to visit Dr. Morgan, but found him dead in a small hovel, surrounded with books and papers and on a light dirty bed. He was attended only by a washerwoman, one of his tenants. . . . What a change from his former rank and prospects in Life! The man who once filled half the world with his name had now scarcely friends enough left to bury him.

Such was the end of John Morgan, who, as a youth, understood the origin of pus and who had founded a medical school with a graduated course of instruction and whose "pre-medical requirements, which had been the most progressive part of Morgan's plan, were thrown on the dump, whence they were salvaged with great *éclat* by the founders of Johns Hopkins University" (Flexner).

William Shippen, Jr., the son of a prominent Philadelphia physician, was born in 1736, graduated with honors at the College of New Jersey, and, at the age of 21, went to Great Britain for his medical education. He studied first with John and William Hunter, imbibing from the latter a great interest in obstetrics. He then went to Edinburgh, where he graduated in 1761, the title of his thesis, *De placentiae cum utero nexu,* indicating his interest in obstetrics but, unlike that of Morgan, showing neither originality nor distinction.

After five years abroad, Shippen returned home with two great ambitions—to teach anatomy and to elevate the status of obstetrics. He immediately began to teach anatomy, holding classes in the State

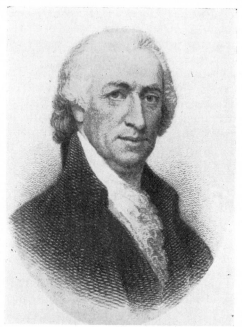

Bull. Soc. M. Hist., Chicago, 1925

WILLIAM SHIPPEN

House and employing in his course a set of anatomical drawings, anatomical models, and a skeleton, all donated to the Pennsylvania Hospital by Dr. John Fothergill of London. For three years, Shippen conducted private courses in anatomy, the first systematic course in anatomy in North America; and, in addition, gave a course in obstetrics, which did much to improve obstetrical practice. On the return of John Morgan in 1765, he joined with him in founding the medical school of the College of Philadelphia and was appointed professor of anatomy and surgery in the new school. He was an excellent teacher, calm, dignified and impressive, who strove to demonstrate facts to his hearers rather than to overwhelm them with his eloquence.

During the Revolution, he succeeded Morgan as surgeon-general of the army in 1777 but, three years later, was court-martialed and, with some difficulty, acquitted. After the war, he resumed his post in the medical school as professor of anatomy over the protests of Morgan and Rush and taught with great success until the year of his death in 1808.

Rush, who attended him in his last illness, noted in the *Commonplace Book* for July 11, 1808:

He had talents, but which from disuse became weak and contemptible. He was too indolent to write, to read, and even to think, but with the stock of knowledge he acquired when young, he maintained some rank in his profession, especially as a teacher of anatomy, in which he was eloquent, luminous and pleasing.

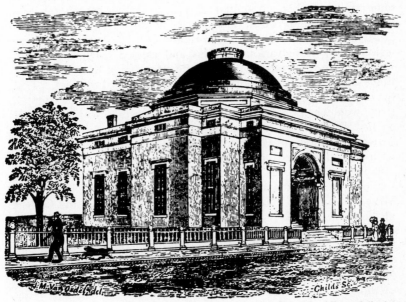

University of Kansas Collection

RUSH MEDICAL COLLEGE, 1843

Rush Medical College was chartered in 1837, when Chicago had only three thousand inhabitants, but courses of instruction began first in 1843. It was a notable institution for more than a half century and numbered many distinguished physicians on its faculty and among its alumni. In 1898, it became affiliated with the University of Chicago as the medical department of that institution.

This verdict by Rush, however, may have been colored by a later passage in the same account—"He was my enemy from the time of my settlement in 1769 to the last year of his life."

Ruschenberger, the historian of medical Philadelphia, noted, "If he contributed anything to the literature of either medicine or science, it has not been found. His claim to the enduring approbation of his fellow citizens mainly rests on his being the pioneer of systematic teaching of anatomy and surgery in Philadelphia." To which should be added "of obstetrics."

BENJAMIN RUSH

Of all the physicians of Revolutionary times, Benjamin Rush was easily the most famous. His fellow citizens were well aware of his presence among them, for he was constantly engaged in public, political or professional controversy and often the champion of some righteous but unpopular and hopeless cause. His writings spread his name abroad so that he was the only American physician of his time with a wide European reputation. His pupils, who were legion, came from various sections and carried his fame far and wide. At one time, more than half the members of the South Carolina Medical Society were former pupils. His medical theories, spread by his students, dominated medical practice for a generation so that, even when in far away Chicago, a new medical school was opened in 1843, 30 years after his death, it was named in his honor Rush Medical College, a tribute to the esteem and affection with which he was still regarded.

Benjamin Rush was born in Byberry, Pennsylvania, in 1746, the son of a gunsmith and farmer. After a preliminary education at West Nottingham, Maryland, he graduated in 1760 at the College of New Jersey—later Princeton. He then began the study of medicine with Dr. Redman as a preceptor, where, in addition to practical work, he became very familiar with the works of Boerhaave and Sydenham. After five years of study with Dr. Redman and attendance on the lectures of Dr. Shippen on anatomy and of Dr. Morgan on materia medica, he sailed for Europe. He spent two years at Edinburgh and received his degree in 1768, presenting a thesis, *De coctione ciborum in ventriculo,* in which he concluded, on the basis of three experiments performed on himself and one on a friend, that gastric digestion is a chemical process resembling fermentation, but not requiring an acid ferment although accompanied by the production of acid.

From Edinburgh, young Rush went to London, where he attended

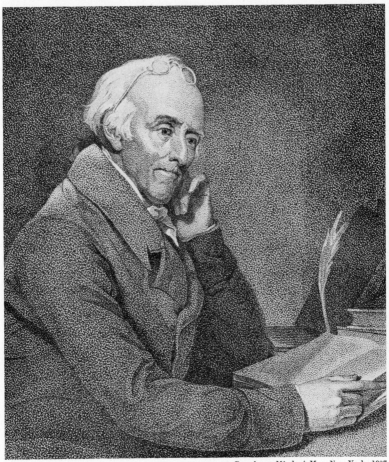

Bromberg, *Mind of Man*, New York, 1937

BENJAMIN RUSH
Engraving by Elwin from portrait by Sully.

the lectures of William Hewson and, thanks to letters from Philadelphia and personal introductions from Benjamin Franklin, met many famous men, including Sir John Pringle, Dr. Fothergill, Samuel Johnson, Oliver Goldsmith, and Sir Joshua Reynolds. After a brief stay in Paris, he returned home, a zealous disciple of his master Cullen in things medical as well as a disciple in things political of a young medical student he had met in Edinburgh, John Bostock. From him, he "heard the authority of Kings called into question," and his arguments convinced Rush of "the absurdity of hereditary rulers" and that "no form of government can be rational but that which is derived from the Suffrages of the people."

Rush settled in Philadelphia in 1769 and tells us, "My shop was crowded with the poor in the morning and at meal times, and nearly every street and alley in the city was visited by me every day." The month after his arrival, he was appointed, through the influence of Morgan, professor of chemistry in the new medical school, and he devoted his efforts to establishing the new medical system of Cullen in place of Boerhaave's, which was then dominant in Philadelphia. This championship of Cullen brought down upon him the wrath of his professional brethren, and Rush writes in his diary, "I do not recollect in the course of the first seven years of my settlement in Philadelphia that any one of my brethren ever sent a patient to me." In 1770, he published "in the newspaper" some observations upon the *Cynanche trachealis,* his first medical paper in the New World, later reprinted in his *Medical Inquiries and Observations.*

Since early youth, Rush was deeply interested in religion and in moral crusades. Baptized and confirmed in the Episcopal Church, he later became a Presbyterian and then a Universalist. Always interested in righteousness, it was but natural that he threw himself body and soul into any cause he considered righteous. In 1773, he published an address on the iniquity of the slave trade, which he said "did me harm by exciting the resentment of many slaveholders against me." But, he could not resist the temptation to express his views and, most of his life, continued his agitation against slavery, against capital punishment, and against alcohol.

An ardent republican, he threw himself into the cause of American independence, assisted Thomas Paine in the production of his pamphlet, for which Rush suggested the name, "Common Sense," was one of the delegates to the Continental Congress, and signed the Declaration of Independence in 1776. He joined the army, was appointed physician-general to the hospitals but, after a controversy with Shippen, resigned and went to live in Princeton. While in the service, he was very critical of George Washington and has been accused, probably unjustly, of activity in the so-called Conway Cabal, which schemed to remove Washington.

In Princeton, Rush was much depressed, so, as the opportunities for practice were meager, he resolved to study law. However, just as he was preparing to begin his studies, the British evacuated Philadelphia, so Rush returned and took up his practice. In 1789, he was appointed to the chair of the theory and practice of physic in the medical school and about this time began to formulate his new theory of medicine.

Before this period, Rush had been a follower of Cullen, who postulated that the nervous system is the source of life and that disease is due to either exaggeration of nervous functions (spasm) or to weakness of this function (atony). Soon after, Brown taught that life was the result of internal or external stimuli and that diseases are of two kinds—sthenic when the excitability is increased, asthenic when it is decreased. Rush, familiar with the writings of both Cullen and Brown, concluded that all diseases, including fevers, are due to debility, which causes an increase of irritability to the point of excess.

According to Rush's theory, there is really only one kind of fever and the logical treatment is one that reduces the excitement of the blood vessels. The proper treatment for fevers is a low diet, heavy purging with calomel and jalap, 10 grains of each, and bleeding to the point of faintness. "The illogicality of treatment which inevitably produces general debility to relieve excitement of blood vessels, supposed to result in the first place from debility, seems never to have occurred to him" (Corner). Rush has been described as a follower of John Brown, but this is incorrect. He was influenced by Brown, as he himself admits, but he was not a disciple. He took pains to point out that, at this period, he followed neither Cullen nor Brown, but had evolved a theory of his own.

The epidemics of yellow fever in Philadelphia in the years 1793 and 1797 gave Rush a golden opportunity to test his theory. He claimed that practically all his patients were cured when they were purged and bled to the limit, whereas William Cobbett, the well-known British radical pamphleteer then living in Philadelphia, observed that Rush's famous cure was "one of those great discoveries which have contributed to the depopulation of the earth." The controversy raged. Cobbett asked for Rush's statistics, but the doctor had none. Cobbett then went to the bills of mortality and claimed there had been a steady increase in the death rate in the city, an increase coinciding with the introduction of Rush's cure. The doctor brought suit for libel and obtained judgment. The jury fined Cobbett $5,000 and $3,000 costs. Cobbett fled to New York and continued his attacks in a book, *The Rush Light,* 1800. Finally he gave up and sailed back to England to become a prominent and somewhat obnoxious political figure.

In his diary, Rush noted,

From the year 1793 'till 1797 my business was stationary in Philadelphia. After 1797 it sensibly declined. I had no new families, except foreigners, added to the list of my patients, and many of my old patients deserted me. Even the cures I performed added to the detraction that had taken place against my character when they were effected by remedies that were new and contrary to the feelings of the citizens.

Probably 10 grains each of calomel and jalap, with bleeding to the limit of endurance, were too much for the feelings of the citizens. In 1797, Rush was appointed Treasurer of the United States Mint by his old friend, John Adams, now President. He died in 1813 and, on his death bed, was bled twice on his own insistence but against the advice of his physicians.

Rush considered his theory of disease his greatest contribution to the science of medicine. Posterity has long since discarded his theories and sees with unanimity that his greatest contributions were his clinical observations printed at various times and later collected and published in his *Medical Inquiries and Observations.* This work, which appeared in five volumes from 1789 to 1812, was reprinted during the course of publication with the addition of new material. In this encyclopedic series, Rush described anew the epidemics of yellow fever in Philadelphia, deciding that the disease was not contagious, not imported, but endemic in origin. He described the epidemics of *cynanche trachealis,* of influenza and of scarlet fever; discussed dropsy, hydrophobia, and pulmonary consumption, diagnosing the earliest stages by "a rapid pulse especially towards evening, slight fever increased by the least exercise, burning and dryness in the palms of the hands, occasional flushing in one or both cheeks." He believed that miasmata caused disease, such as yellow fever and dysentery, and came from decaying vegetable matter in marshes. He suggested the drainage of such marshes. He described cholera morbus for the first time and was the first American physician to describe dengue. In the observation entitled "An Account of the Cure of Several Diseases by the Extraction of Decayed Teeth," he pointed out the relationship between apical abscesses and arthritis, an early, if not the first, contribution to the subject of focal infection. This work also contains a long essay on the habits, diseases and remedies of the North American Indians, noting incidentally, "The small pox and the venereal disease were communicated to the Indians of North America by the Europeans."

The last volume of the series, *Medical Inquiries and Observations upon the Diseases of the Mind,* which was published in 1812, the year before his death, was probably his most important sci-

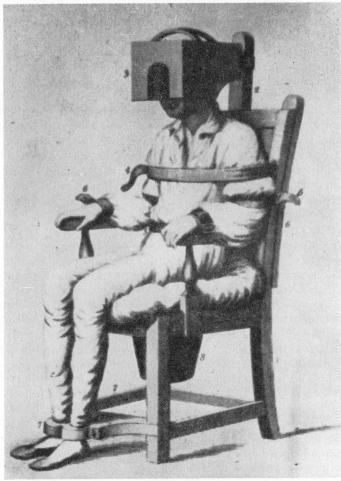

Thacher, *American Medical Biography*, Boston, 1828

THE TRANQUILLIZING CHAIR OF DR. RUSH

Used for the treatment of the insane.

entific work. It was the first American textbook on psychiatry, went through many editions, and remained for 70 years the only American text on the subject. It was based on Rush's personal observations at the Pennsylvania Hospital, where he was in charge of mental patients for 30 years. He noted the role of heredity, injuries and malformation of the brain, diseases of the body, and drugs in the production of mental diseases; advocated humane treatment of the insane; and advised exercise, hydrotherapy, and an adequate diet. He has been called "the first American psychiatrist."

Rush's influence on the medical practitioners of his time and upon those of succeeding generations was immense. Generations of enthusiastic students, after sitting at his feet, went abroad in the land purging their patients vigorously and bleeding them to the limit. Others were not so impressed with his methods, and the controversy which raged during his life continued long after his death. In time, many dismissed him with a shrug as the doctor who treated all his patients with purging and bleeding and believed that yellow fever was caused by putrefying coffee. While these charges may be true in part, yet he was an imposing figure, a man with a brilliant mind who made solid contributions to the progress of medicine.

In 1768, the year the first class was graduated from the Philadelphia Medical School, Dr. Morgan, who was professor of medicine and taught also materia medica and botany, gave up his courses in the latter, and Dr. Adam Kuhn was appointed professor of botany and materia medica. Adam Kuhn (1741-1817) was born in Germantown, Pennsylvania, studied medicine first with his father, and then, in 1761, went to Uppsala, Sweden, where he studied botany under Linné and became one of his favorite pupils. Subsequently, he studied medicine in London and in Edinburgh, receiving his M.D. at Edinburgh in 1767. He lectured on botany only a year but continued his lectures on materia medica for 21 years and was physician to the Pennsylvania Hospital for many years. A staunch follower of Cullen's theories, he became a bitter opponent of Rush. During the yellow fever epidemic in Philadelphia, Kuhn maintained that the disease was imported from the West Indies, attacked Rush's "cure," and proposed in the newspapers his own treatment, which consisted of quinine bark, camomile tea, cold baths and wine. He was subsequently president of the college, professor of chemistry, and professor of the practice of medicine, resigning from the latter chair in 1797, when he was succeeded by his old enemy, Benjamin Rush.

Caspar Wistar (1760-1818) studied medicine under Dr. John Redman and received the degree M.B. from the College of Philadelphia in 1782. He then studied at the University of Edinburgh, receiving the M.D. degree in 1786. On his return to Philadelphia, he became first professor of chemistry, then adjunct professor of anatomy, and, on the death of Shippen in 1808, professor of anatomy, holding this chair until his death. His erudition, combined with his attractive and inspiring methods of teaching, gave him high rank among the anatomists of his time. His *System of Anatomy*, 1811-1814, was the earliest systematic treatise on anatomy published in North America. He assembled a large collection of anatomical preparations, which he bequeathed to the medical school to form the Wistar Museum. His grandson, General Isaac Wistar, presented the University of Pennsylvania with a building to house the anatomical preparations and an endowment to support anatomical research. The new Wistar Institute of Anatomy was formally opened in 1894. Wistar's description of the ethmoid bone has often been praised, and his name has been perpetuated by the wisteria vine, which was named for him by his friend, the botanist Nuttall.

Philip Syng Physick, one of the early notables in the faculty at Philadelphia and a colleague of Rush, has often been called "the father of American surgery." Physick was born in Philadelphia in 1768, the son of a well-to-do father, who was determined that his son should be a doctor. Young Physick received the bachelor of arts degree at the College of the University of Pennsylvania and, after studying with Dr. Adam Kuhn in Philadelphia, went to London, where he became a house pupil of John Hunter and served as a resident at St. George's Hospital. Hunter offered him a position as his personal assistant, but he declined and went on to Edinburgh, where he received his doctor of medicine degree in 1792.

Returning home, Physick opened an office, but practice was slow in coming, and "for several years he trod the alleys and by-ways of his native city before his income was sufficient to pay for his shoe-strings and the powder on his queue" (Gross). He was kept busy, however, during the yellow fever epidemic of 1793 and carried out postmortem studies of the victims. In the great controversy that divided the medical profession, Physick sided with Benjamin Rush, and the two remained friends until Rush's death.

In 1800, Physick began to give lectures on surgery that Rush attended and applauded, and in 1805 was elected professor of surgery, holding this position until his resignation in 1831. During these years as a teacher and as a surgeon, he acquired a great reputation. He introduced buckskin ligatures, devised a successful operation for an artificial anus, invented a tonsillotome, described diverticula of the rectum, and was the first doctor in America to wash out the stomach with a tube and syringe in a case of poisoning. He seemed to have a great aversion to writing and published little. His surgical views and experiences were preserved largely in the surgical treatise of his nephew, John Syng Dorsey. Physick died in 1837.

The second medical school in North America was the Medical School of King's College in the City of New York, which was organized in 1768, only three years after the foundation of the first medical school in Philadelphia. The faculty of the New York school, six in number, were prominent members of the medical profession

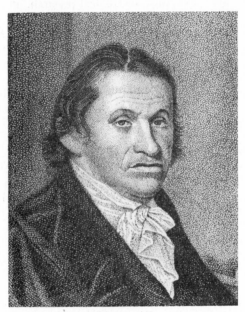

SAMUEL BARD
Drawing by McCleland, etching by W. Main.

and included Samuel Bard, who became professor of the theory and practice of physic at the age of 26.

Samuel Bard was born in Philadelphia in 1742, graduated at King's College in New York, and sailed for Europe in 1760. The vessel on which he sailed was captured by a French privateer, and he was confined at Bayonne for six months. On his release, he went first to London, where he met the Hunters and Dr. Fothergill, and worked at St. Thomas' Hospital; he then proceeded to Edinburgh, where he studied under the Monros and Cullen, receiving his medical degree in 1765. After returning to New York, he was filled, like so many others who had studied abroad, with an ambition to see a medical school in his home town and, because of his brilliant record at Edinburgh, was appointed professor in the new school.

The new medical school was disrupted by the Revolution, and, in 1776, Bard, whose political opinions were unpopular, left New York for Shrewsbury, New Jersey. He returned to New York after its capture by the British and soon regained his practice. He was held in such high esteem, however, that he later became the physician of General Washington during the latter's stay in New York.

After the Revolution, King's College was renamed Columbia College, and, in 1792, the medical college was revived with Dr. Bard as professor of physic and dean of the faculty. The school was not successful, and, in 1807, the regents of the University of New York created in its place the College of Physicians and Surgeons.

Bard was a man of great energy and industry. He was conservative in his views and warned his students, "New names are always deceiving, new theories are mostly false or useless, and new remedies for a time are dangerous." His most noteworthy contribution to medicine was his description of diphtheria in his treatise on *Angina Suffocativa*, published in 1771.

Among the professors of the College of Physicians and Surgeons, the most notable was unquestionably David Hosack (1769-1835). He was a native of New York, the son of a Scotchman, who was an officer in Lord Amherst's army and had settled in New York after the French and Indian War. Hosack graduated at Princeton and studied medicine in New York and Philadelphia, receiving his degree at Philadelphia in 1791. He then practiced for a time at Alexandria, Virginia, but, feeling the need for further study, went to Europe, spending two years in Edinburgh and London, where he worked with Monro, Black, Gregory, Cooper and Abernethy. While in London, he presented before the Royal Society a paper, *Observations of Vision,* which Gross says "made his name widely known on both sides of the Atlantic."

On his return to New York, Hosack was appointed professor of botany in Columbia College and became a partner in practice with Dr. Samuel Bard. He soon numbered many influential men among his patients, including Alexander Hamilton and Aaron Burr. He became a close friend of Hamilton's and stood by his side in the memorable duel on July 11, 1804, when Hamilton fell mortally wounded by Burr's fire. In 1807, Hosack was appointed professor of botany and materia medica in the newly organized College of Physicians and Surgeons as well as professor of surgery and mid- wifery. He held these positions until 1813, when he became profes- sor of physic and clinical medicine, resigning in 1826 to become professor of medicine in the newly formed but short-lived Rutgers Medical College. He retired in 1831 and died four years later.

Hosack was eminent as a physician, surgeon and obstetrician. "Dr. Hosack," wrote Gross,

was a physician worthy to be named with Rush, Physick, Wistar, Chapman, and other savants. . . . I heard him discourse on fevers. He sat in an arm- chair and read from his manuscript; but he frequently indulged in ex- temporaneous flights, accompanied by flashes of his black eyes, and by grace- ful gesticulations, which enchained the attention of his pupils. His manner was delightful; his voice commanding.

In 1808, Hosack performed the first ligation of the femoral artery for aneurysm in America. During the early years of his practice, he did much excellent work in surgery and wrote many surgical papers, but, later, medicine became his chief interest. He wrote on a great variety of topics, the list of his publications filling two columns of the Surgeon-General's Library Catalogue.

In Valentine Mott (1785-1865), the new medical school in New York had one of its most colorful, brilliant and famous professors. He received the degree of M.D. at Columbia College in 1806, went immediately to London, where he became a pupil of Sir Astley Cooper, Abernethy, Cline and Charles Bell, and then went to Edin- burgh, where he studied under Gregory, Monro and Hope. On his return to New York, he was appointed professor of surgery in Co- lumbia College at the early age of 26, and, when this faculty was combined with that of the College of Physicians and Surgeons in 1811, he became professor of surgery in the combined school. He was professor of surgery in the Rutgers Medical School in 1826, was professor again at the Physicians and Surgeons in 1831, became professor of surgery in the newly established University of the City of New York in 1840, then returned to the faculty of the Physicians and Surgeons, and taught there until his death in 1865.

Valentine Mott was the acknowledged leader of American surgery for nearly half a century. His fame began with his ligation of the innominate artery, performed in 1818 when he was 33 years of age, an operation never attempted before. This operation, which made him famous, was followed by a series of notable surgical operations

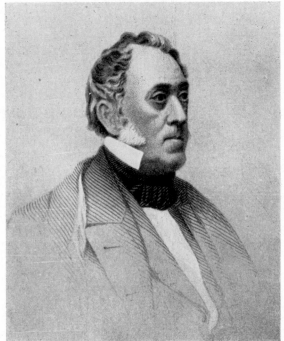

Francis, *Valentine Mott's Surgical Cliniques*, New York, 1860

VALENTINE MOTT

requiring both boldness and consummate surgical skill—removal of the lower jaw, excision of the clavicle, and ligation of the common iliac artery. Samuel D. Gross wrote of him: "No surgeon, living or dead, ever tied so many vessels or so successfully for the cure of aneurysm, the relief of injury or the arrest of morbid growths." Sir Astley Cooper said, "He has performed more of the great operations than any man living." All of these operations were performed without anesthesia.

Gross describes Mott as an excellent pathologist, who "seems to have been as able to diagnosticate a malignant from a benign disease as the most accomplished microscopist of the present day." Gross found him a fair teacher of operative surgery, although egotistical and tiresome at times. His reputation was achieved with the knife and not with the pen. He wrote little. Gross remarks laconically, "He has left us no great work on surgery; indeed, I may say, no work at all."

Harvard College, the oldest college in the United States, was founded for the education of the youth in arts, letters and theology, and almost a half century rolled by before the youth there had an opportunity to study medicine also. The thought, however, that some day Harvard would have a medical school was in the minds of many physicians, such as Dr. Ezekiel Hersey, who, at his death in 1770, left 1,000 pounds to Harvard for the foundation of a chair of anatomy and surgery. In 1780, Dr. John Warren, an alumnus of Harvard College, who had studied medicine under his brother, Joseph, later killed at Bunker Hill, was stationed in Boston as surgeon to a Continental Army hospital. During this period, Warren gave a series of lectures on anatomy, which received such favorable notice that the authorities of Harvard later invited him to draw up a plan for the formation of a medical school. Warren's plan was accepted, and the "Medical Institution of Harvard University" was founded in 1783 with a faculty of three—Dr. Warren, professor of anatomy and surgery; Dr. Waterhouse, professor of the theory and practice of medicine; and Dr. Dexter, professor of chemistry.

For nearly 40 years, John Warren was the foremost surgeon in New England, busy with a large surgical practice but never allowing it to interfere with his dissections or his lectures, which often lasted three hours. He was the first president of the Massachusetts Medical Society, holding this position continuously from 1804 until his death in 1815.

Warren's colleague, Dr. Benjamin Waterhouse (1754-1846), was a very distinguished physician of Boston. He was born in Newport, Rhode Island, his mother being a niece of Dr. John Fothergill of London. In 1775, he went to London, where he became a member of Fothergill's family, attended lectures in London and Edinburgh for three years, then went to Leyden, where he remained four years, taking his medical degree in 1781.

In 1782, after seven years abroad, Waterhouse, probably the best educated physician in North America, returned to Boston. The following year, he assisted Warren in establishing the Harvard Medical School and delivered the inaugural oration, a scholarly address in Latin.

In 1799, he received from his old friend, Dr. Lettsom, a copy of Jenner's *Inquiry* and was so impressed with it that he immediately published in the Boston *Columbian Sentinel* for March 12, 1799, an account of the new discovery with the arresting title, "Something Curious in the Medical Line." He secured some active vaccinae virus and, on July 8, 1800, successfully vaccinated his five year old son, Daniel, the first smallpox vaccination performed in America. Waterhouse, a born fighter and controversialist, began his long fight for vaccination, a crusade that earned for him the title of the "Jenner of America," but resulted in the loss of much medical practice, his resignation from his chair at Harvard, and his impoverishment. He sent some virus to President Thomas Jefferson at Monticello, whose family was vaccinated. Vaccine was sent to Washington, Philadelphia, and New York, and in time the new method of preventing smallpox won its battle. Waterhouse's *A Prospect of Exterminating the Small-pox,* which appeared in 1800, was the first work on vaccination published in the United States.

Dr. Aaron Dexter, the third member of the first Harvard medical faculty, left no permanent impress on medicine. He is perhaps best remembered from the description of one of his chemical lectures, written by a former pupil, Oliver Wendell Holmes:

"This experiment, gentlemen, is one of remarkable brilliancy. As I touch the powder you see before me with a drop of this fluid, it bursts into a sudden and brilliant flame."—which it emphatically does not do as he makes the contact. "Gentlemen," he says with a serious smile, "the experiment has failed, but the principle, gentlemen, the principle remains firm as the everlasting hills."

The progress made by the Harvard Medical School during the first half of the nineteenth century was due in great measure to James Jackson, who succeeded Benjamin Waterhouse as professor of medicine, and to John C. Warren, who succeeded his father as professor of anatomy and surgery.

James Jackson (1777-1867) has been described as "the most conspicuous character in the medical annals of Massachusetts. . . . No physician in the State ever exerted so large and lasting an influence over his professional brethren or his patients" (Green). He was born in Boston, graduated from Harvard College in 1796, and, after studying with Dr. Holyoke of Salem, went to London, where he worked with Cline at St. Thomas' Hospital, with Sir Astley Cooper at Guy's, and studied the new method of smallpox vaccination with Woodville at St. Pancras Hospital. Returning to Boston in 1800, he had obtained a large practice even before he received his M.B. from Harvard in 1802. He was created M.D. by Harvard in 1809 and was the first physician to the Massachusetts General Hospital when it was opened in 1821. In 1812, he succeeded Waterhouse as the Hersey professor of the theory and practice of medicine.

Jackson was an active crusader for vaccination. He wrote a *Textbook . . . on the Theory and Practice of Medicine*, 1825, but his most lasting contributions to medical literature were his *James Jackson, Jr., A Memoir*, 1835, a collection of medical cases by his son, who died soon after his return home from four years spent with Andral and Louis in Paris; and his *Letters to a Young Physician*, 1855, which was very popular and widely read.

John Collins Warren (1778-1856), the eldest son of John Warren, was intended for a commercial career but, deciding upon medicine, went to London in 1799, where he worked for a year in Guy's Hospital under Sir Astley Cooper. He spent a year at Edinburgh, where he received his medical degree, and then went to Paris, where he studied under Dubois, Sabatier, Cuvier, Dupuytren and Corvisart.

On his return home in 1802, he found his father in bad health and immediately took over the greater part of his practice. Trained under Corvisart, he was at first much interested in diseases of the heart and acquired a great reputation as an internist. In 1809, he published *Cases of Organic Diseases of the Heart*, which further increased his reputation. His interests later were more in the field of surgery. In 1806, he was appointed adjunct professor of anatomy and surgery and, on the death of his father, was appointed professor. He was active in the foundation of the *New England Journal of Medicine and Surgery* and in the establishment of the Massachusetts General Hospital, being chosen as its first surgeon.

Warren acquired a great reputation as a careful and skillful surgeon. His *Surgical Observations on Tumors*, published in 1837, is his best work. The outstanding event in his professional career was the operation he performed in 1846 on a patient under influence of ether.

EPHRAIM McDOWELL

While the chief historical events of early American history took place along the Atlantic coast, later American history was not all made on the Eastern seaboard. Nor was all American medical history made in Philadelphia, New York and Boston. Pioneers from the Eastern states were constantly pushing the frontiers westward, and, in their wake, at times in the vanguard, came merchants, ministers, lawyers and doctors. Some of these doctors contributed notable chapters in the history of American medicine.

When Ephraim McDowell, who was born in Rockbridge County, Virginia, in 1771, came to Kentucky, he was 13 years of age. His

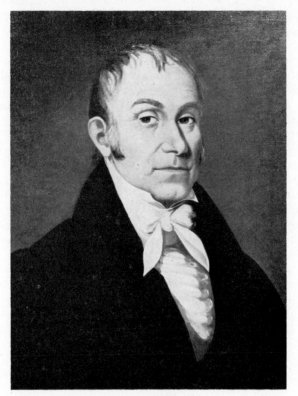

EPHRAIM McDOWELL

Portrait painted by P. H. Davenport in 1829 at Danville, Kentucky.
(Dept. of History of Medicine, University of Kansas.)

father was a judge who settled in 1784 in Danville, a town of some
150 inhabitants. At that time, Kentucky was a somewhat undefined
district, the western fringe of the Virginia colony. In 1790, it was
separated from Virginia, the Attorney General of Kentucky, however,
warning the Governor of Virginia, "Congress did not seem disposed
to protect them, and under the present system she could not exert
her strength." It required men of great courage and self-reliance
to push out into this unknown wilderness, the cockpit of warring
Indian tribes, the "Dark and Bloody Ground." Indeed, it was just
this type of settler who came, courageous, venturesome men, peaceful enough in temperament but with a gun at hand to ward off any
sudden attack of hostile Indians.

It was in this atmosphere that young McDowell grew up, and, like his fellows, he was courageous, enterprising and self-reliant. At the age of 19, he went to study medicine with Dr. Alexander Humphreys of Staunton, Virginia, a graduate of Edinburgh. After two or three years of this preceptorship, McDowell went to Edinburgh, where he attended the sessions of 1793 and 1794, studying chemistry under Joseph Black, anatomy under Monro *secundus,* medicine under James Gregory, and surgery under John Bell—quite a galaxy of noted teachers for a youth from backwoods Kentucky.

McDowell left Edinburgh without a degree and returned to Danville, now a town of about 1,000 inhabitants, and began the practice of medicine in 1795. His practice extended hundreds of miles, and, as these were the days before either roads or stage-coaches, he made his calls on horseback, often through the trackless wilderness. Indians and wolves were plentiful, and distances between homes were great so that McDowell was often absent from home for a week or more. He not only practiced medicine but performed all the operations known to the surgery of his day without any trained assistant, often with a log cabin serving as his operating room.

In 1809, he was summoned to see Mrs. Jane Crawford, who was at first thought to be pregnant but had long since passed the term

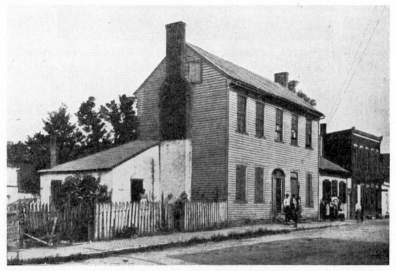

THE HOME OF EPHRAIM McDOWELL
Here the ovariotomy was performed.

of normal gestation. McDowell decided it was an abdominal tumor and proposed an operation if the patient would come to his home in Danville. Mrs. Crawford agreed and made the trip to Danville on horseback, resting the tumor on the horn of the saddle. On December 13, 1809, McDowell, assisted by his nephew James McDowell, M.D., a graduate of Pennsylvania, removed an ovarian tumor weighing 22½ pounds. The operation was performed in "about 25 minutes" without an anesthetic; the patient recovered without any complications and lived 33 years after the operation, dying at the age of 78.

McDowell wrote an account of this and two subsequent operations of the same kind and sent one copy to his old teacher in Edinburgh, John Bell, and a second copy to Dr. Philip Syng Physick of Philadelphia with a request that "it be published if found worthy." The paper was delivered by McDowell's nephew, but, as Physick seemed quite uninterested, young McDowell placed it in the hands of Dr. James of Philadelphia, who, as an editor, published it in the *Eclectic Repertory*, 1817, page 242. The paper created a sensation although it was at first received with great scepticism. It was, however, followed by a second paper in the *Repertory*, dated September, 1819, describing two additional cases. Soon the operation was performed successfully elsewhere—in Edinburgh, in Glasgow, and in London. Later, Sir Spencer Wells, in 1879, somewhat belatedly called McDowell "the Father of Ovariotomy."

McDowell performed eight ovariotomies, the last in 1826. He was also a skilled lithotomist, having performed this operation 32 times with only one death. A quiet, modest, retiring man, he gradually withdrew from his strenuous practice and died in 1830 at the age of 59. He died, as Gross noted, "without probably having dreamed that he had achieved immortality as the father of ovariotomy." Stephen William's *American Medical Biography*, published in 1845, 15 years after McDowell's death, did not contain his name.

Another surgeon of Kentucky, whose local fame during his lifetime exceeded that of McDowell, was Benjamin Winslow Dudley (1785-1870), who, like McDowell, was a native of Virginia and, while still a child, was brought to Lexington, Kentucky, where he spent his entire professional life and where he died. He studied with a local practitioner and, at the age of 19, went to the University of Pennsylvania and received his M.D. in 1806. He wished to study in Europe, but he was poor and lacked funds for further study. Returning to Lexington, he not only doctored patients but also entered business in a small way and, after four years, had saved

enough money to buy a flat-boat and load it with "sundries." He
floated the boat down to New Orleans, sold the boat and its cargo
for a substantial sum of money, which he invested in a cargo of
flour. This he accompanied to Europe, selling it at Gibraltar to the
British for a handsome sum. With the proceeds of the sale, he went
to Paris, where he studied under Larrey three years. Later he went

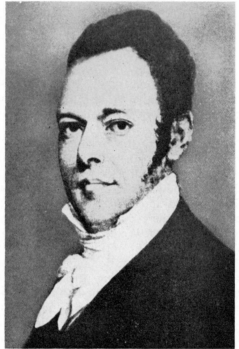

Abell, *Retrospect of Surgery in Kentucky,* 1926
BENJAMIN DUDLEY

from Paris to London, where he saw the work of Abernethy and
Cooper.

Dudley returned to Lexington at the age of 29 and soon had
a large practice. He was original as well as careful. He selected his
patients with care and attributed his great success to the care with
which he prepared his patients for operation. He laid great stress on
the employment of boiled water at operations. Gross, who did not
like him, admitted that he was very skillful but tempers the praise
with the remark that he was "an excellent mechanical surgeon, or,
in other words, operator. Of surgical pathology he knew little or

nothing." Yet, Dudley's experience and skill were unrivalled in his area. He cut for stone 225 times, the first 100 without a death. He successfully ligated the subclavian artery for axillary aneurysm and the common carotid for an intracranial aneurysm. In 1828, he published a report of five successful cases in which he had trephined the skull for the relief of epilepsy due to pressure on the brain. He was probably the first surgeon in America to perform such an operation.

In 1815, the year after his return from Europe, Dudley was appointed professor of anatomy and surgery in the medical department of Transylvania University at Lexington, holding both chairs until 1844, after which he retained only that of surgery. From 1820 until 1840, he was the driving force behind the school, and Transylvania ranked with the schools of Philadelphia, New York, Boston, Hanover and Baltimore. In 1837, the new medical college in Louisville proved too attractive to most members of the faculty, and they migrated to Louisville. Dudley refused to move, but it was the beginning of the end for Transylvania.

Estimates on Dudley's ability as a teacher vary. He is usually described by his contemporaries as having been a clear, concise and interesting lecturer, who had the ability to present briefly facts so that their association was obvious and the impression lasting. Gross, who attended an anatomical lecture of Dudley remarked, "A more puerile discourse I have never listened to. It would hardly have been creditable to a tyro in anatomy." Nevertheless, his ability as a teacher and organizer is nowhere better demonstrated than in his relations with Transylvania University. "The history of the medical department, we may say, represents the history of Dudley's life. With his entrance it rose and prospered, with his exit it faded away" (Schachner). Dudley retired in 1850 and died 20 years later at the age of 85, largely forgotten by the profession.

When Dudley revitalized the medical school of Transylvania University, he did not invite Ephraim McDowell to join the faculty. He did, however, include one man, who, by common consent, was one of the greatest physicians America has ever produced—Daniel Drake.

DANIEL DRAKE

Ephraim McDowell and Benjamin Dudley, while the sons of families in modest circumstances, were both matriculated in medical schools and able to study abroad where they saw the medical élite of the century. Daniel Drake's people were the poorest of the poor. He spent his childhood days in a log cabin, never saw the inside of a medical school until he had practiced for a year and earned enough money to finance a year's medical schooling at Philadelphia, did not receive his medical degree until he had been in practice 12 years, and never went abroad. Yet, he developd into a great teacher, a forceful writer, a founder of medical schools and held during his career 11 different chairs in six medical schools.

Daniel Drake was born in Essex County, New Jersey, in 1785. When he was two and a half years old, his father moved westward and settled in Mason County, Kentucky, with a capital of just one dollar, at that time the price of a bushel of wheat. The father built a log cabin in the wilderness, and here Drake spent the first 15 years of his life, in a community where human life was held cheap and every man was a law unto himself. His early schooling was obtained from itinerant teachers who went from place to place holding classes in reading, writing and arithmetic.

When Drake was 15 his father sent him to study medicine with Dr. William Goforth, one of the most prominent physicians of Cincinnati. Here he read Dr. Goforth's books, Cullen, Cheselden, Haller and Boerhaave, and, surreptitiously, the works of Rush, whom Goforth despised but whom Drake soon came to admire. He also compounded medicines for the doctor, ran errands for him, and saw some of his patients. At the end of four years, he received an autograph diploma from his preceptor signed by Dr. Goforth as "Surgeon General of the First Division of the Ohio Militia." After receiving his diploma, he went to Philadelphia, where he spent five months attending lectures and studying.

On his return from Philadelphia, he practiced for a year and then went to Cincinnati, where he married, took over Dr. Goforth's office during his absence, and began the practice of medicine. He soon developed an extensive practice and found time to publish a book on the *Natural and Statistical View or Picture of Cincinnati and the Miami County,* a treatise on the meteorological and climatic conditions, the plant life, and geological formations of the area, which appeared in 1815 and excited a great deal of interest in the East, and even in Europe. It attracted little attention in Cincinnati, and many of his colleagues ridiculed it. The same year, he went to Philadelphia, where he received his diploma a year later.

Benjamin Dudley was instrumental in starting Drake in his career as a medical teacher when he offered him the chair of materia medica at Transylvania in 1817. He remained in Lexington only one year and returned to Cincinnati fired with the ambition to establish a medical school in his adopted city. His efforts bore fruit, and the Medical College of Ohio opened in 1821 with Drake as lecturer

on the institutes and practice of medicine. Before the year's session
had closed, however, the faculty quarreled, and Drake was expelled.
He then returned to Lexington, where he was appointed professor
of materia medica and later of medicine, holding the latter position
until 1827. In 1830, he was appointed professor of medicine in Jefferson Medical College, Philadelphia, where he created a great

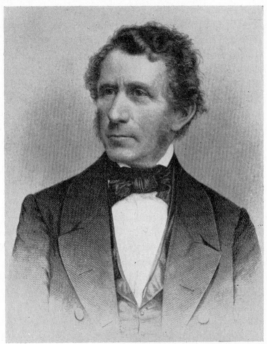

Mansfield, *Memoirs of Daniel Drake*, *M.D.*, Cincinnati, 1855

DANIEL DRAKE

sensation with his brilliant teaching. But, he remained only a year
in Philadelphia, then he went back to Cincinnati, where he founded
the medical department of Miami University. But, receiving a subordinate position, he resigned and devoted himself to his private
practice.

Drake's passion for teaching would not be quenched. He next
organized the medical department of Cincinnati College, which was
eminently prosperous but fell apart when Drake accepted a chair
at the University of Louisville, for, as his friend Gross remarked,
"He was possessed of the demon of restlessness." After five years,

he returned to Cincinnati as professor of the practice of medicine, but, a year after, we find him in Louisville and, two years later, again with his first love, the Medical College of Ohio. "Medical colleges have consumed me," he often said. He died soon after his return to Cincinnati in 1852.

"Dr. Drake," said Gross, "was a great lecturer. His voice was clear and strong, and he had a power of expression which amounted to genuine eloquence." He also, according to Gross, "wielded a pen of rare power." He was a voluminous writer, but his crowning achievement was his *Diseases of the Interior Valley of North America,* the first volume of which was published in 1850. When the American Medical Association met in Cincinnati in 1850, Dr. Alfred Stillé, chairman of the committee on medical publications, spent most of his time in praise of this work. The audience stamped and cheered until Drake arose, when a veritable pandemonium ensued. Drake tried to thank his colleagues but could not speak, sank back in his chair, covered his face with his hands, and wept. The second volume of this work appeared in 1854, two years after his death. It is an extensive treatise on topography, hydrography, climate and meteorology of the Mississippi Valley, including an account of the diet, habitat and occupations of the people, with a description of their diseases and their relation to the topography of the country and the climate. As Garrison stated, "There was nothing like this book in literature, unless it might be Hippocrates on Airs, Waters, and Places, and even Hippocrates made no attempt to map out or triangulate the geographic locale of disease."

Drake had many enemies in his own profession because of his aggressive disposition. He was an outspoken opponent of slavery and was profoundly dissatisfied with the state of medical education. Yet, he was extremely modest. In 1850, he declined to allow his name to be presented before the nominating committee of the American Medical Association although it was a foregone conclusion that he would have been elected president. His friend Gross often asked him why he did not go abroad where his fame was such that he was sure to be received with respect and deference. But Drake invariably answered,

I don't care to be brought into contact with the great physicians on the other side of the Atlantic, men of university education, whose advantages were so much greater than my own. I think too much of my country to place myself in so awkward a position.

Gross added, "And he never swerved from his purpose; never saw the Atlantic Ocean."

WILLIAM BEAUMONT

The year 1785, that saw the birth of Benjamin Dudley and Daniel Drake, also saw the birth of William Beaumont, the first great American physiologist, whom Osler once called "a backwood physiologist."

William Beaumont was born in Lebanon, Connecticut, received a common-school education, tilled the soil, and went to church

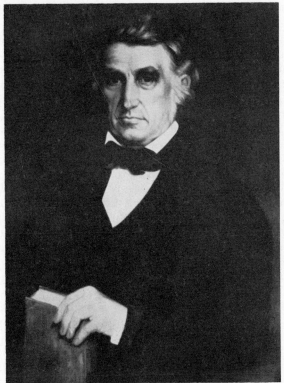

Myer, *Life and Letters of Dr. William Beaumont,* St. Louis, 1912

WILLIAM BEAUMONT

regularly. In 1806, at the age of 21, he determined to see the world, so, setting out with a horse and cutter, a barrel of cider, and $100, he drove northward without any definite destination. Arriving at Champlain, New York, near the Canadian border, he was favorably impressed with the place, applied for and received the position of village schoolmaster, and taught there for three years. During these

years, he decided to study medicine. He crossed Lake Champlain to
St. Albans, Vermont, and became an apprentice and student of
medicine under Dr. Benjamin Chandler. He remained with his
preceptor for two years, preparing drugs, sweeping out the office,
and assisting the doctor in his practice.

At the completion of his apprenticeship, the medical society of
Vermont granted Beaumont a license to practice, this document
bearing the date of "the 2nd Tuesday of June A.D. 1812." The same
month, war was declared against England, and, in September, 1812,
he joined the American Army as surgeon's mate.

During the war, Beaumont kept a diary of his experiences, which
is most interesting reading. He describes "the Surgeons wading in
blood, cutting off arms, legs, and trepanning heads" after the Battle
of Little York and notes, "I cut and slashed for 48 hours without
food or sleep." He saw much fever in the army and criticizes one
regimental surgeon who gave emetics and purges followed by tonics
and lost 26 out of 400, while the next regiment with a diametrically
opposite treatment lost no cases out of 600. He adds, "No! depletion
by blood-letting and antimonial sudorifics and diaphoretics, and an
entire disuse of all tonic medicines, is the proper plan of cure."
Obviously, young Beaumont was a disciple of Benjamin Rush.

Beaumont resigned from the army in 1815, formed a partnership
with Dr. G. Senter, another army surgeon, and began practice at
Plattsburgh, New York, where they also opened a store "containing
a general assortment of drugs, medicines, groceries, dye-woods, etc.,"
according to their advertisement in the Plattsburgh *Republican*.
Five years later, he took a commission as a post surgeon and was
immediately ordered to Fort Mackinac on the northwestern frontier.
He continued his diary, describing in it his trip to Mackinac and
his early impressions of the new country with observations on various patients he saw.

In June, 1822, Alexis St. Martin, a young French-Canadian voy-
ageur, was standing in front of the American Fur Company's store
with a group of men when a shot-gun, held by one of the party,
was accidentally discharged. The muzzle of the shot-gun was not
over three feet from St. Martin's body. He fell to the ground with
a hole in his upper left abdomen that would have admitted a man's
fist. Dr. Beaumont was immediately summoned and, after extracting
some of the shot, pieces of clothing and dressing the wound, left
with the remark, "The man cannot live 36 hours." The next day,
the patient was better, and Beaumont expressed the opinion that
he would recover. Genuinely touched by the youth's misfortune,
Beaumont took him into his family, nursed him, fed him, and

clothed him—a real act of charity since Beaumont's salary at this time was only $40 a month with two to four rations daily, out of which he had to supply his own needs, those of Alexis and support his own family as well. Alexis recovered completely in two years, but the large fistula into his stomach remained.

The idea of carrying out some experiments on St. Martin occurred to Beaumont in 1825. He wrote in his notebook,

When he lies on the opposite side, I can look directly into the cavity of the Stomach, and almost see the process of digestion. . . . I have frequently suspended flesh, raw and wasted, and other substances into the perforation to ascertain the length of time required to digest each. . . . This case affords an excellent opportunity for experimenting upon the gastric fluids and process of digestion.

Soon after beginning his experiments, Beaumont was ordered to Fort Niagara and took Alexis with him, continuing his experiments. His first four were published in the *Medical Recorder,* January, 1826, p. 94. In these experiments, he noted the length of time required for the digestion of various articles of food when suspended in the stomach by a silk string, also when placed in vials containing gastric juice, which he had extracted. These few experiments convinced him that the old theories of maceration and fermentation did not correctly explain digestion. He concluded that the gastric juice possessed innate solvent powers.

Beaumont continued his experiments, later taking St. Martin to Plattsburgh with the intention of showing him to medical groups. At Plattsburgh, however, St. Martin took an unceremonious departure, returned to Canada, and married. Four years later when Beaumont was stationed at Fort Crawford in the Upper Mississippi, he learned of Alexis's whereabouts and persuaded him to come to the fort. After considerable delay and at much expense, Beaumont transported him some 2,000 miles from lower Canada. Alexis arrived in 1829 in good health and with the aperture still open. Beaumont carried on his experiments for two years, after which Alexis returned to Canada. In 1832, he agreed to return for further experiments, and Beaumont, having received a six months' leave, drew up a legal contract with Alexis and took him to Washington, where he spent his furlough carrying out further experiments. He succeeded later in having Alexis enrolled in the army as a sergeant, subject to his orders. This third set of experiments was interrupted by Alexis's absence in Canada because of the death of a child, but, on his return, Beaumont began his fourth group of experiments. His last recorded experiment was November, 1833.

Realizing his ignorance of chemistry, Beaumont enlisted the assistance of Robley Dunglison, professor of physiology in the University of Virginia, and of Benjamin Silliman, professor of chemistry in Yale University. Dunglison made valuable suggestions regarding his experiments, and Silliman examined the gastric juice and reported, "Its free acid is chiefly hydrochloric acid."

The indomitable experimenter, having now carried out his observations on gastric digestion for eight years, decided to publish a book summarizing his work, and, in 1833, *Experiments and Observations on the Gastric Juice and the Physiology of Digestion* by William Beaumont, Surgeon, U.S.A., was printed at Plattsburgh. This work is a classic in physiology. The author described clearly the appearance and properties of gastric juice, proved that the active acid in the gastric juice is hydrochloric acid, pointed out that gastric juice and mucus are separate secretions, demonstrated the profound

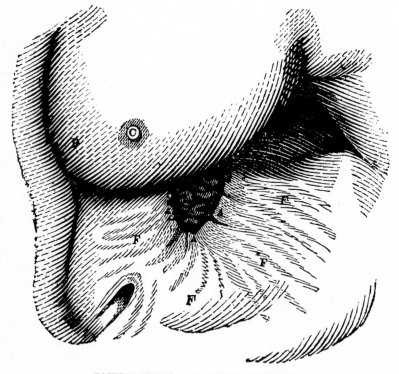

GASTRIC FISTULA OF ALEXIS ST. MARTIN
From Beaumont, William, *Experiments and Observations on the Gastric Juice.*

influence of mental disturbances upon the secretion of the gastric juice, and carried out the first study on gastric motility. He studied further the digestibility of various foods, work which remains today one of the greatest contributions to the subject of dietetics.

In 1839, Beaumont resigned from the army and went into practice in St. Louis, Missouri, where he died in 1853. Alexis St. Martin, his famous patient, lived until 1880, when he died at the advanced age of 83.

The operations of McDowell and the experiments of Beaumont created a sensation in medical circles in Europe, who were not quite prepared to expect medical research from the wilderness of Kentucky or from the frontiers of Michigan territory. The next medical discovery from America had an even greater impact upon the medical world of Europe, which received it without reservation and recognized it immediately as one of the great medical discoveries of all time. It was the discovery of ether anesthesia. While there has been some controversy regarding the credit for this discovery, there has been no controversy that it was an American discovery and that the contestants for the honor of discoverer were all Americans.

THE DISCOVERY OF SURGICAL ANESTHESIA

The search for an anesthetic which would give relief from pain in surgical operations had been an age old endeavor. Anesthesia is a Greek word and was employed by Plato in philosophical discussion and by Dioskorides in the first century A.D. in the modern sense, when he recommended mandragora to produce anesthesia before operations or cauterizations. The Arabians, a millennium later, employed a soporific sponge to produce anesthesia. Then we read of the "soporific sponge" at Salerno and in the writings of Hugo of Lucca.

Through the centuries, anesthesia is a constantly recurring theme in surgical literature, although there is much reason to believe that it was found more frequently in surgical texts than seen in surgical practice. In the sixteenth century, Hans von Gerssdorff probably described the practice of most surgeons when he wrote, "There has been much said and often written how you give a drink and make one sleep whom you wish to cut. I leave it alone. I have never used it or seen it even and at that I have cut off a hundred or two members." Ambroise Paré performed his operations without anesthesia, as did Wiseman, Cheselden, Fabry, John Hunter, Larrey, Bell, Abernethy, Cooper and McDowell. In 1839, Alfred Velpeau, the distinguished French surgeon, wrote, "To escape pain in surgical operations is a chimera which we cannot expect in our time."

With the development of chemistry in the nineteenth century, scattered references to the anesthetic effects of certain chemicals appear. Joseph Priestley discovered nitrous oxide in 1772, and Sir Humphry Davy described the analgesic and exhilarating effects of this gas in 1798. Ether, which was synthetized as early as 1540 by Valerius Cordus, was studied by Michael Faraday in 1818 and found to produce "effects very similar to those occasioned by nitrous oxide." In 1824, Hickman carried out a series of operations on animals which had inhaled carbon dioxide and found that this gas produced insensibility to pain. He suggested its use in surgical operations on human patients, but, receiving no encouragement from Sir Humphry Davy, asked the Paris *Académie de Médecine* to investigate his claims. Larrey supported Hickman, but his colleagues outvoted him, and the matter was dropped.

Meanwhile in America, William E. Clark, a young student at Berkshire Medical College, administered ether in January, 1842, to a patient whose tooth was then extracted by Dr. Elijah Pope of Rochester, New York. This was apparently the first use of ether anesthesia on record. A few months later, Crawford W. Long of Jefferson, Georgia, performed a memorable operation. After attending a public demonstration of the effects of nitrous oxide, Long began to consider the possibility of operating upon patients made insensible to pain by the administration of an anesthetic. He knew little about nitrous oxide, but, while a medical student at Pennsylvania, where he graduated in 1839, he had attended "ether frolics" and, upon the insistence of his friends, had arranged some similar parties in his own office. While his companions were interested only in the exhilarative effect produced by the ether, Long himself noted that, after these parties, he often had bruises on his body, the result of injuries he must have received but which he totally failed to remember.

On March 30, 1842, he persuaded one of his patients, James W. Venable, to inhale ether and then allow him to remove a small tumor from his neck. Venable agreed, Long poured some ether over a towel, the patient inhaled the ether and soon became unconscious, and Long then removed the tumor.

With the exception of use in dental extractions, Crawford Long was unquestionably the first man to employ ether to produce surgical anesthesia. He continued to perform minor operations under

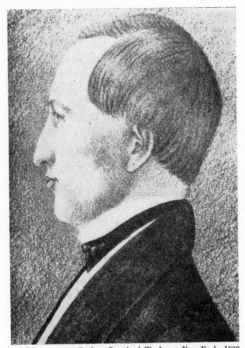

Taylor, *Crawford W. Long*, New York, 1928

CRAWFORD W. LONG

A crayon portrait drawn a few months after his first employment of ether as an anesthetic.

ether anesthesia and hoped to perform a major operation under its effect. But Jefferson was a small town, and no opportunity came. Seven years later, Long reported his operations in the *Southern Medical and Surgical Journal* for December, 1849. Long's pioneer work attracted little attention and was virtually unknown until after the spectacular demonstration of ether anesthesia by Morton in 1846.

William Thomas Green Morton (1819-1868) was a native of Charlton, Massachusetts. While it is often stated that he graduated from the Baltimore College of Dentistry, a search of this school's records reveals no evidence that Morton graduated or even studied there. In 1849, three years after the demonstration of ether anesthesia, Washington University of Baltimore, a medical school which had a somewhat checkered career, granted him an honorary degree in medicine. Morton began the practice of dentistry with Dr. Horace Wells, who had learned of the anesthetic effects of nitrous oxide anesthesia, remarking after the operation, "I didn't feel so much as the prick of a pin." Wells obtained permission to demonstrate his method before a class at Harvard Medical School, but the anesthesia was incomplete, the patient screamed, the students hissed and called the so-called discovery a hoax.

Morton had witnessed the unsuccessful demonstration of Wells. He had meanwhile entered the Harvard Medical School with the purpose of obtaining a medical degree and had as a preceptor Dr. Charles T. Jackson, who suggested to him the local application of ether to relieve pain in filling teeth. This application proving successful, Morton then thought of ether inhalation, and, after experiments on some puppies which were completely anesthetized by the fumes, he administered it to a patient with an ulcerated tooth and extracted the tooth without pain.

He was now convinced that he had a great discovery. He wrote to Dr. John C. Warren, professor of surgery at Harvard and chief surgeon of the Massachusetts General Hospital, asking for permission to administer his new drug to a patient before operation. Warren agreed, and his house surgeon wrote Morton, inviting him to come.

On the morning of October 16, 1846, the members of the surgical staff filled the operating room of the hospital at 10 o'clock, but Morton was not present. Dr. Warren, who strongly suspected that Morton would not appear, prepared to proceed with the operation when Morton, who had been delayed by the instrument maker, just finishing the inhalation apparatus, entered. Morton immediately applied the apparatus to the patient's mouth, and he began to breath the vapor "for about three minutes," as Warren wrote later, "at the end of which time he sank into a state of insensibility." Warren then made an incision on his neck and removed a tumor of the jaw "without any expression of pain" by the patient. Warren was deeply impressed and, turning to the surgical staff, said, "Gentlemen, this is no humbug."

Warren's championship of ether anesthesia doubtless played a large role in its immediate acceptance. Warren, at that time nearing 70, the professor of surgery at Harvard and son of one of the founders of Harvard Medical School, was a commanding figure in the surgical world. Dr. H. J. Bigelow, one of the surgeons of the Massachusetts General Hospital, published an account of the operation in the *Boston Medical and Surgical Journal* for November 18,

1846. This article provoked an attack in the *Philadelphia Medical Examiner* that Boston physicians were encouraging quackery, stating that, if this tendency were not checked, "physicians and quacks will soon constitute one fraternity." However, the method spread, and ether was administered in Paris on December 15, 1846, and in London on December 18, 1846. On December 21, Robert Liston, "the most brilliant surgical operator of his generation in England" (D'Arcy Power), amputated a thigh at University Hospital, employing ether as an anesthetic, and, on January 12, 1847, Malgaigne reported to the Paris *Académie de Médecine* three cases successfully operated upon under ether anesthesia.

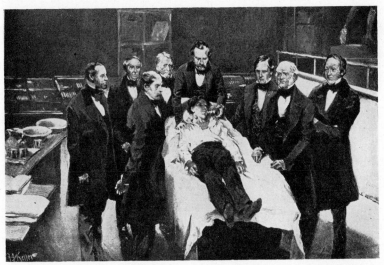

THE FIRST PUBLIC DEMONSTRATION OF SURGICAL ANESTHESIA
From painting by Keller.

Morton called his preparation "letheon" and planned to patent it but changed his mind when he learned of Dr. Warren's opposition. He then petitioned Congress to grant him compensation for his discovery, but this failed. Jackson now claimed the discovery as his own, and a bitter fight began between him and Morton. The latter became involved in a series of lawsuits which ruined him financially, and he died impoverished in 1868, aged 49. Horace Wells, after his unsuccessful demonstration at Harvard in 1845, returned to Hartford and later used nitrous oxide successfully in his practice. However, he became depressed and took his own life in 1848 when

33 years of age. Crawford Long, by contrast, continued his practice in far-away Georgia and died in 1878 at the age of 63.

There has long been a controversy as to whether Long or Morton discovered surgical anesthesia. Most impartial investigators agree with William H. Welch when he said,

We need not withhold from Dr. Long the credit of independent and prior experiment and discovery, but we cannot assign to him any influence upon the historical development of our knowledge of surgical anesthesia or any share in its introduction to the world at large.

On November 21, 1846, Oliver Wendell Holmes wrote to Morton,

Everybody wants to have a hand in the great discovery. All I will do is to give you a hint or two as to names. The state should, I think, be called anaesthesia. This signifies insensibility more particularly . . . to objects of touch. . . . I would have a name pretty soon, and consult some accomplished scholar such as President Everett, or Dr. Bigelow, Sr., before fixing upon the terms which will be repeated by the tongues of every civilized race of mankind.

Thus, Holmes suggested the name "anesthesia." He neither created it nor invented it. Plato and Dioskorides had employed it more than a millennium before.

OLIVER WENDELL HOLMES

Oliver Wendell Holmes is so well known as a poet and as a man of letters that the reading public is sometimes unaware of the fact that he belongs also to the world of medicine, where he rendered distinguished service.

Holmes was born in Cambridge, Massachusetts, in 1809, son of the Rev. Abiel Holmes, minister of the First Church of Cambridge. He was sent to Phillips Academy at Andover and then entered Harvard College, graduating in 1829. The year after graduation, he spent studying law, and it was during this period that the Government announced that the old frigate "Constitution" lying in Boston harbor would be scrapped. Holmes, in a moment of inspiration, dashed off the poem, "Old Ironsides," which swept Boston and the rest of the nation like wildfire and created such a wave of indignation against the proposed destruction of the vessel, that the Government reversed its decision.

Presently, Holmes decided that he preferred medicine to law and entered the Harvard Medical School in 1830. After two and a half years, he went abroad, going on the advice of Dr. James Jackson, to Paris. Here he studied under Andral "the eloquent," Dupuytren, Broussais "the old volcano," Lisfranc "drawer of blood and hewer

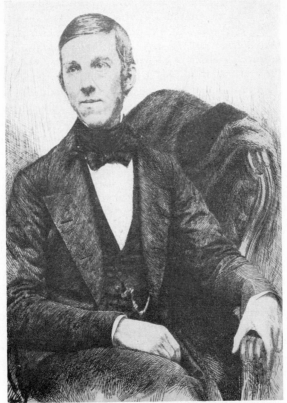

Morse, *Life and Letters of Oliver Wendell Holmes*, Boston, 1896

OLIVER WENDELL HOLMES IN 1850

This picture shows Holmes at the height of his fame, four years after he had suggested the term, "anesthesia," and three years after he had become professor of anatomy and dean of the Harvard Medical School.

of members," who regretted the disappearance of Napoleon's guard because "they had such magnificent thighs to amputate," Ricord "the Voltaire of pelvic literature," the great sceptic who believed that even the Vestal Virgins would have been improved by a course of mercury. But most of all, he admired Louis, who constantly told his pupils, *"Formez toujours les idées nettes."* Holmes's descriptions of his old teachers remain interesting and valuable commentaries—witty, trenchant and pithy—on medical life in Paris, then the undisputed world center of medical activity and progress.

On his return to Boston, Holmes took his medical degree in 1836, joined the Massachusetts Medical Society, and began practice. The same year, he won the Boylston prize with his essay on *Intermittent Fevers in New England* and, the following year, two prizes for his papers on the *Nature and Treatment of Neuralgias* and on the *Utility and Importance of Direct Exploration in Medical Practice*. In spite of these distinctions, he achieved only moderate success in practice. The reason he mentioned in a later address to medical students, in which he warned them: "Do not dabble in the muddy sewer of politics, nor linger in the enchanted streams of literature nor dig in far-off fields of alien sciences. The great practitioners are generally those who concentrate all their powers on their business."

Holmes did not dabble in politics or "dig in far-off fields of science," but he did linger all his life "in the enchanted streams of literature." In 1836, his first volume of *Poems* appeared, marking his entrance into the field of literature. However, he did not desert medicine for literature but wrote in 1842 an essay on *Homeopathy*, which still ranks as the most brilliant exposé of that system of healing. The following year, 1843, he wrote an epochal essay on the *Contagiousness of Puerperal Fever*, a medical classic. In this, he pointed out that the disease was frequently carried by the physician from one patient to another, or from a case of erysipelas to a mother recently delivered of a child. This essay was his greatest contribution to medical science and appeared five years before the work of Semmelweiss. Holmes' views were vigorously attacked by the leading obstetricians of his day, but their correctness is a matter of history.

In 1847, Holmes was appointed Parkman professor of anatomy and physiology at Harvard Medical School, was dean of the Medical School from 1847 to 1853, and held his professorship until 1882, when he resigned. He was not a scientific anatomist; he made no anatomical discoveries; but he was a delightful lecturer, an excellent demonstrator; and his wit, fund of general knowledge, and interesting anecdotal method of presentation made him a great favorite among the students. As a physician, he was a great believer in the healing powers of nature and a strong opponent of the overdosing with drugs—so prevalent in his day. His views on the latter were well expressed in his oft-quoted remark to the effect, "If all the drugs in the Pharmacopoeia, with a few exceptions, were thrown into the sea, it would be all the better for mankind and the worse for the fishes."

His literary labors, his articles in the *Atlantic Monthly, The*

Autocrat of the Breakfast Table, The Professor at the Breakfast Table, Elsie Venner, and his poems have won for him a permanent place in American literature. He died in 1894 at the age of 85.

William W. Gerhard (1809-1872), born the same year as Holmes, spent, like him, an exhilarating year in Paris working under Chomel, Andral and Louis. He was born in Philadelphia, graduated from the University of Pennsylvania in 1832, and, after a year abroad, returned to Philadelphia, where he became resident physician to the Pennsylvania Hospital. He demonstrated that the prevalent common continued fever of Philadelphia was identical with the typhoid fever he had studied in Paris. In 1836, during an epidemic of typhus fever in Philadelphia, Gerhard had an opportunity of studying hundreds of cases and showed by clinical and anatomical studies that typhus fever and typhoid fever are two distinct and separate diseases. His article, *On the Typhus Fever,* published in the *American Journal of Medical Sciences,* 1837, is the first description "in any language which gives a full and satisfactory account of the clinical and anatomical distinctions we now recognize" (Osler).

Gerhard had great success as a teacher and, in 1838, was appointed assistant professor of medicine at the Medical School of the University of Pennsylvania. His book, *On the Diagnosis of Diseases of the Chest,* published first in 1836, was an early and very successful treatise on physical diagnosis. He retired from practice in 1868 and died in 1872.

AUSTIN FLINT

Austin Flint (1812-1886), the son and grandson of physicians, was born in Petersham, Massachusetts, and graduated at Harvard Medical School in 1832. He began practice in Boston but soon moved to Buffalo, New York, where he was active in founding the Buffalo Medical College, of which he was appointed professor of medicine. In medical school, young Flint was a pupil of James Jackson, who was an enthusiastic admirer of Laennec and was rarely seen without his stethoscope. Flint later became a vigorous champion of the new methods of diagnosis and spent most of his professional career studying and expounding physical diagnosis. Gross remarked of him: "I know of no one who is so well entitled as Austin Flint, Sr., to be regarded as the American Laennec."

Flint was a brilliant and inspiring teacher and, during his career as a teacher, was professor of medicine at Buffalo, Chicago, Louisville, New Orleans, and New York. He kept extensive clinical records, which he began in 1833 and which filled 16,992 pages. He was an excellent and voluminous writer, essays and monographs literally pouring from his pen. His best known works are his *Physical Exploration and Diagnosis of Diseases affecting the Respiratory Organs,* 1856; *Compendium of Percussion and Auscultation,* 1864, which went through five editions; *A Manual of Percussion and Auscultation,* 1876, which went through eight editions; *A Practical Treatise . . . of Diseases of the Heart,* 1859; and *A Treatise on the*

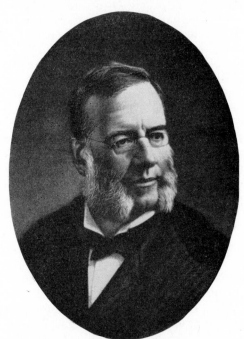

Atkinson, *Physicians and Surgeons of the United States,* Philadelphia, 1878

AUSTIN FLINT

Principles and Practice of Medicine, 1866, a classic in the history of American medicine. His description of the Flint murmur was published in 1862. In 1875 to combat the theory of Niemeyer, who had attacked the doctrine of Laennec that phthisis was caused by tubercles, Flint published *On Phthisis,* analysing 670 cases and supporting vigorously the views of Laennec. A list of Flint's writings contains 200 articles and six books. No man had a greater influence in his time on American medicine. He died in 1886.

Two contemporaries of Gerhard and Flint—Sims and Gross—have equal claim to pedestals in America's medical hall of fame. Both achieved their fame in the field of surgery.

JAMES MARION SIMS

James Marion Sims (1813-1883) was born in South Carolina and attended the Charleston Medical School for one year, after which he entered Jefferson Medical College in Philadelphia, from which he graduated in 1835. After a discouraging experience in practice and army service during the Seminole War, he located in Montgomery, Alabama, where his skill and boldness as a surgeon attracted such a large clientele that he established a private hospital.

In 1852, Sims published a paper in the *American Journal of Medical Sciences,* which startled the medical world by announcing the cure of vesico-vaginal fistula by an original method. Up to that time there was not on record a single authentic cure of this distressing condition. In his practice, Sims had seen three cases, had taken them into his hospital, where he gave them free treatment and board, and, after four years of patient experiment and observation, had cured them. In the development of his operation, he devised the "Sims' position," introduced the silver wire suture, and invented the duck-bill speculum. His announcement was followed by astonishment and often by incredulity.

Locating in New York in 1853, Sims established the State Hospital for Women and, because of his work there, has been considered "the founder of gynecology in this country." In 1861, he visited Europe and demonstrated his operation before the leading surgeons of Paris, including Velpeau, Nélaton and Civiale. In Paris, he created a furor, was called either into consultation or to operate in all the European countries, and on one occasion was the guest of the Emperor Napoleon III. He remained abroad until 1868. At the outbreak of the Franco-German War, he hurried back to Paris to become surgeon-in-chief of the Anglo-American Ambulance Corps, serving with the French Army and was decorated Commander of the Legion of Honor. From this time until his death in 1883, he lived alternately in America and in Europe, carrying out his practice on both continents. For many years, he had the ambition to be professor of gynecology in some great medical school, such as Jefferson, his alma mater. But, when an opportunity at Jefferson appeared probably in 1822, he wrote Gross, "My health will not permit my acceptance of so onerous a chair." So, as Gross remarks, "Sims has never worn a professor's gown."

SAMUEL D. GROSS

The life span of Samuel David Gross witnessed a great number of notable events in the history of medicine, both at home and abroad. He was but a boy of 11 when McDowell published his first three cases of ovariotomy and a youth of 14 when Laennec's *Traitè*

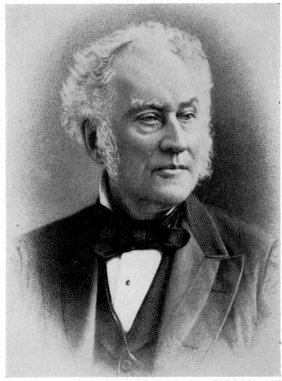

Autobiography of Samuel D. Gross, Philadelphia, 1887

SAMUEL D. GROSS

appeared. He was, however, a mature surgeon, indeed, a professor of surgery, when Holmes wrote his paper on puerperal fever, when Morton introduced ether anesthesia, when Sims devised his operation for vesico-vaginal fistula, and when Lister introduced antisepsis. He lived in stirring medical times and made his contribution to them.

Gross was born in Easton, Pennsylvania, in 1805 and, from earliest childhood, had the ambition to be a doctor. At 17, he began to study medicine under a country doctor but, soon recognizing his educational deficiencies, obtained his release and entered the academy at Wilkesbarre, studying especially Latin, mathematics, English and Greek and where, as he wrote later, "I generally slept with a book under my pillow." At 19, he recommenced the study of medicine under Dr. Swift, a physician of Easton, who urged him to matriculate at the University of Pennsylvania. But Gross, attracted by the fame of Dr. George McClellan of Jefferson, entered the "new school" instead in 1826 and graduated two years later.

Immediately after graduation, Gross began practice in Philadelphia, employing his leisure time in study and in translating French and German medical works. In 1830, young Gross at the age of 25 wrote his first book, *The Anatomy, Physiology and Diseases of Bones and Joints.* "The title," says Gross, "was unfortunate; it should have been *A Practical Treatise on Fractures and Dislocations.*" But the book did well, and 2,000 copies were sold.

Gross now returned to Easton, where he soon obtained a good practice. In 1833, he went to Cincinnati as demonstrator of anatomy in Ohio Medical College and, two years later, became professor of pathology and anatomy at Cincinnati Medical College. In 1839, he published his *Elements of Pathology and Anatomy,* the first exhaustive treatise on pathological anatomy in the English language. This work, he tells us, was based on his "dissections, from an elaborate course of reading, and from numerous visits to the pork and slaughter houses of Cincinnati." The book was an immediate success, went through three editions, and was highly praised by Virchow. In 1840, he was called to the chair of surgery at the University of Louisville, where he spent, excepting one year, 16 happy years, teaching, operating, and carrying out physiological investigations. During this period, he wrote an authoritative *Treatise on Diseases . . . of the Urinary Bladder, the Prostate Gland, and the Urethra,* 1851; and *A Practical Treatise on Foreign Bodies in the Air-passages,* 1854, the first systematic treatise on that subject.

In 1856, Gross was called to the chair of surgery at Jefferson Medical College and accepted. "One of the chief motives which induced me to remove to Philadelphia," he writes, "was to get rid of a large and annoying family practice at Louisville and to write an elaborate *System of Surgery.*" This work, the composition of which he had commenced in Kentucky, was completed in 1859, when his *System of Surgery* appeared in two octavo volumes numbering 2,360 pages and profusely illustrated with engravings on wood. In 1870, it had passed through four editions, the last edition being of 6,000 copies. "What compensation," asks the author at this time, "did I obtain for this hard work, this excessive toil of my brain, including original composition, the correction and improvement of new editions and the proof-reading . . . extending over a period certainly not less than 15 years? Eighty-five cents a copy, all told, and no extra dividends!"

In Philadelphia, Gross found no leisure and continued teaching, working and writing. His fame became world wide, honors came his way in increasing numbers, including the degrees of D.C.L. from Oxford and LL.D. from Cambridge. He died in 1884, "the greatest American surgeon of his time" (Garrison).

In addition to his purely surgical writings, Gross found time to write authoritative histories of Kentucky surgery and of American surgery. His *Autobiography*, published in 1887 after his death, is fascinating reading, and the appended *Sketches of Contemporaries* is a collection of notable biographies written with great skill and charm. In these sketches, he had his favorites and his *bêtes noires*, praising the first group with all the adjectives at his command, damning the latter with faint praise or none at all. His descriptions of McDowell, Drake and Flint are enthusiastic panegyrics, whereas his description of Dudley rather grudgingly allows him some ability as a surgeon, and, in describing Holmes, he remarks, "If he had remained faithful to his early love, he would, there is no doubt, have gained great distinction at the bar." He makes amends, however, by adding, "His forte was literature, and, as the author of *The Autocrat of the Breakfast Table, Elsie Venner, Songs in Many Keys,* of many charming magazine articles, and of many delightful poems, his name is indelibly impressed upon our age and country."

American medicine at the middle of the nineteenth century had come of age. In its youth, it was but a reflection of what was thought in London, Edinburgh, Leyden and Paris. It had now produced its own physiologists and clinicians whose contributions to medical science were recognized everywhere and its own surgeons who had performed operations never before attempted and who had taught the world to operate under anesthesia. American medicine now merged with world medicine, not in the subordinate role of a pupil, but as an equal. Yet, it remained noticeably free from chauvinism, sought the best wherever it was to be found, and presently followed the spectacular advances in Germany with the same interest and profit as it had formerly followed those of Edinburgh, London and Paris.

Biographical Addenda

THE RISE OF AMERICAN MEDICINE

1679-1766—Zabdiel Boylston was born in Muddy River (Brookline), Massachusetts, and received his medical education from Dr. John Cutter of Boston. Boylston is chiefly remembered as the first inoculator for smallpox in the colonies. He was induced to try this method by Cotton Mather, who had received accounts of it from Europe. This new method was violently opposed by the other physicians and by most of the populace of Boston, and feeling was so intense that Boylston's life was often in danger. He was the author of *Some Account of What is said of Inoculation . . .* , Boston, 1721; and *An Historical Account of the Smallpox Inoculation in New England,* London, 1726.

1708-1779—Thomas Cadwalader was born in Philadelphia and later went abroad, where he studied medicine at Rheims and anatomy under Cheselden in London. Returning to Philadelphia, he established a dissecting room, where he taught anatomy, popularized inoculation against smallpox, acquired a large practice, and became an influential citizen. He was the author of *An Essay on the West India Dry Gripes, to which is added an extraordinary case in physic,* Philadelphia, 1745, printed by his friend, Benjamin Franklin. The "dry gripes" was later shown to be lead colic, and the "extraordinary case" was an example of osteomalacia.

1712-1784—Thomas Bond was a native of Calvert County, Maryland, and studied medicine under Dr. Alexander Hamilton of Annapolis, then traveled in Europe, and studied at the Hôtel Dieu, Paris. He settled in Philadelphia about 1734 and was active in founding the Pennsylvania Hospital and the medical school in Philadelphia. He wrote two interesting articles—"A Worm and a Horrid One found in the Liver" and "A Letter to Dr. Fothergill on the Use of Peruvian Bark," published in *Medical Observations and Inquiries;* and was the author of *Introductory Clinical Lectures.*

1722-1808—John Redman.

1735-1789—John Morgan.

1736-1808—William Shippen, Jr.

1741-1817—Adam Kuhn.

1742-1821—Samuel Bard.

1745-1813—Benjamin Rush.

1750-1829—Aaron Dexter.

1753-1815—John Warren.

1754-1846—Benjamin Waterhouse.

1760-1818—Caspar Wistar.

1760-1834—David Hosack.

1762-1829—Nathan Smith, born in Rehoboth, Massachusetts, was a farmer's son, spent his boyhood in Chester, Vermont, and received a very desultory education. At the age of 21, he saw an operation performed by Dr. Josiah Goodhue of Putney, Vermont, and became interested in medicine. A year later, he came to Putney, studied three years with Dr. Goodhue, and then settled down to practice at Cornish, New Hampshire. He soon saw his own deficiencies and went to Harvard, where he attracted the attention of Dr. John Warren, the professor of surgery, who encouraged him and aided him in his work. After a year at Harvard, he received the degree of M.B. and returned to Cornish, where he was impressed more than ever with the crude methods of the local doctors and decided to devote himself to raising the standards of medical practice by establishing a medical school.

Smith turned to Dartmouth College with his project, and, receiving encouragement from President Wheelock, he went to Europe for further study. He worked in Glasgow, Edinburgh and London, sending home from Edinburgh several boxes of books and from London chemical, anatomical and surgical apparatus. He returned to Dartmouth in 1797, and the medical school was opened in 1798 with Dr. Smith as lecturer on anatomy, surgery, chemistry, and the theory and practice of physic, filling as Holmes remarked not a chair but "a whole settee of professorships."

His lectures were extremely popular, and, on one occasion, President Wheelock, coming from a lecture of Smith to hold evening prayers in the chapel, was so inspired by the lecture that he prayed, "Oh Lord! we thank Thee for the Oxygen gas, we thank Thee for the Hydrogen gas; and for all the gases. We thank Thee for the Cerebrum; we thank Thee for the Cerebellum, and for the Medulla oblongata."

Smith taught for 12 years at Dartmouth, gave all the lectures, quizzed all the classes, held all the examinations, and made all the recommendations for graduation. In 1813, he was called to the newly founded Yale Medical School as professor of medicine but continued to lecture at Dartmouth and at the University of Vermont. In 1821, he was called to the new Bowdoin Medical School to teach anatomy, surgery, medicine and obstetrics. As these courses at Bowdoin were held in summer, they did not interfere with his work at Yale.

Nathan Smith was both physician and surgeon, a great organizer and teacher. His *Practical Essay on Typhus Fever,* 1824, was a notable work on typhoid fever. In 1821, he performed an ovariotomy, an original conception as he did not know of McDowell's previous work. He also devised an improved method for reduction of dislocations of the thigh, was a skilled lithotomist, and performed probably the first staphylorrhaphy in North America.

1764-1831—Samuel L. Mitchill was a native of North Hamstead, New York, received the degree of M.D. at Edinburgh in 1786, but, disliking medicine, began the study of law, which he abandoned for natural science. He was professor of chemistry in Columbia College and later professor of natural history, botany, and materia medica. He wrote numerous articles on geology, biology, chemistry, botany, and materia medica and, entering politics, served as representative in Congress and later United States Senator from New

York. He was an able naturalist and a man of great erudition, possessed much knowledge in many fields, and was called by John Randolph the "Congressional Library."

1766-1815—Benjamin Smith Barton was born in Lancaster, Pennsylvania, and studied medicine in Edinburgh, London and Göttingen, receiving his M.D. at Göttingen. In 1789, he returned to Philadelphia, began the practice of medicine, and, the same year, was appointed professor of natural history and botany in the College of Philadelphia. On the death of Benjamin Rush, Barton was appointed professor of the theory and practice of medicine. He had given but two courses when he became ill. He took a sea voyage for his health but died soon after returning home. He was one of America's foremost botanists.

1768-1841—William Potts Dewees was born in Pottstown, Pennsylvania, attended medical lectures at the University of Pennsylvania, and began practice at 21 without a diploma. After practicing for a time, he entered the medical school again and received his M.D. in 1806. Four years later, a chair of obstetrics was established at the University of Pennsylvania with the proviso that "an attendance should be optional for graduation." Dewees hoped to receive the chair, but James was appointed.

Dewees built up a large obstetrical practice in Philadelphia and "patients, it was said, postponed their confinements until he was at leisure" (Waterson). In 1824 was published his *System of Midwifery,* which ran through 12 editions; in 1825, *A Treatise on the Physical and Medical Treatment of Children;* in 1826, *On the Diseases of Females,* both books running to 10 editions.

1768-1837—Philip Syng Physick.

1770-1843—Nathaniel Potter, founder of the University of Maryland, was born in Easton, Maryland, studied medicine under Benjamin Rush, and graduated at the University of Pennsylvania in 1796. He settled in Baltimore and remained in practice there. He was active in the organization of the College of Medicine of Maryland in 1807 and was appointed professor of medicine, holding the chair until his death. He was a great believer in the efficiency of drugs, especially calomel, and was very partial to bleeding. He had little faith in the healing powers of nature and is said to have told his students that, if nature came in the door, he would throw her out the window. Believing that yellow fever was not contagious, he experimented upon himself with the secretions of yellow fever patients to prove his contention. He remained well after these inoculations. His later years were embittered by poverty, and the expenses of his funeral were borne by his friends.

1771-1843—Elisha North, born in Goshen, Connecticut, studied medicine at home under local doctors and later under Dr. Lemuel Hopkins of Hartford. He began practice in his home town and, after accumulating some money, studied two years at the University of Pennsylvania but did not graduate. He practiced in Goshen until his removal to New London in 1812. In 1817, he established in New London the first eye infirmary in the United States. Ten years before that, while he was still in Goshen, a new disease, spotted fever, or epidemic cerebrospinal meningitis, descended on the town "like a flood of mighty waters, bringing along with it the horrors of a most dreadful plague." His experiences are described in *A Treatise on a Malignant Epidemic, commonly called Spotted Fever* . . . , New York, 1811, an early American medical classic.

1771-1830—Ephraim McDowell.

1774-1844—John C. Otto was born in New Jersey, the son, grandson, and great-grandson of physicians. His grandfather emigrated from Germany and served in the American Army during the Revolutionary War. Otto received his B.A. at the College of New Jersey (Princeton) in 1792 and his M.D. from the University of Pennsylvania. As a student, he worked in the office of Dr. Benjamin Rush and became a favorite pupil of this eminent physician. On the death of Rush, Otto succeeded him as physician to the Pennsylvania Hospital. At the age of 29, Otto wrote an article in the *Medical Repository,* "An Account of an Haemorrhagic Disposition existing in certain Families," pointing out that hemophilia is a familial affection, that males are subject to it, whereas females are not, although it is transmitted by the latter to their children.

1778-1856—John C. Warren.

1775-1821—Lyman Spalding was born in Cornish, New Hampshire and, as a boy of 11, attracted the attention of Dr. Nathan Smith, and, following his advice, later went to Harvard, where he graduated in 1797. After graduation, he went to Dr. Smith's new medical school at Dartmouth as a lecturer on chemistry for two years. He then moved to Portsmouth, New Hampshire, where he demonstrated the efficacy of vaccination against smallpox in the pest house of Portsmouth Harbor. In 1808-1809, he went to Philadelphia and worked with Rush but especially with Wistar in anatomy. He located in New York City, was active in the establishment of the United States Pharmacopeia, and would probably have succeeded Wistar as professor of anatomy when he died as the result of an accident, the cause of death being traumatic meningitis.

1777-1867—James Jackson.

1779-1864—Benjamin Silliman, a native of Connecticut, received his A.B. and A.M. degrees from Yale in 1796 and 1799. From 1802 to 1858, he was professor of natural science at Yale and was considered one of the leading chemists in America.

1783-1818—John Syng Dorsey was born in Philadelphia, the son of a successful merchant and the nephew of the illustrious Philip Syng Physick. He received his doctor's degree from Pennsylvania at the age of 19 and was appointed resident physician at the City Hospital during the yellow fever epidemic, which he studied carefully at the bedside, carrying out also many autopsies. In 1803, he went to London, where he worked in John Hunter's anatomical school, and later went to Paris, where he studied surgery under Boyer at La Charité. He noted, however, in his diary, "As to French surgery, I have learned nothing from it."

Returning to Philadelphia in 1804, he began the practice of surgery and, in 1807, was appointed adjunct professor of surgery. His *Elements of Surgery,* published in 1813, with illustrations mainly by the author, received world wide recognition. In 1813, he was made professor of materia medica and, in 1818, succeeded Wistar as professor of anatomy, but died the same year of typhus fever at the age of 35.

1785-1865—Valentine Mott.

1785-1852—Daniel Drake.

1785-1870—Benjamin Dudley.

1785-1853—William Beaumont.

1790-1872—Samuel Jackson, a native of Philadelphia, graduated from the medical department of the University of Pennsylvania in 1808. He began practice in Philadelphia in 1815, and, during the yellow fever epidemic of 1820, he was chairman of the Board of Health. He wrote several articles on yellow fever, maintaining that it was of local origin due to filth and putrefying animal and vegetable matter. In 1821, he became professor of materia medica and, in 1835, professor of the "institutes of medicine," a broad term covering the entire field of medicine, except anatomy, surgery, and materia medica, but practically a synonym for physiology. He lectured very well and wielded a facile pen. His best work was his *Principles of Medicine founded on the Structure and Functions of the Animal Organism,* 1832.

1793-1853—William Horner was born in Warrenton, Virginia, and, in 1809, began to study medicine under Dr. John Spence, an Edinburgh graduate, meanwhile attending two sessions at the medical school of the University of Pennsylvania. In 1813, he enlisted in the army and, after serving a year and seeing active service at the Battle of Bridgewater, he returned to the medical school, where he graduated in 1814. He settled in Philadelphia and, in 1831, succeeded Physick as professor of anatomy. He wrote several anatomical treatises and discovered the *tensor tarsi,* often called the muscle of Horner. He assembled a notable collection of anatomical specimens.

1804-1873—Josiah C. Nott, a native of Columbia, South Carolina, graduated at the University of Pennsylvania in 1827, practiced in Columbia for five years, and, after further study in Paris, settled in Mobile, Alabama, where he soon achieved a reputation as a physician and obstetrician. After the Civil War, he went to Baltimore and later to New York, where he practiced for several years, returning to Mobile the year before his death. He was well known in New York as a physician and gynecologist and is said to have been the first physician to describe coccyodynia. In a paper published in the *New Orleans Medical and Surgical Journal,* 1848, he advanced the theory that yellow fever was of "insect or animalcular origin."

1807-1895—William W. S. Ruschenberger, a native of New Jersey, graduated from the medical department of the University of Pennsylvania in 1830 and, the following year, was commissioned a surgeon in the United States Navy. A number of books on his cruises were written by him, and they were widely read. One of his best known works was *An Account of the Institution and Progress of the College of Physicians of Philadelphia During 100 Years,* 1887, a valuable source book on the early medical history of Philadelphia. His *First Books on Natural History* "contributed more than any other work to popularize the natural sciences in this country" (Allemann).

1809-1872—William W. Gerhart.

1809-1894—Oliver Wendell Holmes.

1811-1859—Thomas D. Mütter was a native of Richmond, Virginia, and, at the age of 20, graduated in medicine at the University of Pennsylvania. He then spent a year in Paris, attending the clinics of Larrey, Dupuytren, Velpeau and Chomel, and returned to Philadelphia to practice surgery. Philadelphia at that time had several prominent surgeons, and, as Gross relates, "Mütter crept along slowly, notwithstanding that he made himself conspicuous by his tall gray horse, his low carriage, and his servant in livery as he drove through the fashionable streets of our city." In 1841, he was appointed professor of surgery in Jefferson Medical College and soon became a popular and distinguished teacher.

Mütter was a skillful surgeon and gained a deserved reputation for his operations on clubfoot, on harelip, and for the correction of deformities caused by injuries and bones. He was not a facile writer, and his somewhat loosely written treatise on "Clubfoot" in Liston's *Operative Surgery* is his only surgical contribution. His greatest monument was the gift of his museum to the Philadelphia College of Physicians, with a sum of money for its upkeep and for a lectureship on some scientific subject.

1812-1886—Austin Flint.

1813-1883—James Marion Sims.

1813-1848—Horace Wells.

1813-1900—Alfred Stillé received his A.B. at Yale and the University of Pennsylvania, later receiving the degrees A.B., M.D. and LL.D. from the University of Pennsylvania. In 1835 he became house physician under W. W. Gerhard at Old Blockley. Following this, he went abroad and studied at Paris, spending two years in Europe. On his return to Philadelphia, he taught at the Pennsylvania Medical College and, in 1864, succeeded Dr. Pepper in the chair of medicine at the University of Pennsylvania. He was active as a teacher and writer and in the formation of the American Medical Association, serving as its first secretary and later becoming president. His most important writings were his *Elements of General Pathology,* 1848; and his monographs on *Cerebrospinal Meningitis* and *Cholera.*

1814-1874—Jeffries Wyman was born in Chelmsford, Massachusetts, and graduated from Harvard Medical School in 1837. Following graduation, he became a demonstrator of anatomy at Harvard. He subsequently traveled extensively and, in 1847, was appointed Hersey professor of anatomy at Harvard College, the chair at this time being transferred to Cambridge while a new professorship, the Parkman, was established at the Medical School and bestowed upon Oliver Wendell Holmes. In his new position, Wyman lectured on embryology, anatomy and physiology and assembled an extensive museum. His work on comparative anatomy and paleontology was outstanding.

1818-1878—Adam Hammer was a native of Mingalsheim, Baden, and received his M.D. from the University of Heidelberg in 1842. He became involved in the revolution of 1848, had to flee Germany, and emigrated to America, settling in St. Louis. He saw the deficiencies in American medical education and established in 1850 a medical college with high requirements for preliminary education, a graded curriculum, and four courses of lectures. It lasted but one year. In 1859, he established the "Humboldt Institute," with the same requirements and with all instruction in the German language. It survived 10 years. In 1878, Hammer described the first authentic case of coronary occlusion confirmed by necropsy findings.

1819-1868—William Thomas Green Morton.

1823-1891—Joseph Leidy was born in Philadelphia, wished first to become an artist, but then turned to medicine, and entered the University of Pennsylvania, where he graduated in 1844. In 1853, he succeeded Horner as professor of anatomy and held this position for 38 years, attaining a great reputation as anatomist, botanist, paleontologist and zoologist. A prodigious worker, he was the author of 553 books, papers and communications.

1831-1893—Crawford W. Long.

1835-1900—Hunter H. McGuire was born in Winchester, Virginia, graduated in medicine at the Winchester Medical College in 1856, and, the following year, matriculated at both the University of Pennsylvania and Jefferson Medical College. At the outbreak of the Civil War, he enlisted as a private soldier but was later commissioned a surgeon and became medical director of the Army of the Shenandoah under General "Stonewall" Jackson. After Jackson's death, he served under General Ewell and General J. E. B. Stuart. He headed a movement to establish a college of medicine at Richmond and was active in practice and in medical education until his death.

1837-1889—Samuel D. Gross.

The Nineteenth Century—
The Second Half

IT HAS SOMETIMES been said that medicine made more progress during the first half of the nineteenth century than during the entire eighteenth century, more during the second half of the nineteenth than during the first half. Such comparisons are, however, broad generalizations, both inaccurate and unfair. Discoveries in medicine are poor objects for comparison. We can say neither that auscultation, a discovery of the nineteenth century, was a greater discovery than percussion, discovered in the eighteenth, nor that asepsis, a discovery of the latter half of the nineteenth was of greater importance than anesthesia, introduced during the first half. Medicine is a vast edifice resting on a foundation of many stones. Some centuries have contributed more stones but not necessarily larger ones. The second half of the nineteenth century contributed a great number of stones, and some of them were very large ones.

PARIS

Paris, the unquestioned leader of world medicine during the first half of the nineteenth century, continued to hold this position although she was beginning to share it with others.

In clinical medicine, Armand Trousseau (1801-1867) of Tours, an old pupil of Bretonneau, was an outstanding personality in Paris. He graduated at Paris in 1825 and became *agrégé* in 1826. His work on yellow fever, published in 1830, attracted much attention and was followed by a treatise on laryngeal phthisis, 1837, which won the grand prize of the *Académie de Médecine*. In 1850, he became professor of medicine and physician to the Hôtel Dieu. He was the first physician in Paris to perform a tracheotomy and wrote an excellent treatise on that subject in 1851. His *Traité . . . de thérapeutique,* published first in 1836, went through eight editions and was translated into English, Spanish and Italian, but he is best remembered for his *Clinique Médicale de l'Hôtel-Dieu de Paris,* 1861, which was translated into German and English, English editions appearing in both London and in Philadelphia in 1867 and carry-

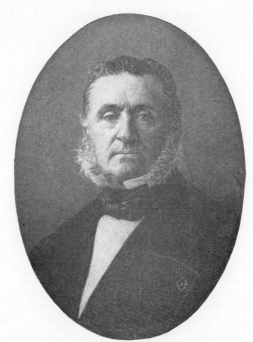

University of Kansas Collection

ARMAND TROUSSEAU

Photo by Trinquart in the *Académie de Médecine*, Paris.

ing his reputation to English and American physicians. Trousseau was an outstanding clinician and an excellent teacher, endearing himself to his pupils and colleagues by his integrity and generosity. Because of his high qualities of mind and character, he has been described as the counterpart of Richard Graves across the channel in Dublin.

Alfred-Armand-Louis-Marie Velpeau (1795-1867), the son of a blacksmith and, early in life, a blacksmith's apprentice, came to Tours at the age of 20 and began the study of medicine under Bretonneau. Like Trousseau, he praised his master to the end of his days. After four years in Tours, he went to Paris, where he graduated in 1823 and, two years later, laid the foundation of his success by publishing his *Traité d'anatomie chirurgicale*, which passed through four French, two German, two English, and three Italian

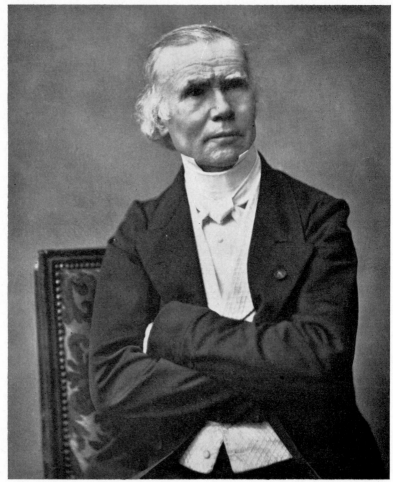

ALFRED-ARMAND-LOUIS-MARIE VELPEAU

editions. Professional success now came rapidly. In 1834, he became chief of the surgical clinic in the Charité and held this position until his death 33 years later. He was such a voluminous writer that Gurlt estimated his collected articles and books would easily fill 20 large volumes. On his death-bed, he murmured the words which may well have served as his motto: "Il ne faut pas être paresseux; travaillons toujours" (One must not be idle, we should always work).

Joseph François Malgaigne (1806-1865), the son of a poor country doctor, received his doctor's degree in Paris in 1831. After service in the army during the Polish Revolution of 1831, he returned to Paris and presently became one of its outstanding surgeons. His *Manuel de médecine operatoire,* 1834, went through eight editions and was translated into five languages, including Arabic. His edition of Ambrose Paré, published in 1840, contains a scholarly account of the historical development of French surgery as well as an admirable biography of Paré. Billings called Malgaigne "the greatest surgical historian and critic whom the world has yet seen."

During the first half of the nineteenth century, Paris, while preeminent for its clinicians and surgeons, was lagging in experimental physiology and pathology. Magendie, the sole representative during this period of experimental physiology, was a busy physician in charge of a service at the Hôtel Dieu as well as professor of medicine at the Collège de France. He carried out his experiments during the scant leisure time snatched from his duties as an active clinician and a teacher of medicine. Yet, Magendie accomplished much in physiology, founded the new science of pharmacology, and trained and inspired a young man, Claude Bernard, who became the greatest physiologist of modern France and one of the great names in the history of that science.

CLAUDE BERNARD

Claude Bernard was born in the village of St. Julien in 1813 and, while still a youth, obtained a position in a pharmacy, where he remained some two years. He found his work somewhat dull so spent his free evenings at the theatre. Presently he himself wrote a comedy, *La Rose du Rhône,* which was played at the theatre and had a certain success. Encouraged by this venture, he wrote a five act tragedy, *Arthur de Bretagne,* and, at the age of 21, took it to Paris, where he showed it to the great critic, Saint-Marc Girardin, professor at the Sorbonne. Girardin received him kindly, read his manuscript with great care, and, although recognizing that the young man had unusual literary powers, advised him to pursue literature in his leisure moments and turn to something else to earn his daily bread. "You have studied pharmacy," Girardin said, "study medicine, you will thereby much more surely gain a livelihood."

Bernard followed his advice and threw himself heart and soul into the study of medicine. Meanwhile, as his financial means were very meagre, he taught natural history in a girls' school. Five years later,

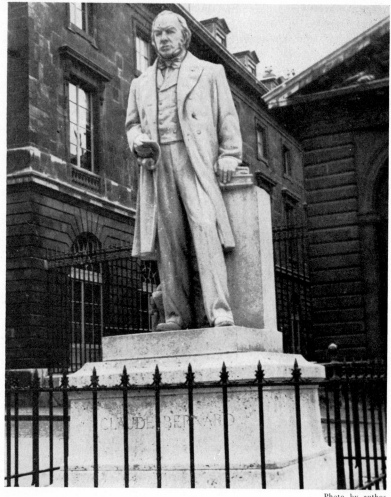

Photo by author

CLAUDE BERNARD
Statue in front of Collège de France, Paris.

he became *interne* under Magendie at the Hôtel Dieu in 1839 and, in 1841, became Magendie's *préparateur,* charged with the preparation of his experiments which were demonstrated before the students. Here his great skill in experimentation became evident. After the third or fourth demonstration, Magendie is said to have remarked, "Well, you're better than I am." This was the beginning of his fruitful years of association with Magendie, assisting the latter in his experiments, collaborating at first with him in his scientific papers, then working on his own problems, writing his own papers, and slowly, but surely, proving the correctness of Magendie's estimate of his ability. Magendie, while making great discoveries, usually went about his work in a haphazard fashion, like one groping in the dark. Bernard, by contrast, followed the advice he gave:

> Put off your imagination, as you take off your overcoat, when you enter the laboratory; but put it on again, as you do your overcoat, when you leave the laboratory . . . put it right away from you during the experiment itself lest it hinder your powers of observation.

All of Bernard's great discoveries were based upon isolated facts, accidentally discovered, but he had the rare ability to correlate them and to build them into larger, physiological generalizations, the correctness of which he later proved by experiments. His first paper was on the anatomy of the chorda tympani nerve; his second, which was his thesis for the degree of M.D. in 1843, described those experiments in which he showed that cane sugar, when injected into a vein, appears in the urine. This does not occur, however, when the sugar is treated with gastric juice previous to the injection. After receiving his degree, he transferred his activities from the hospital wards to the laboratory. He never practiced medicine.

Bernard's three outstanding contributions to physiology were the demonstration of the role played by the pancreatic juice in digestion, his discovery of the glycogenetic function of the liver, and the demonstration of the vaso-motor mechanism. The first discovery was the result of experiments carried out between the years 1846 and 1849. In these he showed that digestion was not entirely a matter of gastric action but that the pancreatic juice renders neutral fats absorbable, digests proteins, and converts starch into sugar. The second discovery was the result of a long series of experiments in which he set up many hypotheses, later found to be wrong, and made many experiments which he at first misinterpreted. Finally he arrived at the correct explanation that sugar is stored in the liver in the form of glycogen but, when released, is again transformed into sugar. In the course of his work, he succeeded in isolating glycogen. He referred to glycogen as the "internal secretion" of the liver, the first use of this term in physiological literature. Later he included the thyroid and adrenal among the glands having internal secretions. This entire concept gave offense to many physiologists who could not conceive of a ductless gland producing a secretion. His research on vasomotor nerves was finished in 1858, when he proved by experiments on the blood vessels of the submaxillary gland, using galvanization of the cut end of the nerves, that "the sympathetic is the constrictor nerve for the blood vessels, the tympanicolingual is their dilator."

In addition to these major pieces of research, Bernard made other interesting discoveries. He found that a slight wound, *piqûre,* in the floor of the brain near the cerebellum produced a transient diabetes in animals. He had carried out this experiment not haphazardly but in an attempt to produce irritation of the vagal nuclei. Cutting the vagus nerve interrupted the secretion of sugar by the liver so Bernard reasoned that irritation of the vagus should cause increased sugar production and glycosuria. When this striking experiment was successful, he considered his theory proved but found, to his dismay, that the glycosuria occurred after his *piqûre,* even when the vagus nerve was cut. From 1846 to 1854, he studied carbon monoxide poisoning and found that carbon monoxide displaced oxygen in the red blood corpuscles. He also investigated curare and, in 1850, showed that it destroys the communication between nerve and muscle but that the muscle still responds to stimuli, thus proving the doctrine of Haller that contractility is a specific property of muscular tissue.

Honors came to Bernard as he progressed in his work. In 1849, he was made a Chevalier of the Legion of Honor, the citation reading, through an amusing error, "for his excellent work on the musical properties of the pancreas." In 1855, on the death of Magendie, Bernard was appointed his successor as professor of medicine at the Collège de France, was elected in 1861 to the *Académie de Médecine,* was elected in 1868 to the *Académie Francaise,* and, in 1869, was created a senator by an imperial decree of the Second Empire. He died in 1878 at the age of 64.

At the time of his death, Bernard was working on fermentation. After his death his notes on fermentation were published, which contained, among other notations, the sentence, "Alcohol is formed by a soluble ferment outside of life." This statement gave great offense to Pasteur, who maintained there could be no fermentation without life. A bitter scientific controversy ensued, Pasteur and his followers maintaining that fermentation involved life, and the followers of Bernard holding that fermentation was simply a chemical reaction. In 1895, 17 years after Bernard's death, Büchner separated from yeast cells under pressure a substance which, added to sugar, fermented it with the production of alcohol and carbon dioxide.

CHARLES EDOUARD BROWN-SÉQUARD

Bernard's successor at the Collège de France, Charles Edouard Brown-Séquard (1817-1894), presented many contrasts to him in origin, life, disposition, and methods of work. Unlike Bernard, Brown-Séquard was born, not in France, but on the island of Mauritius, formerly French but British at the time of his birth,

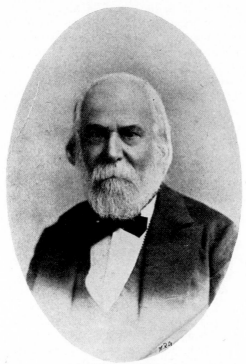

Münchener Mediz'n'sche Wochenschrift
CHARLES EDOUARD BROWN-SÉQUARD

making him a British subject. Unlike Bernard, who spent his entire professional life in Paris and never practiced medicine, Brown-Séquard, the son of an American sea captain and a French woman, speaking and writing both English and French with equal facility, was of a roving disposition and practiced medicine in the course of his life in such widely separated places as Paris, Mauritius, London and New York. For good measure, he gave lectures at various times in Philadelphia, New York, Boston, London and Dublin, and, before he was called to the chair at the Collège de France, he had already been a professor at the Medical College of Virginia in Richmond and at Harvard Medical School.

He went to Paris in 1838 and enrolled in the medical school. He also enrolled as a pupil in the private laboratory of Dr. Martin-Mageon, who gave a course in physiology, and, in 1842, he became an *interne* on the service of Trousseau. His medical course was interrupted by a sojourn on the island of Mauritius, after which he returned to Paris and took his medical degree in 1840 with a thesis on the study of reflex movements and the functions of the columns of the spinal cord. In this thesis, he noted "the inexcitability of the longitudinal fibers of the anterior columns."

After graduation, Brown-Séquard began practice, continued his experiments, and was active, together with others interested in physiology, in forming the new *Société de Biologie*. "The index of speakers and topics at the sessions of the new society during its first year, 1849, makes it appear almost as if Brown-Séquard had kept up a running monologue with occasional interruptions by Claude Bernard and still rarer ones by Robin and by Rayer, the president" (Olmsted). The same year, Brown-Séquard gave a summary of his work on transverse hemi-section of the spinal cord, describing the well-known Brown-Séquard syndrome, loss of sensation below the lesion on the opposite side of the body with retention and augmentation of sensation on the same side.

In 1852, he gave in Philadelphia a series of lectures, in which he described contraction of the blood vessels of the face following galvanic stimulation of the cervical sympathetic. This discovery later proved embarrassing to Claude Bernard, who reported the same discovery unaware of Brown-Séquard's work.

Returning to Paris, Brown-Séquard became discouraged and sailed for Mauritius, where he found an epidemic of cholera raging. After the epidemic, he received a call to the professorship of physiology at the Medical College of Virginia, which he accepted. The post proving uncongenial, he went back to Paris, established with his friend, Charles Robin, a small laboratory, took pupils, and continued his experiments. In 1856, he published a series of experiments showing that the adrenal glands are necessary for life.

Brown-Séquard had now, at the age of 39, done his best work and had made three discoveries sufficient to insure the permanence of his name in physiology—his demonstration of the effects produced by hemisection of the cord, the effects on the blood vessels caused by stimulation of the cervical sympathetic, and the effects of removal of the adrenals. He continued experimenting, however, until the end of his seventy-seventh year. During his tenure of the professorship at the Collège de France, he became interested in the study of testicular extracts, which he thought built up "nervous force." This led to many abuses, the commercialization of the products, and much unfavorable publicity.

Brown-Séquard's work gave a great stimulus to the study of internal secretions. The thought, even the term, was not his own but the creation of Claude Bernard. Nevertheless, Brown-Séquard became convinced from his imperfect experiments that not only the thyroid but also the adrenal, pancreas, liver, spleen and kidneys had internal secretions which could be employed in the treatment of diseases of those organs.

THE NEW VIENNA SCHOOL

While Paris was still the Mecca of medicine, signs of new activity became apparent in Vienna, where the traditions of the Old Vienna School had not entirely died out. The embers were fanned into flame by the activity of three remarkable men who became the nucleus of a group, since designated as the New Vienna School, who raised Vienna once more to the position of a great medical center. These men were Rokitansky, Skoda and Hebra.

Carl Rokitansky was a Czech born in Königgrätz in 1804, who studied medicine first at Prague and then at Vienna, where he received his degree in 1828. At this time, German medicine was deeply influenced by the *Naturphilosophie* of Schelling and has been trenchantly described by Wunderlich: "They had much industry and few results, they made many words and few observations, they created phantasies in profusion and philosophized very well." The New Vienna School, by contrast, made many observations and initiated a new era in German medicine.

After graduation, Rokitansky became an assistant in pathological anatomy and by degrees climbed the ladder of professional rank, becoming assistant professor in 1833 and full professor in 1844. He did not practice medicine but spent his entire professional life in the Pathological Institute. His first autopsy was performed in 1827, and, when he resigned in 1875, after 48 years of service, the number of autopsies performed by him or by assistants under his direction had reached the astounding number of 59,786! In addition, according to Schönbauer, there were at least 25,000 medicolegal autopsies! Probably no one, before or since, has had so great pathological experience, and no one of his time equalled him in gross pathological diagnosis or in the description of pathological lesions.

Rokitansky was the first to differentiate between lobar and broncho pneumonia and to describe in detail acute yellow atrophy, amyloid disease of the kidney, and spondylolisthesis. He also described the microscopic appearance of emphysema of the lungs, wrote an extensive monograph on diseases of the arteries, 1852, and on defects in the septum of the heart, 1875. His treatise on pathological anatomy, *Handbuch der pathologischen Anatomie,* which appeared in 1842, contained a wealth of material, with excellent, clear-cut descriptions, illustrated with drawings of pathological lesions, both gross and microscopic, and with such a clear and logical classification of disease from the pathological standpoint that Virchow called him the "Linné of pathological anatomy." The book was, however, marred by Rokitansky's humoral theories and his doctrine of "crases" and "stases," which drew down upon the work the severe criticism of Virchow. Rokitansky died in 1878, honored by his colleagues for his astonishing knowledge of pathological anatomy and loved as a genial, cheerful, kind and generous man.

Josef Skoda, a colleague of Rokitansky, was, like him, also a Czech but presented a contrast in certain respects. Rokitansky was genial and sparkling, Skoda reserved and rather pedantic. Rokitansky talked and wrote with charm and wit, whereas Skoda was rather dull and matter-of-fact.

Josef Skoda, whose name was written Škoda, indicating the pronunciation, "Schkoda," was born in 1805 in Pilsen. His father was a locksmith in poor circumstances, but his three sons became successful men. Josef's elder brother, Franz, studied medicine, became a prominent health official, and was later raised to the nobility, while his younger brother, Johann, became an industrialist and founded the famous Skoda works in Pilsen.

After studying first at Pilsen, Josef Skoda went to Vienna, walking the entire distance on foot in six days. There he worked at various positions while studying medicine and received his degree in 1831. Following some two years' practice in Bohemia, he returned to Vienna and obtained a position as second physician *(Sekundararzt)* in the Allgemeines Krankenhaus with no salary. He lived simply, obtained some practice, but spent most of his time in the hospital and in the autopsy room, where, as he said later, he enjoyed the "incomparable teaching" of Rokitansky. Here he had constant opportunity to examine patients with the new methods of percussion and auscultation, make his diagnoses, and later check their correctness with Rokitansky. In 1839, the last year of his service as *Sekundararzt*, he wrote his *Abhandlung über Perkussion und Auskultation*, his chief claim to the attention of posterity.

In this remarkable book, he corrected certain errors of Laennec and introduced some new and better terms into the nomenclature of physical diagnosis. He stressed particularly the point that the changes which produce physical signs are physical changes, that the same disease may produce a variety of signs while a variety of diseases may produce the same signs. The book did not evoke much praise from most of his professional brethren, who were still talking about a "stationary asthenic-nervous Genius" to explain the prevalent epidemic of influenza and who were otherwise immersed in the mystical jargon of *Naturphilosophie*.

About this time, Skoda was asked by Baron von Türkheim of the Imperial Chancellory to see in consultation the French minister, the Duc de Blacas. The other physicians made the diagnosis of liver disease, but Skoda, after examining the patient carefully, said the supposed liver disease was an aneurysm of the abdominal aorta. The patient died shortly afterwards, and the autopsy proved the accuracy of Skoda's diagnosis. Türkheim was deeply impressed with Skoda and shortly afterwards created for him a department for chest diseases in the Allgemeines Krankenhaus. In 1841, Skoda was appointed *Primararzt* (first physician) and, in 1846, Professor of the Medical Clinic.

Skoda was an excellent teacher, and his pupils soon held the leading positions in the hospitals of Vienna. His skill in physical diagnosis became almost legendary; in therapeutics he was described by his contemporaries as a "nihilist." "Medicine," write Kussmaul, "appeared to him as a chaos, a dismal swamp, out of which rose up only two islands with a rich soil, pathological anatomy and physical diagnosis." Skoda opposed bleeding, purges and emetics and often maintained that more patients with pneumonia would recover if left alone instead of being bled copiously and dosed with purges and emetics.

Ferdinand Hebra (1816-1880) was born in Brünn in 1816 and graduated in medicine at Vienna in 1841. He was appointed *Sekundararzt* in Skoda's department for chest diseases at the Allgemeines Krankenhaus, and Skoda, seeing his interest in diseases of the skin, turned over to him the entire division for skin diseases and encouraged him to study dermatology intensively.

Skoda's new division consisted mainly of patients suffering from scabies, and, in the first year of his incumbency, Hebra had 2,700 cases, of which 2,200 were scabies. However, in the course of time, he saw many skin diseases other than scabies and threw himself into the study of dermatology with great enthusiasm. The study of dermatology, as well as a reasonably clear idea of the classification of skin diseases, was practically non-existent in Vienna as elsewhere. Most skin diseases were considered to be the result of dyscrasias and, therefore, to be treated with laxatives and antimony; skin eruptions, ulcers and fistulae were thought to be due to impurities in the blood. Hebra began his work believing these theories correct but presently found by experience that they were false.

Scabies, he found, was not a dangerous humoral disease with metastases but a local, self-limited disease transmitted from person to person by the itch-mite, the destruction of which cured the disease. Eczema, he found, could be produced locally by certain irritants, notably croton oil, and could be healed by local therapy. He worked in close association with Skoda, the clinician, and Rokitansky, the pathologist, and acquired new knowledge and techniques.

His first book, *Versuch einer auf pathologische Anatomie gegründeten Eintheilung der Hautkrankheiten* (An attempt to classify skin diseases on the basis of pathological anatomy), which appeared in 1846, shows the influence of Rokitansky and is the first clear systematic classification of skin diseases based on the pathology of the lesions. He became *Primararzt* in 1848 and professor of dermatology in 1869. His reputation as a teacher and lecturer spread far and wide; students came from all over the world to study dermatology at Vienna.

His chief literary monument was his *Lehrbuch der Hautkrankheiten,* 1860-1876, a monumental textbook of skin diseases, the first part of which was written by Hebra himself but which was completed by his pupil, Kaposi. It was translated into English, French, Italian and Russian. Many honors and titles were bestowed on Hebra. He was elevated to the nobility and died in 1880.

The leading spirits of the New Vienna School—Rokitansky, Skoda and Hebra—drew other notable young men to Vienna, among them Joseph Hyrtl (1810-1894), the greatest teacher of gross anatomy in his time. Hyrtl was born in Eisenstadt, the son of a musician who came to Vienna as an oboist in the famous orchestra of Prince Esterhazy and later played in Haydn's orchestra. Young Hyrtl, himself, was very musical and was a chorister in his youth but chose a medical career, studied at Vienna, and, after graduation, was appointed prosector in anatomy. In 1837, he was named professor of anatomy at Prague but returned to Vienna in 1845 as the first professor of anatomy, holding this chair for 30 years, the most popular and fascinating lecturer on anatomy in all Europe. His lectures were concise, clear and interspersed with innumerable witty epigrams, classic quotations, and historical anecdotes.

In his teaching, Hyrtl followed the strict Vesalian tradition of gross anatomy, did not venture into histology, and made no great anatomical discoveries. His *Lehrbuch der Anatomie,* a text of gross anatomy, was first published in 1846, contained no illustrations until it reached its twentieth edition in 1880, but was immensely popular because of the author's remarkable style and interesting method of presentation. "Hyrtl," as Zuckerkandl remarked, "spoke like Cicero and wrote like Heine."

Hyrtl was also a philologist and a great scholar. After his retirement from his professorship in 1874, he wrote three masterpieces— on Arabic and Hebraic elements in anatomy *(Das Arabische und Hebräische in der Anatomie,* 1879), on anatomic terminology *(Onomatologia anatomica,* 1880), and on old German anatomical terminology *(Die alten deutschen Kunstworte der Anatomie,* 1884). "Hyrtl ranks with Émil Littré as one of the greatest of modern medical scholars" (Garrison).

Another notable character in Vienna at this period was the brilliant and unhappy Ignaz Philipp Semmelweis (1818-1865). Semmelweis was born in Ofen, Hungary, a town with a large German population, and his own family is thought to have been descended from German immigrants to that region. He spoke both Hungarian and German, but his Hungarian is said to have been tinged with a curious accent and his German very uncertain in its grammatical construction and orthography.

After studying law at Pest, he came to Vienna for a time as a law student, then returned to Pest, and came once more to Vienna in 1840, taking his medical degree in 1844. He decided to devote himself to obstetrics and, in 1846, became assistant in the First Obstetric Clinic at the Allgemeines Krankenhaus. He soon noted that the mortality rate in the first clinic was much higher than in the second clinic. In the first clinic, he further observed that the students often came directly from the autopsy room and made vaginal examinations without washing their hands, whereas, in the second clinic, devoted mainly to the instruction of midwives, much greater attention was given to personal cleanliness. Semmelweis noted also that the mothers who had their children while en route to the hospital rarely suffered from puerperal fever. In 1847, he was present at the autopsy of one of the professors, Prof. Kolletschka, who had died from infection, the result of a small scalpel wound received during an autopsy. Semmelweis noticed that the pathological findings were the same as those he had seen in so many postmortems of puerperal fever victims and became convinced that puerperal fever was due to infection transmitted to the mother by the unclean hands of the examining physician. He was also deeply perturbed by the conviction that he, himself, had caused the death of many of these unfortunate women.

Semmelweis now introduced in 1847 the regulation that all the attendants who examined pregnant women or attended them during labor must first wash their hands in a solution of calcium chloride. This was unquestionably the first application of antisepsis. The effect was astounding. The mortality, which in May had been 12.24 per cent, fell to 2.38 in June and to 1.20 in July. In March and April of the following year, there was not a single death from puerperal fever in the wards of the First Obstetrical Clinic.

Professor Klein, the chief of the clinic, was unimpressed by Semmelweis's observations and declared that the reduction in mortality was due to a change in the *Genius epidemicus*. Rokitansky, Skoda and Hebra, however, became vigorous champions of Semmelweis. Hebra published a paper in his *Zeitschrift der k. k. Gesellschaft der Ärzte* for December, 1847, describing the remarkable results obtained by Semmelweis. This paper begins with the observation that the editor of the journal, Dr. Hebra, "feels it is his duty to communicate to the medical profession . . . the following observations made by Dr. Semmelweis" and was the first publication on the subject. It unleashed a great controversy, with most of the obstetricians following the lead of Klein and either passing over the discovery in silence or attacking Semmelweis bitterly.

Semmelweis was admitted to the medical faculty as docent in 1850, and the catalogue for the winter semester of 1850-1851 announced his lectures "on obstetrics with practical demonstrations on the mannikin." But he suddenly left Vienna five days after his appointment and went to Budapest, where he received a hospital appointment and, in 1855, was appointed professor of theoretical and practical obstetrics in the University. In 1860, he published his first work on the subject, the immortal treatise, *Die Ätiologie, der Begriff und die Prophylaxis des Kindbettfiebers* (The Etiology, Concept, and Prophylaxis of Puerperal Fever), in which he not only presented his views but attacked his old enemies with renewed vigor. Battle was again joined, and the fight became fiercer after his scathing *Offener Brief an sämmtliche Professoren der Geburtschilfe,* 1862 (Open Letter to all Professors of Obstetrics).

In 1864, Semmelweis showed unmistakable signs of mental trouble and died the following year from an infected finger.

The New Vienna School did not, like the Old Vienna School, disappear from the stage of medical progress with the death of its leaders. Rokitansky, Skoda and Hebra did more than bring glory to the Vienna of their day. They left disciples who carried on their traditions of accuracy, industry and honesty throughout the century. Billroth, Toldt, Tandler, Zuckerkandl, Wenckebach, von Noorden, Escherich, von Eiselsberg, and von Pirquet were their spiritual heirs. Laryngoscopy was introduced by the New Vienna School as well as rhinoscopy. The specialties of ophthalmology, otology and laryngology were all created near the middle of the century and participated in the great spirit of scientific enthusiasm, which was the warp and woof of Vienna medicine. In the latter half of the nineteenth century, Vienna became the Mecca of young American doctors studying abroad, just as Paris once had been. The New Vienna School had left to its descendants, among other things, the precious heritage of excellent instruction.

THE RISE OF GERMAN MEDICINE

While Vienna was writing a brilliant chapter in the history of German medicine, a chapter ironically written not by Germans but mainly by Czechs and Hungarians, a new generation was growing up in Germany. This generation was slowly forgetting the miseries resulting from the Napoleonic wars and from the French occupation and was recovering from the offspring of this mental and physical degradation—the romantic, mystic and soothing precepts of *Naturphilosophie*. For a quarter of a century, German medicine had been groping along in the metaphysical fog of *Naturphilosophie*. The new generation turned from philosophizing about nature to the study of nature and, in time, shifted the center of medical activity to Berlin. Unlike French medicine and Austrian medicine, which were sharply circumscribed by the limits of Paris and of Vienna, German medicine was not limited to the confines of Berlin but soon spread to all Germany with the development of numerous centers of medical activity.

JOHANNES MÜLLER AND HIS PUPILS

The pioneer in this movement was Johannes Müller, born in Coblenz in 1801 while the town was occupied by French troops. His father was a cobbler, poor but not penniless, and, as his son early showed the unmistakable evidence of an unusual mind, he gave

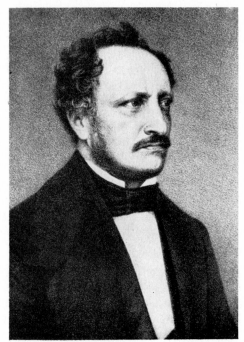

Sigerist, *Grosse Ärzte*, München, 1932

JOHANNES MÜLLER

"About his mouth with the drawn lips a trait of sternness, about the brow and eye the expression of profound thought, in every line of his face the remembrance of a complete work." (Virchow.)

him a good education. He matriculated at Bonn in 1819 with the idea of studying Roman Catholic theology but decided on medicine and, while still a student, won a prize for his essay on the respiration of the fetus. Like most students at Bonn, he was infected with the prevailing *Weltschmerz* and found much comfort in *Naturphilos-*

ophie. With increasing maturity, however, he wandered from natural philosophy into natural science, and his later work, with that of his pupils, did more than any one single factor to drive out the speculative *Naturphilosophie* and to replace it with the methods of accurate experimentation, followed by careful deduction.

He graduated at Bonn in 1822 and then spent a year and a half in Berlin with Rudolphi, who inspired him to devote his life to anatomy and also convinced him that experiment and observation, not philosophical speculation, were the keys which would unlock the mysteries of natural science. Freed, as it were, from the last vestiges of *Naturphilosophie,* Müller returned to Bonn, where he became successively *Privatdozent,* assistant professor, and professor of anatomy and physiology. On the death of Rudolphi, he went to Berlin in 1833 as his successor and as professor of anatomy, physiology and pathology. He held this post for 25 years until his sudden death in 1858.

Müller was an unusually stimulating and inspiring teacher, as well as a man of remarkable industry and versatility. He was equally eminent in biology, embryology, comparative anatomy, physiology, chemistry, psychology and pathology. He was the author of more than 200 articles and monographs. While he made no epochal discoveries, he enriched every field he touched.

In anatomy, he discovered the Müllerian duct, worked out the finer structure of glands, bones and cartilage, described the uriniferous capsule (also described by Bowman), and discovered the lymph heart in the frog. In physiology, he studied color sensation produced by pressure on the retina, studied the vocal cords and the voice, explained color contrasts, and formulated the Law of Specific Nerve Energy, i.e., that each sense organ, however it may be stimulated, produces it own peculiar sensation. In chemistry, he isolated chondrin and glutin. In pathology, he employed the microscope and called attention to the microscopic differences in the appearance of various tumors, but did not live to complete his work in this field. In 1834, he founded the *Archiv für Anatomie und Physiologie,* better known as *Müllers Archiv,* and, in 1833-1840 appeared his monumental *Handbuch der Physiologie des Menschen,* which contained many of his own and his pupils' discoveries reported for the first time and every statement in it is said to have been checked by the author's own experiments. This went through four editions. "It is a rich mine of novel facts and original ideas and introduces two new elements into physiology—the comparative and the psychologic" (Garrison).

Müller was a man of rare charm and magnetic personality. "He became," said Virchow,

as he had said of his predecessors, an abiding priest of nature; the cult which he served also bound his pupils to him, as if by a religious bond; and the earnest priestly manner of his speech and movements completed the impression of reverence with which everyone looked up to him. About his mouth with the drawn lips a trait of sternness, about the brow and eye the expression of profound thought, in every line of his face the remembrance of a complete work—so stood this man before the altar of nature, freed by his own strength from the fetters of training and tradition, a witness of personal independence.

Müller shared with Bernard the reputation of being the greatest physiologist of his time. Yet, Bernard left no great pupils and no disciples; he was the last of his line. By contrast, Müller was the first of his line, his pupils bringing great honor to their master as well as to themselves. Among them were Schwann, Henle, du Bois-Reymond, Virchow and Helmholtz, each a great man in his own right, who had a powerful influence upon the later course of German and of world medicine, the germ of whose work we usually find in some earlier experiment, thought, or stimulus of which Müller was the father.

Johannes Müller had a definite mystical element in his nature and, as a young professor in Bonn, published in 1826 a remarkable work on apparitions, *Phantastische Gesichtserscheinungen*. He was also a deep student of philosophy, which colored his biological and physiological thinking. He was a firm believer in "Vitalism" and shared Stahl's view that a reasoning soul is the *primum movens* of life and that "the structure of the forms of nature has not arisen through chance . . . it has proceeded from the creative spirit of God." He drew a sharp distinction between organic substances which were imbued with life and inorganic, or dead, chemical compounds. These "vitalistic" views were combated by the "physical" school, which showed that many processes of life explained on a vitalistic basis were capable of explanation by physical and chemical phenomena. A leader in this school was Ludwig, an outstanding rival of Müller in the field of physiology.

CARL LUDWIG

Carl Ludwig (1816-1895) was a native of Witzenhausen, graduated at Marburg in 1839, and was prosector and professor there until

1849, 10 fruitful years. During this period, he worked on the secretion of the urine and stated his well-known theory that the glomerular epithelium acts as a passive filter, a theory still accepted by most physiologists. In 1847, he invented the kymograph, that indispensable instrument of physiological research employing this instrument in his fundamental studies of the circulation. He was professor in Zürich from 1849 until 1855, and in Vienna from 1855 until 1865. During the Viennese period, he studied the gases of the blood and described his well-known *Stromuhr*. Under his direction, his pupil Cloetta discovered inosite, taurin, leucin, and uric acid in the animal body. In 1865, he was called to Leipzig, where his Physiological Institute soon became the Mecca of Europe for students of physiology from all over the world. It has been estimated that at least 200 men, who later became prominent scientists, were pupils of Ludwig.

In his inaugural address at Leipzig, Ludwig described his method of perfusing organs outside the body, another epochal contribution to physiological methods. However, most of Ludwig's energies there were directed towards stimulating his students, many of whom, according to von Kries, sat in the window while Ludwig and his assistant carried out the experiments. Ludwig planned the experiments in the laboratory, often carried them out himself, usually wrote the draft of the report, and then published it under the pupil's name.

"All who met Ludwig," wrote Kronecker, "came under the influence of his enchanting personality." He was genial, kindly, sympathetic, and utterly free from selfish aims and ambitions. He was a splendid draftsman and a passionate lover of music. All of his pupils revered his memory and never tired of recalling his charming personality and innate honesty.

Another contemporary whose work touched medicine at many points and left its impression was Justus Liebig (1803-1873), the chemist. He was a native of Darmstadt who, after studying chemistry at Bonn and Erlangen, went to Paris, where he studied in the laboratory of Gay-Lussac. Returning to Germany, he decided to become a teacher of chemistry and was appointed associate professor of chemistry at Giessen in 1824 and, two years later, became full professor. He persuaded the government to provide a laboratory for instruction in chemistry. This laboratory, unique at the time as the first university laboratory of chemistry, together with Liebig's unrivaled gifts as a teacher, drew throngs of enthusiastic hard-working students and soon became the most famous chemical school in the world.

Here Liebig made many important discoveries in inorganic chemistry, devised new methods of organic analysis, discovered hippuric acid, chloral and chloroform, studied uric acid, devised a method of estimating urea, and carried out investigations on blood, fat, bile,

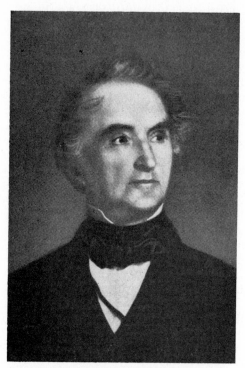

JUSTUS VON LIEBIG

and meat juice. In opposition to many physicians of the time, he taught that animal heat was the result of combustion and oxidation in the body. His book, *Die organische Chemie in ihrer Anwendung auf Physiologie und Pathologie* (Organic Chemistry in its Application to Physiology and Pathology), published in 1842, was the first book on the subject and introduced the concept of metabolism (*Stoffwechsel*).

Liebig studied fermentation and putrefaction, but his results were vitiated by a materialistic conception of the processes as catalytic processes and his disbelief in such living agencies as bacteria or living ferments. Pasteur, after proving that a few yeast cells when placed in a solution of sugar multiplied and fermented the solution, went to Liebig's laboratory to discuss the experiments. Pasteur relates, "The tall old man in a long frock coat received me with kindly courtesy," but, when he tried to discuss the matter, Liebig, "without losing his amenity, refused all discussion, alleging indisposition" (Vallery-Radot).

In 1845, Liebig was created a baron and, in 1852, went to Munich as professor of chemistry, remaining there until his death in 1873. Most of his best work was done in Giessen and published in the *Annalen der Pharmazie*, later the *Annalen der Chemie und Pharmacie*, a journal he founded in 1832.

One of the most famous papers in the history of chemistry, that on benzaldehydes, was published in 1832 by Liebig in collaboration with Wöhler. Friedrich Wöhler (1820-1882) was a graduate of Heidelberg, later a student of Berzelius, and from 1836 to 1882 professor of chemistry at Göttingen. In 1824, when 24 years of age, he discovered that benzoic acid taken with food appears in the urine as hippuric acid, a fundamental discovery in physiological chemistry, since it showed that animals, as well as plants, can synthetize complex chemical substances. Four years later, he made one of the striking chemical discoveries of the century—the synthesis of urea by heating ammonium cyanate. This was the first time an organic substance had been formed from an inorganic compound without the intervention of any vitalistic process and was a severe blow to the "Vitalists," as it indicated a complete similarity between the structural chemistry of life and of inanimate nature.

JOHANN LUCAS SCHÖNLEIN

While Johannes Müller was laying the foundation of scientific medicine in Germany, Johann Lucas Schönlein was performing the same service in clinical medicine. Like Müller, he came from outside Berlin, his father being an artisan. Unlike Müller, who was a voluminous writer, Schönlein, aside from his doctor's dissertation, published only two papers—one of three pages, the other 20 lines. His *Allgemeine und Specielle Pathologie und Therapie,* which was first published at Würzburg in 1832 and passed through six editions, was, as stated on the title-page, "written down from his lectures and published by some of his hearers." His great influence

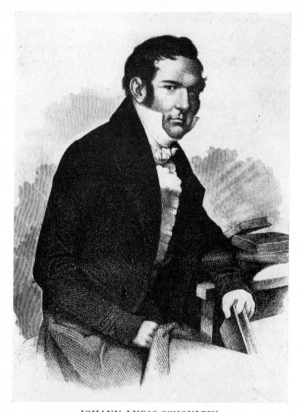

JOHANN LUCAS SCHÖNLEIN
Engraving by Karl Meyer. (From Schönlein, J. L., *Allgemeine und specielle Pathologie und Therapie,* St. Gallen, Litteratur–Comptoir, 1841.)

was wielded not by his writings but by his lectures, clinical demonstrations, and methods of examining patients. He was indisputably the founder of modern German clinical medicine.

Schönlein was born in Bamberg in 1793, the son of a rope-maker and, in 1811, entered the University of Landshut, where he found *Naturphilosophie* and *Brunonism* struggling for the medical souls of the students. Here also he found von Walther, who taught that medicine "can make true progress only by employing physics, chemistry, and all the natural sciences." Walther later went to Bonn, where he taught the same precepts to young Johannes Müller.

From Landshut, Schönlein went to Würzburg, where he received his doctor's degree in 1816. His doctor's dissertation, *Von der Hirn-metamorphose* (Concerning metamorphosis of the brain), 140 pages long, showed, as Virchow remarks, "a certain natur-philosophical tint, particularly such sentences as 'Light in wedlock with water gives birth to the organic. While the spherical form of the priestly green material becomes algae, the infusoria takes the form of zo-ophytes'!" Schönlein became *Privatdozent* at Würzburg in 1817 and professor of medicine in 1824.

During this period, Schönlein, influenced by de Candolle, the Swiss botanist who had founded a "natural" botanical classifica-tion as opposed to Linné's "artificial" classification, became the founder of the so-called Natural History School, one ambition of which was to classify disease as botany classified plants and zoology classified animals. This system led Schönlein to the classification of tuberculosis and phthisis as separate families, gangrene of the uterus and hydrocephalus as members of the same family of "neurophlogases," and to other patent absurdities.

The new Natural History School, which had now broken with *Naturphilosophie*, accomplished much more than this arbitrary and somewhat ridiculous classification of diseases. Schönlein introduced the new methods of percussion and auscultation into his clinic; the microscope took its place by the bedside; and the urine and blood of the patients were examined both microscopically and chemically. Students swarmed in great numbers to his clinic. One of his old students wrote enthusiastically, "Has he not made Würzburg a place of pilgrimage for German physicians, just as Rome is for artists. . . . Schönlein has left no writings, but his words will remain immortal."

From Würzburg, Schönlein went to Zürich in 1833 as professor of medicine, from Zürich in 1839 to Berlin. There he revitalized and quickened the medical clinic, as he had in Würzburg and in Zürich, and his lectures and clinics were thronged with enthusiastic students and young doctors. He suffered from a goitre for years, his health becoming so poor in 1859 that he resigned and went to his old home in Bamberg, where he died in 1864.

Schönlein was the first to describe *peliosis rheumatica,* or Schön-lein's disease, and discovered the parasitic nature of favus. His literary activity, however, pales beside his great capacity as a teacher and organizer. His medical career was a series of interesting transi-tions. He began as an adherent of *Naturphilosophie,* but, finding its speculations sterile and leading to no real enlightenment in medi-cine, he founded his Natural History School. Here he attempted to fit all diseases into the strait jacket of his new classification, but, with further study of natural history, which his school claimed as its *leitmotiv,* he saw the futility of the plan of "systems" and realized that medicine was built on a foundation of facts and experience. During his Berlin period, the general verdict on his teaching, according to Virchow, was "little system, many facts."

One of Johannes Müller's pupils who attained great fame during the lifetime of the master was Theodor Schwann (1810-1882), the co-founder of the cell-theory, one of the greatest biological discoveries of all time. Schwann was born in Neuss, a town in the Rhineland near Düsseldorf, and studied at Würzburg under Schönlein, in Bonn under Müller, and again under Müller in Berlin. After graduation at Berlin in 1834, he was appointed assistant in the Anatomical Museum. In Berlin, he was in close and constant contact with Müller, Henle, and Matthias Schleiden, a young man who had studied law and had practiced it in Hamburg but who had become dissatisfied with that profession and was now studying botany in Berlin. Later, Schleiden became a noted botanist and professor at Jena.

In 1838, Schleiden published in *Müllers Archiv* a paper, *Beiträge zur Phytogenesis,* in which he pointed out that all plants are formed of cells and that they grow through changes which take place in their nuclei. The following year, Schwann published an extensive monograph, *Mikroskopische Untersuchungen über die Uebereinstimmung in der Struktur und dem Wachsthum der Thiere und Planzen* (Microscopic Investigations on the Accordance in the Structure and Growth of Plants and Animals), describing his observation that both animal and vegetable tissues are composed of cells and that the cells of each tissue have a characteristic appearance. Both Schleiden and Schwann published their papers at about the same time, and the discovery is usually referred to as the Schleiden-Schwann cell-theory.

Cells of plants had been seen as early as the seventeenth century by Robert Hooke (1665), Malpighi (1675), and Nehemiah Grew (1682), and the cell nucleus by the botanist, Robert Brown, in 1831. Müller, Henle and Purkinje had described cells in animal tissues. Indeed, Oken in 1805, Mirbel in 1808, Lamarck in 1809, Dutrochet in 1824, Turpin in 1826, and Meyen in 1828, according to Karling and Conklin, all antedated both Schleiden and Schwann in this discovery. However, the observation of Schleiden and Schwann had a much more powerful impact upon the scientific thought of this period and they have been usually described as the discoverers of the cell theory, even though subsequent investigations have shown that they really share this distinction with others.

During the five years of association with Müller, Schwann made several capital discoveries. He showed that air was necessary for the development of the embryo and that putrefaction was caused by living bodies which could be destroyed by heat. He described the sheath of the axis cylinder of nerves, demonstrated striped muscle in the upper part of the esophagus, showed that the yeast plant causes fermentation which can be prevented by heating the culture medium, and discovered pepsin in the stomach. Later, in 1841, while at Louvain, he showed that bile is essential to proper digestion.

Following the publication of his *Mikroskopische Untersuchungen* in 1839, Schwann went to Louvain as professor of anatomy, then in 1848 to Liège, where he taught until 1880, when he retired. He died in 1882. From the viewpoint of scientific activity, the 40 years spent in Belgium contrast unfavorably with the five years in Berlin. He probably missed the masterly directing hand of Müller and the stimulating atmosphere breathed by Müller's pupils.

Jacob Henle, one of Müller's favorite pupils, is often described as one of the great anatomists of all time and as the man who rendered to microscopic anatomy, the same service that Vesalius performed for gross anatomy. Henle was born in Fürth in 1809, the son of a prosperous mechant, and received an excellent education. He studied medicine in Bonn, where he joined a *Burschenschaft,* a student organization which was considered radical since it was liberal in its political principles, worked for the unification of Germany, and fought the despotic power wielded by some of the princes ruling the numerous German principalities and dukedoms. Here he also met Johannes Müller, who was much impressed by the young man, who, in turn, was inspired and charmed, as all others were who came in contact with the master.

Afterwards Henle went to Heidelberg, where he received his degree in 1832, took a trip to Paris with Müller, and then went to Berlin to take his state examination. Meanwhile, Müller had been called to Berlin, and Henle, deciding to remain there with his old teacher, made application for an appointment as *Privatdozent.* Ordinarily this was a routine matter, but, in Henle's case, his old connection with the *Burschenschaft* was brought up, and his appointment seemed doubtful until Alexander von Humboldt successfully intervened. Henle remained but two years in Berlin working with Müller and Schwann, but they were remarkably fruitful years.

During this period, Henle published in 1840 his remarkable monograph, *Von den Miasmen und Contagien und von den miasmatisch-contagiösen Krankheiten* (On Miasmas and Contagions and concerning miasmatic-contagious Diseases), "which contains the first clear statement of a *contagium animatum*" (Garrison). In this work, after reviewing the studies of Schwann on yeast fermentation, of Bassi on silk worm disease, and of many others, he concluded, "The material of contagions is not only an organic but a *living* one and is indeed endowed with a life of its own, which is, in relation to the diseased body, a *parasitic organism.*"

Henle discussed smallpox, rabies, syphilis, tuberculosis and exanthemata and points out that they are best explained on the basis of this theory. He studied the exudates in various diseases and saw "vibrions," infusoria, and many microscopic forms of life but was unable to assign an etiological role to them. His paper is now considered a landmark in the history of bacteriology; at the time, however, it attracted little attention.

In 1840 at the age of 30, Henle left Berlin to become professor of anatomy at Zürich. He remained there four years, leaving to go to Heidelberg, where he was professor eight years. From Heidelberg, he was called to Göttingen in 1852. Three years later, he was offered, after the death of Müller, the post of his old master but declined, remaining in Göttingen, fresh, active and vigorous until his death in 1884 at the age of 75. Like his friend Schwann, Henle did some of his best work in Berlin as a young man. Unlike Schwann, his productivity seemed to increase with the years, his last paper being published only six months before his death.

Henle was a great figure in medicine who, as an investigator, practically created the science of histology and who, as a teacher, inspired generations of students with remarkably clear, penetrating, fascinating and interesting lectures and demonstrations. In his *Habilitations-schrift,* presented when he was appointed *Privatdozent,* he was the first to describe the epithelium of the skin and intestines, to define columnar and ciliated epithelium, and to point out the importance of epithelium as the lining membrane of all free surfaces of the body and of its tubes and cavities.

In 1841 his *Allgemeine Anatomie* was published, the first systematic treatise on microscopic anatomy. In this, he describes many of his important discoveries. His larger *Systematische Anatomie,* 1866-1871, is an exhaustive three volume scientific treatise of the highest order, describing many of Henle's own discoveries and illustrated with drawings by Henle himself. In the field of pathology, he wrote a *Handbuch der rationellen Pathologie,* 1846-1853, which, like all his books, is a mine of information. During his Zürich period, Henle founded in 1842, with his friend Pfeufer, the *Zeitschrift für rationelle Medizin,* which was published until 1869 and, during these years, contained some of the best scientific work in medicine of that period.

Henle was a skillful artist, drawing his own illustrations for his articles and books and using this gift to illustrate his inspiring lec-

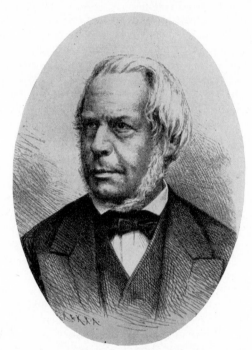

Sigerist, *Grosse Ärzte*, München, 1932

JACOB HENLE

tures. He was also an accomplished musician, playing the violin, viola and violincello so well that he could, at a moment's notice, take his place in any string quartet. Personally, he was much loved for his charm, modesty, and innate integrity.

For 23 years, Johannes Müller occupied three academic chairs simultaneously. He was professor of anatomy, physiology and pathology. Two years before his death, the chair of pathology passed to one of his students, Virchow. After his death, two more of his pupils were rewarded—Reichert became professor of anatomy, and du Bois-Reymond professor of physiology.

Karl Bogislaus Reichert (1811-1884) was a native of Rastenburg in East Prussia, who, after studying at Königsberg as a pupil of von Baer, "the father of embryology," went to Berlin, where he came under the influence of Johannes Müller and, on the departure of Henle in 1840, became prosector at the Anatomical Institute. He went to Dorpat three years later as professor of anatomy, then to Breslau, and, on the death of Müller in 1858, returned to Berlin as professor of anatomy, where he remained until his death. He made many contributions to the histology of organs and of tissues and introduced the cell theory into embryology, proving that the segments of the fertilized ovum in the "mulberry" stage develop into cells and that all the organs develop from these cells. He was a very popular teacher but, in later life, lost some of his standing among biologists by his opposition to the Darwinian hypothesis of evolution and to the doctrine of transmutation.

Emil du Bois-Reymond was born in Berlin in 1818, the son of a French Swiss father from Neufchâtel and of a mother descended from a French Huguenot family who had taken refuge in Germany after revocation of the Edict of Nantes. Du Bois-Reymond studied at the Collège Français in Berlin, later at Neufchâtel, and, at the age of 18, entered the University of Berlin as a student of philosophy. Later he turned to the natural sciences, became pupil of and later assistant to Müller, who directed his interest to the study of electro-physiological problems. His doctor's dissertation was on the subject of electrical fishes. He now devoted all of his energies to the study of electro-physiological problems, and in 1848 appeared the first volume of his *Untersuchungen über thierische Elektricität* (Investigations on animal electricity), which marked the creation of a new science—electrophysiology, the physics of muscles and nerves. In 1858, when he became professor of physiology, a new laboratory was built for him, the finest and most complete of its time, where he worked until his death in 1896.

In addition to his numerous physiological studies, du Bois-Reymond wrote many fascinating essays and biographical studies. These showed much erudition and were written with that rare combination—French clarity of presentation combined with German thoroughness in preparation.

Karl von Vierordt (1818-1884), although never having enjoyed the close association with Johannes Müller that had been the privilege of Schwann, Henle and du Bois-Reymond, nevertheless was Müller's pupil at Berlin in the years of 1839 and 1840. In addition to studying under Müller in Berlin, where he also attended the clinics of Schönlein, he studied in Göttingen under Wöhler, who first synthetized urea, and learned physical diagnosis under Skoda and pa-

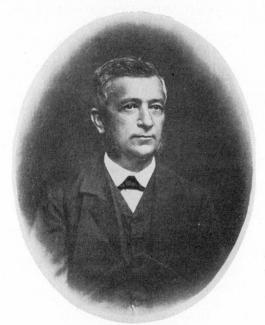

von Vierordt, *Die Schall-und Tonstaerke*, Tübingen, 1885

KARL VIERORDT

thology under Rokitansky in Vienna. In Heidelberg, where he received his degree in 1841, he had as teachers Gmelin and Tiedemann, the chemists, Naegele, the obstetrician, and Chelius, the surgeon.

A native of Baden, where he was born in the little town of Lahr, he began practice at Karlsruhe in 1842, but also found time for investigation and published a paper on strabismus and on respiration. Both papers attracted much attention, and, in 1849, he was called to Tübingen as associate professor of theoretical medicine. Henceforth his life for 35 years was closely bound up with the fortunes of that little Swabian university.

In 1852, Vierordt published in the *Archiv für physiologische Heilkunde* an important paper on a *Neue Methode der quantativen mikroskopischen Analyse des Blutes* (New Method of Quantitative Microscopic Analysis of the Blood), in which he described the first exact method of counting the blood cells. He employed a graduated capillary tube to measure the exact amount of blood used. This blood was then dropped upon a glass plate covered with a thin film of egg albumin and allowed to dry. A micrometer, marked in squares, was placed over the dried film, and the erythrocytes counted under the microscope. He states in a second paper on this subject that a blood count made upon himself on October 6, 1851, showed 5,010,000 red cells per cubic millimeter.

In 1853, he became professor of physiology at Tübingen and, the same year, demonstrated at the annual meeting of the *"Naturforscher"* a sphygmograph, the first instrument with which a tracing of the human pulse could be made. By adding weights to little pans attached to a lever, he attempted to estimate the blood pressure. His instrument was cumbersome and his measurements were inexact, but he established the principle that the estimation of the blood pressure can be accomplished by measuring the outside pressure necessary to obliterate the pulse—the method we employ today.

Every year important papers came from his pen. He studied the rate of the blood flow in 1858, giving figures that are still quoted. In 1868, he studied the sensation of time, time perception, and speed perception, the first accurate observations in a field later known as physiological psychology. In 1875, he applied the principles of spectral analysis to the study of urine, blood and bile. And, during the last years of his life, he made fundamental observations on the intensity and conduction of sound.

Vierordt has suffered from a certain neglect at the hands of medical historians, but every physician who makes a blood count, estimates the hemoglobin, and takes the blood pressure owes a great debt to the patient, accurate and modest physiologist of Tübingen. His industry found expression in his advice to students: "Make it a rule to say as rarely as possible, *'Diem perdidi'* (I have lost a day)."

HERMANN VON HELMHOLTZ

One of the most brilliant of all the remarkable pupils of Johannes Müller was Hermann von Helmholtz. He was born in Potsdam near

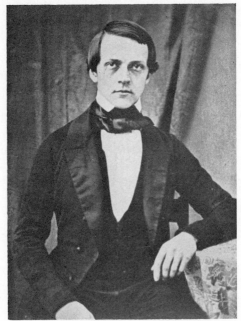

Koenigsberger, *Hermann von Helmholtz*, Oxford, 1906

HERMANN VON HELMHOLTZ

The photograph shows Helmholtz at the age of twenty-seven, one year after the publication of his memoir on the conservation of energy.

Berlin in 1821, the son of a teacher in the Gymnasium, a very intelligent and cultured man. His mother was the daughter of a Hanoverian artillery officer named Penne, a lineal descendant of William Penn, the great Quaker, who founded Pennsylvania, and his maternal grandmother was of French descent. Thus, German, English and French blood flowed in his veins. He was a precocious child, learned languages at an early age, reading Homer in the original Greek and the fables of Luqmān in the original Arabic when 12 years of age. He also showed unusual mathematical ability when very young.

As a youth, Helmholtz wished to devote his life to the study of physics, but his father pointed out their slender financial resources and persuaded his son to study medicine instead. So, Helmholtz was admitted as a bursary student at the Friedrich-Wilhelm Institut

in Berlin, an institution for the education of Prussian army surgeons. The students at the Institute attended the regular courses
at the University, so Helmholtz became another pupil of Johannes
Müller. In later years, Helmholtz said,

> I recall my student days and the impression made upon us by a man
> like Johannes Müller, the physiologist. When one feels himself in contact
> with a man of the first order, the entire scale of his intellectual conception
> is modified for life; contact with such a man is perhaps the most interesting
> thing life has to offer.

Receiving his medical degree in 1842, he described in his doctor's
thesis an important discovery—the anatomical connection between
nerve cells and the nerves themselves. After graduation, he served
for a time as an army surgeon in Potsdam, but Alexander von Humboldt, recognizing his unusual ability, succeeded in having him
released from military duties, and he was appointed assistant in the
Anatomical Museum, lecturer on anatomy at the Academy of Art,
and associate professor of physiology at the University. At this time,
he carried out some important experiments on fermentation, showing that living organisms in the air and in yeast cause fermentation
and putrefaction. The following year, he proved that animal heat,
produced by muscular contraction, arises from chemical phenomena
occurring in the muscle.

In 1847, in his twenty-sixth year, Helmholtz read before the
Physical Society of Berlin his famous essay, *Über die Erhaltung der
Kraft* (On the conservation of energy), one of the epoch-making
scientific papers of the century. He showed mathematically that all
forms of energy, such as heat, light, electricity, and chemical phenomena, can be transformed from one form to another but are in-
destructible as well as impossible of creation. He proclaimed as the
fundamental principle of physics the conservation of energy, just
as Lavoisier had previously shown that the fundamental principle
of chemistry was the persistence of matter. Unknown to Helmholtz
Robert Mayer had previously expounded this principle, but with
so little experimental proof that it had no influence on science. "The
science of energy would have progressed much as it had done had
Mayer never lived" (McKendrick).

This paper established Helmholtz's reputation as a scientist. In
1849, he was appointed professor of physiology and pathology at
the University of Königsberg, where he spent six busy years. In
1850, he measured the velocity of the nerve impulse although his
old teacher, Johannes Müller, had stated 10 years previously, "We
shall probably never attain the power of measuring the velocity

of nervous action." Another great achievement of the Königsberg years was Helmholtz's invention of the ophthalmoscope in 1851, an instrument which revolutionized ophthalmology and was of untold value in medical diagnosis. He followed this with the invention in 1852 of the phakoscope, an instrument for studying the changes in the lens during accommodation, and the ophthalmometer, an instrument for measuring the refractive powers of the eye. With these instruments as his tools, he began an intensive study of the mechanism of accommodation and initiated the studies which later found expression in his *Handbuch der physiologischen Optik,* 1856-1866. While in Königsberg, he also began his investigations on color sensation, examined carefully the color theory of Thomas Young, and, in later researches, concluded that there are three fundamental color sensations—red, green and blue. This theory is now universally known as the Young-Helmholtz theory of color sensation.

Helmholtz went to Bonn as professor of physiology in 1856. Here he became interested in the subject of hearing, studied the anatomy and the mechanism of the ear, and began his researches on sound. After three years in Bonn, he went to Heidelberg, where he continued his studies on sound and published in 1863 his great work, *Die Lehre von den Tonempfindungen,* which remains today a fundamental work on the physics and physiology of sound.

In 1871, he was called to Berlin as professor of physics. After more than 30 years, he had realized his youthful ambition to become a physicist. True, during all the years of his activity, his physiological researches had been dominated by a physical concept, but now he was at last free to devote himself wholly to physics. He made further fundamental discoveries in thermo-dynamics, in electro-dynamics, in physical optics, and in sound. He received innumerable honors and the insignia of various orders and was ennobled by Wilhelm I. In his later years, he traveled extensively in Europe, visited the Chicago Exposition in 1893, and saw the natural scenery of the United States and Canada. He died in 1894.

During his entire scientific life, Helmholtz was, he tells us, deeply influenced by Müller's doctrine of specific nerve energy. He never lost his interest in medicine despite his preoccupation with physical problems; and, in his address on *Das Denken in der Medicin* (Thought in Medicine), delivered in 1877, he made the oft-quoted statement: "Medicine was once the intellectual home in which I grew up; and even the immigrant best understands and is best understood by his native land." All of his contemporaries testify to his absolute sincerity, his amazing natural intelligence, his courteous manners, his personal charm, and his nobility of character. The scope of his knowledge and the breadth of his scientific activities and achievements raise him to the rank of one of the greatest minds of his century.

RUDOLF VIRCHOW

In Hermann Helmholtz, Johannes Müller had trained one of the greatest minds of the period. In Rudolf Virchow, he trained a man who was unquestionably the outstanding physician of his generation, a man who stands aloof in the select company of Hippocrates, Galen, Morgagni, Auenbrugger and Laennec. He was the creator of the modern science of pathology, in which subject he had among his precursors only one rival, Morgagni, and among his successors none.

Rudolf Virchow was born in Schievelbein in Pomerania in 1821, the son of an official. After finishing the Gymnasium as Köslin, he came to Berlin in 1839 and entered the Friedrich Wilhelm Institut, taking his medical courses at the University. Virchow's letters written to his parents describe with vividness the life of a German student at that time and tell how he received his degree on October 21, 1843, from the hands of "the dean of the medical faculty, the most famous physiologist in the world, Johannes Müller." Young Virchow was appointed Frorieps' prosector at the Charité in 1845, became full prosector and began teaching courses in pathological anatomy in 1846. He was released from military service, became a *Privatdozent* in 1847, and, the same year, founded with Benno Reinhardt, another young physician, the journal since known as *Virchows Archiv*. In the first issue, he wrote,

The point of view which we shall take and whose aim appears in the first issue is simply that of natural science. Practical medicine as applied to theoretical medicine, theoretical medicine as to pathological physiology is the ideal for which we shall strive insofar as our strength permits. Pathological anatomy and clinical medicine, whose justification and independence we fully recognize, are valuable to us particularly as the sources of new problems whose answers lie in pathological physiology.

So spake the young man of 26. This ideal of the close union of clinical medicine, pathological anatomy and physiology, he followed until he closed his eyes at the age of 81.

In 1848, a commission of which Virchow was a member was sent to investigate the epidemic of typhus fever raging in Silesia. He saw that the epidemic was largely the result of the miserable conditions under which the workers lived and worked. His report was a severe indictment of the government for permitting such conditions to exist, noting, "The proletariat is the result, principally, of the introduction and improvement of machinery" and adding, "Shall the triumph of human genius lead to nothing more than to make the human race miserable?" This report did not please the government, and Virchow further incurred official displeasure by his action in helping construct some barricades during the Berlin uprising of 1848 and his participation in a movement of physicians to appoint a minister of health and to secure greater professional rights for doctors. He received notice from the Minister of Health that he was relieved of his official duties; later he was informed that he was still the prosector but must give up his room and board. At this juncture, a call came from the University of Würzburg to become professor of pathology. He accepted promptly.

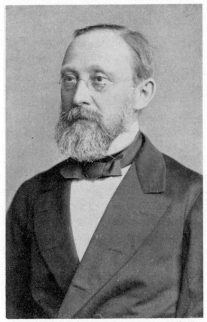

Photograph in University of Kansas Collection

RUDOLF VIRCHOW

Virchow went to Würzburg in 1849 and remained there seven years. Here he established a brilliant reputation as a teacher and added to this reputation by writing numerous articles. In 1856, a separate chair of pathological anatomy was established in Berlin. He was called to the position and returned to Berlin as a full professor and director of the new Pathological Institute, which had just been completed. He remained in Berlin until his death.

In 1858, Virchow published his unforgettable *Cellularpathologie,* one of the great books in medicine. Morgagni had pointed out the importance in pathology of an organ as the seat of disease; Bichat had celled attention to the importance of the tissues; Virchow now pointed out the fundamental role of the cell. In the preface to his book, Virchow presents the new view "of the cellular nature of all life-processes, both physiological and pathological . . . in opposition to the humoral and solidar views which have been transplanted from the myths of antiquity down to our own time." He states his famous dictum—*Omnis cellula e cellula* (Every cell from a cell), that every "pathological form has its physiological prototype" *(Jedes pathologische Gebilde hat ein physiologisches Vorbild)*—in other words, pathological cells are derived from and are only modifications of physiologic types, "every form of new growth . . . assumes preexisting cellular elements as its origin."

This work caused a revolution in medical thinking. Diseases no longer had a personal individuality; a ruling *Archaeus,* in the terminology of van Helmont and the age-old theories of humors and crases, now seemed childish and foolish. Organic diseases were due to pathological lesions formed by pathological cells, which arose from normal physiological cells as the result of irritation or stimulation. In a brief time, the medical world *in toto* became disciples of Virchow.

His book on tumors, *Die krankhaften Geschwülste* (1863-1867), was a study from the morphologic standpoint. It is a mine of information, is the model for all later works on the subject, and can still be read with great profit. A very large number of tumors are described and named here for the first time. Virchow's later studies on embolism and thrombosis and on endocarditis were also epochal.

The following 44 years of Virchow's life were years of intense activity. He lectured, performed autopsies, worked at his microscope, and edited his *Archiv,* in which he published hundreds of communications on a variety of medical, anthropological and historical topics. He became well known as an anthropologist, as an archeologist, as a sanitarian who secured a good sewage system for Berlin, and as an "old parliamentary hand," serving from 1880 until 1893 in the Reichstag, where, as a liberal, he was recognized in political circles as an able and often effective opponent of Bismarck. He also found time to write historical and biographical articles, his essays on Morgagni, Müller and Schönlein being especially noteworthy.

It has often been said that Virchow in his youth was a liberal in politics; whereas, in his old age, he became a reactionary in science. Yet, while he often seemed prejudiced in his views as he grew older, he was open-minded and generous when proved wrong. His seventieth and eightieth birthdays were the occasions of celebrations in which scientists from the entire world took part. His death in 1902 marked the close of a long life of phenomenal activity.

THE ADVANCE OF SCIENCE AND MEDICINE IN GREAT BRITAIN

While science and medicine were advancing on the Continent by leaps and bounds, Britain was by no means playing the role of a passive bystander. She also produced some outstanding scientists in the fields of chemistry and physics and a group of distinguished physicians and surgeons.

Humphry Davy (1778-1829), the son of a poor woodcarver, was early in life apprenticed to a surgeon-apothecary. At the age of 19, he obtained a position at the Medical Pneumatic Institution of Bristol, an institution which had been established by Dr. Thomas Beddoes to investigate the medicinal properties of various gases. The following year, Davy discovered that nitrous oxide was respirable and produced great exhilaration. This discovery attracted much attention, so, when Benjamin Thompson, Count Rumford, established the Royal Institution, Davy was chosen as lecturer on chemistry. A few years later, a young man named Michael Faraday (1791-1867), who had been apprenticed to a book binder, where he read the scientific books his master bound, enrolled in Davy's class in chemistry. He later became Davy's assistant and, on Davy's death, professor of chemistry.

Davy's studies with gases led to the development in 1816 of the Davy safety lamp, an oil lamp covered with wire gauze, this wire gauze absorbing the heat of the flames so that it did not cause an explosion when brought into contact with an inflammable gas. This type of lamp has since been extensively employed in coal mines.

"If Count Rumford's establishment, the Royal Institution," said Lenard, "had no other result than to provide a working place for Davy and Faraday, this would have brilliantly justified for all time the establishment of the institute." Davy's investigations were mainly in the field of electro-chemistry and gases. In his *Researches, Chemical and Philosophical, chiefly concerning Nitrous Oxide . . .*, published in 1799, he described not only the exhilarating effect of the gas but also its anesthetic properties, and suggested its use in surgical operations. Davy, in collaboration with Faraday, also made fundamental investigations on the liquefaction of gases. In 1831, Faraday gained scientific immortality by his discovery of electro-magnetic induction and by the invention of the induction coil. The term, "faradic," has since been employed for an induced current.

John Dalton (1766-1844), the son of a poor farmer, himself a farm laborer and then a school teacher, made fundamental studies on the properties of gases. He also described color blindness and made important contributions to the atomic theory, working out a table of atomic weights. His great merits won increasing appreciation so that, at the time of his death, this man, whose formal schooling ceased at the age of 11, was a D.C.L. of Oxford, a LL.D. of Edinburgh, a fellow of the Royal Society, and a member of the Royal Academies of Science of Paris, Berlin and Munich.

Among the eminent men of science was also Richard Owen (1804-1892), who studied medicine first at Edinburgh and then at St. Bartholomew's Hospital, London, where he came under the influence of John Abernethy, the eminent surgeon. He, himself, planned to become a surgeon and accepted an appointment as assistant curator of the museum of the Royal College of Surgeons. He spent several years cataloguing and studying the Hunterian Collection and acquired an unrivaled knowledge of comparative anatomy. He became subsequently professor at the Royal College, conservator of the museum, and, in 1856, superintendent of the natural history department of the British Museum. He wrote many papers on comparative anatomy, on fossils, on mammals, and on prehistoric animals. He was one of the founders of modern comparative anatomy.

CHARLES DARWIN

In 1859, Charles Darwin published his *On the Origin of the Species*. Few books in the history of science have had more influence upon biology, philosophy, religion and sociology. Darwin, who was born in Shrewsbury in 1809, the son of a doctor and the grandson of Dr. Erasmus Darwin, was a "truant" from both medicine and theology, having studied medicine at Edinburgh and theology at Cambridge. From 1831 to 1836, he went on the brig, the "Beagle," as naturalist with a surveying expedition to several Atlantic islands, the coast of South America, and islands in the Pacific and Indian Ocean. This long voyage, during which he studied many animals, some still numerous and others recently extinct, was the preparation and stimulus for his life work. He read *Malthus on Population* in 1838, and, as he became impressed by the struggle for existence, it struck him "that, under these circumstances, favourable variations would tend to be preserved and unfavourable ones to be destroyed. The result of this would be the formation of new species." He

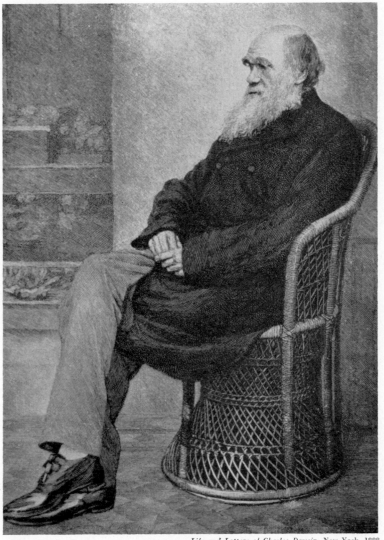

Life and Letters of Charles Darwin, New York, 1888

CHARLES DARWIN

worked constantly on this new theory, collecting data and analysing it, and presently wrote out an essay on the subject. In 1844, he wrote his friend, Sir Joseph Hooker, the botanist, "I am almost convinced (quite contrary to the opinion I started with) that species are not (it is like confessing a murder) immutable."

Darwin now began the draft of his book and had completed about one-half when he received from A. R. Wallace an essay, which had been sent to him for his opinion. On reading Wallace's essay, he was startled to find in it a complete summary of his own theory of natural selection. He placed the essay in the hands of Lyell, the geologist, and of Hooker, the botanist, who sent it together with an abstract of Darwin's work to the Linnean Society, which published both together in 1858. Darwin now completed his own work, *On the Origin of the Species* . . . , which was published on November 14, 1859, the whole edition of 1,250 copies being sold out the day of publication. The circumstances of the publication after the communication from Wallace led to a controversy regarding their respective claims to priority, but a careful study of all the circumstances has established the rights of Darwin as the creator of the theory of natural selection and evolution. Darwin's *Origin* demolished, once for all, the Linnean concept of the fixity of species as well as the various attempted explanations of this assumed fixity. Although the idea of evolution was expressed by Aristotle and by other Greeks, suggested by Bacon, Erasmus Darwin, Goethe, and many others, Darwin's systematic and lucid marshalling of facts made it a fundamental concept of biological science, much as Copernicus, three centuries earlier, had made his heliocentric theory the fundamental concept of astronomy.

Darwin's *Descent of Man*, 1871, fulfilled the prediction he had made in his *Origin* that, through his theory, "light would be thrown on the origin of man and his history." This work made an end to the ancient theory that the universe was created for man, a theory already tottering, since Galileo had shown the immensity of the universe and the relative insignificance of the earth.

The revolutionary concepts of Darwin aroused much bitter opposition among some men of science and particularly among the clergy, many of whom felt that the new theory attacked the fundamental tenets of the Church. Bishop Wilberforce of the Church of England denounced the *Origin* as "atheistical." Many other Protestant divines followed his example. Pope Pius IX in a personal letter referred to "the aberrations of Darwinism. . . . A system which is repugnant at once to history, to exact science, to observation, and even to reason itself . . . a tissue of fables." But Darwin's books were not placed on the *Index*. Darwin, himself, refused to be drawn either into controversy or into polemical writing and lived quietly at Down until his death in 1882 at the age of 74. He was buried in Westminster Abbey, Canon Farrar, one of the noted divines of the Church of England and the famous author of *The Life of Christ,* delivering the funeral sermon.

THOMAS HENRY HUXLEY

While Darwin himself was not fond of controversy, Thomas Henry Huxley thrived on it and devoted much of his energy to a militant championship of the Darwinian hypothesis, on one occasion remarking, "I am Darwin's bull-dog." One of the best known occasions when he broke a lance for Darwin was his public debate at Oxford with Bishop Wilberforce, who, after talking for half an hour, turned to his opponent and asked whether it was through his grandfather or grandmother that he claimed his descent from a monkey. Huxley answered that he was not ashamed to have a monkey for his ancestor; but he would be ashamed to be connected with a man who used his great gifts to obscure the truth.

Although Huxley is remembered for his controversies and popular lectures, these were but a small part of his scientific activity. Born in Ealing in 1825, he was the son of an assistant-master in a semi-public school, whom Huxley described as "rather too easy going for this wicked world." Thomas Huxley's earlier education seems to have been rather desultory. He speaks of "two years of a Pandemonium of a school and after that neither help nor sympathy in any intellectual direction till he reached manhood." During these years, however, he developed a passionate love of reading, particularly scientific books. At 16, he became assistant to a Dr. Chandler, was then apprenticed to his brother-in-law, Dr. Scott, and secured a scholarship at the medical school of Charing Cross Hospital, receiving his M.B. from the University of London in 1845. The next year, he sailed as assistant surgeon to the "Rattlesnake," which went out to survey the eastern shores of Australia.

The voyage of the "Rattlesnake" lasted three years and gave Huxley, as the voyage of the "Beagle" had previously given Darwin, an opportunity to study a great variety of animal and vegetable life. He studied birds, reptiles, mammalia, fish, marine animals and plants, invertebrates, and even geology. He carried a microscope with him and studied the microscopic appearance as well as the gross appearance of the innumerable specimens. A paper on the Medusae, or jelly-fish family, sent back to England was published in the *Transactions of the Royal Society* and led to his election as a Fellow at the early age of 26.

After his return to England, his fame and reputation grew rapidly. He received the gold medal of the Royal Society in 1852, was appointed professor of natural history in the Royal School of Mines in 1857, was chosen professor of comparative anatomy at the Royal Institution, and was elected in 1862 professor of anatomy at the Royal College of Surgeons. During this period, he wrote many papers and books on comparative anatomy, physiology, biology and geology. He became well known for his popular lectures on science, and, when the *Origin of the Species* appeared in 1859, his mind was already prepared to accept the theory because of his own extensive observations in those fields. Darwin sent an advance copy of the book to Huxley, who knew of the proposed publication but still had some doubts on the validity of the theory. After reading the *Origin,* Huxley wrote the author that he was "prepared to go to the stake, if requisite" for the doctrine of natural selection and added, "I am sharpening up my claws and beak in readiness for defense of the noble book." Darwin replied, "Like a good Catholic who has received extreme unction, I can now sing 'Nunc dimittis.'"

In his *Collected Essays,* Huxley wrote,

It must be admitted that the popularization of science, whether by lectures or by essays has its drawbacks. . . . The "people who fail" take their revenge by ignoring all the rest of a man's work and glibly labelling him a mere populariser.

Huxley was also labelled a popularizer by some of his enemies, particularly theological, and was so considered by others unaware of his solid and original contributions to science. His lectures on the origin of the skull in vertebrates, delivered in 1806, demolished the theory that the skull is formed of a series of expanded vertebrae joined together, as maintained by Owen. His *Manual of the Anatomy of Vertebrated Animals,* 1871, which passed through 30 editions, and his *Elementary Lessons in Physiology,* 1866, were masterpieces in their field. His *Evidence as to Man's Place in Nature,* 1863, remains one of the best expositions of Darwin's ideas, a book written in the charming and lucid style, which is characteristic of all his writings.

Huxley received a LL.D. degree from Edinburgh in 1866 and from Cambridge in 1879. In 1833, he was elected president of the Royal Society. Oxford, which had seen little of Huxley since his

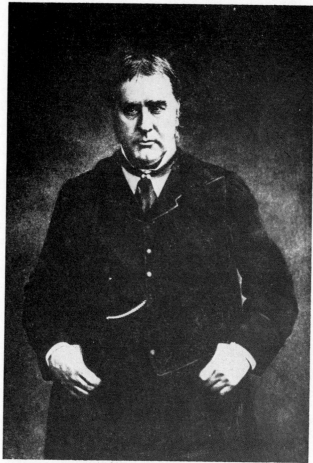

Published Writings of William Withey Gull, London, 1896

WILLIAM WITHEY GULL

famous duel with Bishop Wilberforce of Oxford, awarded him a D.C.L. in 1885. He was a man of deep convictions, kindly and charitable by nature, respected alike by friend and foe for his intellectual honesty and uncompromising integrity. From early youth until his death in 1895 at the age of 70, he believed and taught, "Science commits suicide when it adopts a creed."

In William Withey Gull (1816-1890), the great men of Guy's Hospital—Addison, Bright, Hodgkins and Cooper—found a worthy successor. Gull, a native of Colchester, came to London in 1837 at the age of 21, obtained a position at Guy's, and became so attached to this institution that he lived within its walls or in adjacent lodgings for 15 years. In 1841, he received the degree of M.B. from London University and, in 1846, that of M.D. He taught successively materia medica, natural philosophy, physiology and anatomy at Guy's and, in 1858, became physician to the hospital. He was elected a Fellow of the Royal Society in 1858 and received the degrees of D.C.L. from Oxford in 1868, LL.D. from Cambridge in 1880, and LL.D. from Edinburgh in 1884. In 1871, he attended the Prince of Wales, who was ill of typhoid fever, and, on the prince's recovery, he was created a baronet.

Gull was a brilliant and forceful speaker, his addresses bristling with aphorisms and epigrams. His own impartial attitude toward medicine, he expressed by saying, "We have no system to satisfy, no dogmatic opinions to enforce. We have no ignorance to cloak, for we confess it." He was a great opponent of the polypharmacy prevalent in his day and remarked, "I do not say no drugs are useful; but there is not enough discrimination in their use." He early developed a large practice and was, without question, the foremost physician of London in his time. At his death in 1890, he left a fortune of 344,000 pounds, unprecedented in the history of medicine.

In addition to being one of the greatest practitioners of his time, Gull was a brilliant and attractive lecturer. He also published a number of excellent papers. He was one of the first to describe the pathological lesions in tabes dorsalis (1856), described intermittent hemoglobinuria (1866), and described, with Sutton, arterio-capillary fibrosis, since known by their name, in chronic nephritis. His description of myxedema in 1873 is easily the clearest and best published up to that time.

James Paget is called by Bettany "the foremost surgical philosopher and orator of his day." He towered above his surgical colleagues, as Gull did above his medical colleagues. Paget, like Gull, was brilliant and learned, but he had a great dislike for cleverness and an antipathy towards epigrams and proverbs. "To be brief," he said, "was to be wise; to be epigrammatic was to be clever." One of his favorite sayings was "as false as most proverbs." His love for brevity was well known; he never used two words where one was sufficient.

Born in Yarmouth in 1814, Paget was apprenticed to a surgeon at the age of 16 and, in 1834, came to London, where he began study at St. Bartholomew's Hospital. During his first year's study, he found, while dissecting a subject, some small white specks in the muscles. On examining one of these specks under the microscope, he saw it to consist of a small worm surrounded by a capsule. The specimen was shown to Richard Owen, who named it *Trichina spiralis*. This was the first demonstration of trichinosis in man.

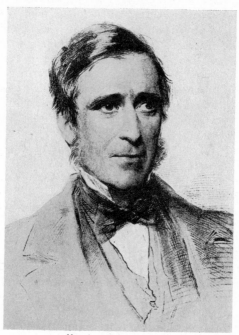

Memoirs and Letters of Sir James Paget, 1901

JAMES PAGET
Portrait by George Richmond, 1867.

Paget passed the examination of the Royal College of Surgeons, then coached pupils, worked as a sub-editor on medical journals, and was appointed curator of the pathological museum in 1837, holding this position for six years. He became a demonstrator of morbid anatomy and later in anatomy. In 1847, he was chosen professor in the Royal College of Surgeons and, in 1851, was elected a Fellow of the Royal Society and, the same year, began private practice—15 years after his graduation. At the time of his election to the Royal Society, Sir Richard Owen remarked that Paget had his choice either to be the first physiologist in Europe or to have the first surgical practice in London with a baronetcy.

Paget's rise in practice was phenomenal. Charming in person, dexterous and skillful with his hands, and learned with 15 years' study in pathology and anatomy, he had an exceptional combination of talents, inherited and acquired. In a few years, he was earning 10,000 pounds a year. Paget never allowed his large practice to dull his scientific interest; indeed, it seemed to increase with his practice. His best known works are his *Lectures on Tumours*, 1851; *Surgical Pathology*, 1863; and *Clinical Lectures and Essays*, 1875. Two diseases bear Paget's name—eczema of the nipple with subsequent mammary carcinoma, which he described in 1874; and the disease of the bones, osteitis deformans, which he first noted in 1876, seven additional cases of which he described in 1882. He was created a baronet in 1871 and appointed Serjeant Surgeon to the Queen in 1877.

Paget was literally worshipped by his patients and admired and trusted by every member of his profession. He had a great capacity for friendship and, apart from his hosts of friends in the English medical life, numbered among his close friends Gladstone, Cardinal Newman, Ruskin, Tennyson, Robert Browning, George Eliot, Tyndall, Huxley, Darwin, Virchow and Pasteur. He died in 1899 at the age of 85.

The bustling metropolis of London always seemed to have an especial attraction for young Scotsmen who came down to the city and made their fame and fortune there. This was particularly true of medicine, such leaders of London medicine as William Hunter, John Hunter, Matthew Baillie, Charles Bell, William Smellie, and Robert Liston, all coming from north of the English border. One physician, however, James Simpson, who achieved an international reputation, was born in Scotland, died in Scotland, and lived practically his entire life there.

James Young Simpson (1811-1870) was born in Bathgate, one of the seven sons of the village baker. At the age of 14, aided by a stipend and financial assistance from an elder brother, he entered Edinburgh University and, two years later, began the study of medicine, receiving his M.D. in 1832. Soon after, he was appointed assistant to John Thompson, professor of pathology, also becoming an extracurricular teacher of obstetrics. In 1835, he published an article on diseases of the placenta, following this with noteworthy papers on peritonitis in the fetus (1838), hernia in the fetus (1839),

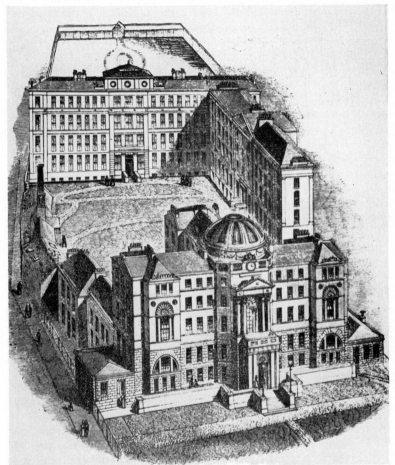

Lister and the Lister Ward in the Royal Infirmary of Glasgow, Glasgow, 1927.

THE GLASGOW ROYAL INFIRMARY IN 1861

and an exhaustive article on hermaphrodism, which appeared in the
Cyclopaedia of Anatomy and Physiology, 1839. The following year,
at the age of 29, he was elected by a majority of one vote, professor
of midwifery in the University of Edinburgh.

Young Simpson took up his new duties with characteristic energy,
and his lectures and demonstrations soon became very popular. His
course on obstetrics rose from the former rank of the dullest course
in the curriculum to the most sought after and best attended. As

a practitioner, his skill, combined with his charm, tenderness, and sympathetic manner, soon made him the busiest obstetrician in all Scotland.

Ether anesthesia was first administered by Morton in Boston on October 16, 1846, and Robert Liston operated under ether anesthesia in London on December 18, 1846. On January 19, 1847, Simpson introduced ether into obstetrical practice, but, later, because of its disagreeable qualities, particularly its persisting odor and its tendency to cause bronchial irritation, he sought a substitute. This he found in chloroform, the anesthetic properties of which had been already demonstrated by Flourens, the French physiologist. After some preliminary experiments on himself and on two assistants, Simpson began to use chloroform in obstetrical practice. On November 10, 1847, he read before the Edinburgh Chirurgical Society a paper describing the employment of chloroform anesthesia in labor.

The Scottish Calvinist clergy opposed Simpson's innovation as unscriptural since it was written in Genesis III:14 that the Lord God had said to Eve, "In sorrow thou shalt bring forth children." However, Simpson was also well versed in Scripture and pointed out that in "the first surgical operation ever performed on man," according to the account in Genesis, "the Lord God caused a deep sleep to fall upon Adam; and he slept; and he took one of his ribs, and closed up the flesh instead thereof." For good measure, he pointed out to the Calvinists that John Calvin himself in his *Commentaries* wrote, "It ought to be noted, that Adam was sunk into a profound sleep, in order that he might feel no pain." The controversy continued for several years, but, when Queen Victoria received chloroform during the birth of her eighth child in 1853, the respectability of chloroform anesthesia in childbirth was assured.

Simpson was created a baronet in 1866 and, the same year, was awarded the degree of LL.D. by the University of Oxford. In addition to papers on obstetrical subjects, he also made contributions to archeology and to medical history. In 1869, he received the freedom of the City of Edinburgh, a signal honor not often bestowed.

Simpson's chief claim to fame was unquestionably his introduction of chloroform anesthesia in obstetrics, but this was not his only achievement. He introduced iron wire sutures, particularly in the operation for vesicovaginal fistula and for hydrocele, the long obstetrical forceps, "acupressure"—the method of arresting hemorrhage by drawing together the edges of the wound with needles inserted into the tissue—and dilatation of the cervix uteri for diagnostic purposes. He was much interested in what he termed "Hospitalism," writing several papers on this subject. He collected statistics on some 2,000 amputations in hospitals and the same number in country practice, finding that the mortality in these operations was not only much higher in hospitals than in private homes but that it increased exactly in proportion to the size of the hospital. He stated, "The man laid on the operating table in one of our surgical hospitals is exposed to more chances of death than the English soldier on the field of Waterloo. . . . Why is this hospitalism so dangerous to the sick?" Because, he continues, "There exists, I think, evidence on this question, tending to show that the constitution of the patient in the surgical wards is liable to be endangered sometimes by the influence of morbific contagious materials from the bodies of other inmates."

However, Simpson, who had embraced the discovery of anesthesia with such enthusiasm, proved to be one of the most bitter opponents of the practice of antisepsis when introduced by Lister and waged until his death in 1870, an active warfare against what he called rather contemptuously the "carbolic acid treatment." Why Simpson opposed Lister has been a matter for much speculation. Simpson and Syme, Lister's father-in-law, had been in conflict for years, and Lister may have inherited some of its aftermath. Simpson may have had a certain jealousy towards a new method of treating wounds which might threaten to supersede acupressure. He was a good lover and an equally good hater. Edinburgh had never witnessed a greater funeral than that of Simpson, a tribute to the esteem and love so many had for him. Yet, as Godlee said, "Few men who could claim so many friends had so many detractors. For the former he was the embodiment of all the virtues; the latter were unable to speak of him with moderation."

ANTISEPSIS AND ASEPSIS

Joseph Lister was born in London in 1827, the son of a prosperous wine merchant. For generations, the family had been Quakers, and young Joseph received his early education in Quaker schools and became, on the insistence of his father, quite proficient in French and Latin. He decided early in life to study medicine and, in 1844, entered University College, London, a non-sectarian institution, called by some of the most orthodox "the godless college" since students could receive degrees there, in contrast to Oxford and Cambridge, without taking an oath and subscribing to the Thirty-nine

Articles of the Church of England. Dissenters from the Established Church were not given degrees from Oxford and Cambridge until 1858.

In 1847, Lister was graduated Bachelor of Arts and, in 1852, received his M.B. As a student, he was much impressed by Wharton Jones and Sharpey, who encouraged him to carry out some investigations, which were published the following year in the *Quarterly Journal of Microscopical Science*. In this first paper, he demonstrated two distinct muscles in the iris—the dilator and the sphincter —which respectively enlarged and diminished the size of the pupil. The second paper described the involuntary muscles of the skin which elevate the hairs and produce the well-known phenomena of "goose skin." These papers, which confirmed some previous observations of Kölliker, pleased the celebrated German anatomist very much and was the beginning of a life-long friendship between the two.

In 1853, Lister went to Edinburgh to visit the clinic of Professor Syme, then considered by many to be the best and most original surgeon in the British Isles. Impressed by Syme's ability, he gladly accepted the post of "supernumerary clerk" to him and, the following year, was appointed resident house surgeon. The next year, 1855, he applied for and received the position of lecturer on surgery at the College of Physicians and assistant surgeon to the Royal Infirmary.

Lister continued to assist Syme in his operations and had great respect for his chief, whose skill, judgment, and original mind he constantly praised in his letters home. He wrote weekly summaries of Syme's lectures to the *Lancet* in 1855. His relationship to Syme became closer when, in 1856, he married Syme's daughter, Agnes. This was, on the personal side, a very serious step for Lister. He was a Quaker, and Quakers who married outside their own persuasion either resigned from membership in the Society of Friends or were disowned. Lister resigned from the society, joined the Episcopal Church, the church of his bride, and ordered his first door-plate inscribed "Mr. Lister," instead of plain "Joseph Lister," according to Quaker custom. His family regretted his action, but his good old father, with characteristic Quaker humility, wrote to his own daughter, "I trust we shall be very careful to say nothing in disparagement of those whom we shall probably find on acquaintance to be our superiors."

Lister soon became a very busy man, taught surgery at the College of Physicians, operated at the Royal Infirmary, and worked in the

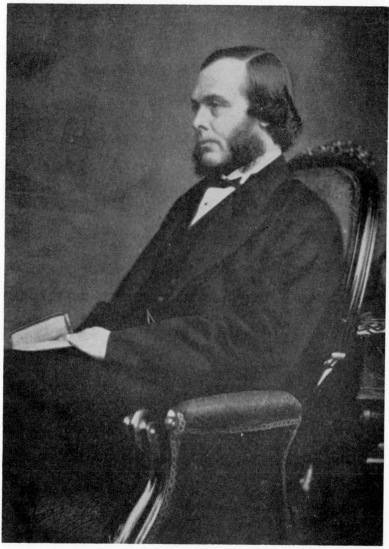

Lord Lister, London, 1918

JOSEPH LISTER

This picture was taken about the time Lister discovered antisepsis.

laboratory, studying particularly inflammation, gangrene, and the coagulation of the blood and publishing papers on these subjects. He employed the microscope extensively and illustrated his papers with camera lucida drawings. In 1860, he was appointed Regius Professor of Surgery at the University of Glasgow and, the same year, was elected Fellow of the Royal Society. He went to Glasgow at the age of 33, in the prime of life, full of energy and ambition and intellectually prepared to take full advantage of his opportunities. His predecessors in the chair had been doctors with a large general practice. Lister limited his work to surgery.

In Glasgow, he found the same scourges haunting the surgical wards, suppuration and gangrene. About 1861, he began to teach his classes, "The occurrence of suppuration in a wound under ordinary conditions and its continuance . . . are determined simply by the influence of decomposition." He was struck by the fact that simple fractures healed without complications, whereas compound fractures with laceration of the skin were followed by suppuration and often gangrene and death. He also recognized that inflammation, or even suppuration, was sure to follow any wound made by the surgeon. While this had been true since the beginnings of surgery and even welcomed by some surgeons who spoke of "laudable pus," Lister saw that sepsis was the principal obstacle to any great advance in surgery. Finally, noting that closed wounds did not suppurate while open ones exposed to the air did, he concluded that suppuration was in some unexplained manner due to contact with the air but that the air alone did not cause suppuration.

Lister discussed his problems in 1865 with Dr. Thomas Anderson, professor of chemistry, who called his attention to the work of Louis Pasteur on fermentation and putrefaction. Here Lister found the solution of his problem; it was not the air but the germs in the air that produced suppuration. He saw at once that putrefaction was fermentation and that putrefaction could only be avoided by preventing germs from gaining access to wounds. At the Glasgow Royal Infirmary, notorious for the unhealthiness of its wards, he had an unusual opportunity for testing the validity of his theory. He next looked around for a suitable antiseptic, and, remembering that carbolic acid had been used successfully as an antiseptic in treating the sewage in Carlisle, he chose carbolic acid.

Lister employed carbolic acid in the treatment of a compound fracture in March, 1865, but his first striking success was obtained in May, 1866, and is described in a letter to his father. His method was simple—a piece of calico or lint was soaked in crude carbolic acid and then introduced into the wound with forceps, a piece of lint also soaked in carbolic was placed over the wound, and over this was placed a slightly larger piece of thin block tin or lead to prevent evaporation. After nine months' experience with this method, there was not a single case of pyemia, erysipelas, or hospital gangrene in Lister's ward although the other wards of the hospital had their customary large number of cases.

The first papers of Lister describing his method on 11 patients appeared in the *Lancet* between March and July, 1867, with the title, "On a New Method of Treating Compound Fractures." In August of the same year, he read at the annual meeting of the British Medical Association a paper which was later published. His papers attracted a great deal of attention, and the newspapers and magazines gave the discovery much publicity, confusing, however, the discovery of a great and new principle in surgery with the discovery that carbolic acid was an antiseptic, even the authoritative *Lancet* committing this error. The new discovery made little headway. In Glasgow, the senior surgeons opposed the new method, the same was true in Edinburgh, in London, and in Dublin. On the Continent, it met with better success. Professor Thiersch of Leipzig, in 1867, the same year that Lister's papers appeared, introduced the method in his clinic, and, in the course of 12 months, hospital gangrene disappeared from his hospital.

In 1869, Lister returned to Edinburgh as professor of clinical surgery, remaining in Edinburgh nine years. His bitter opponent, Simpson, died the following year as well as his father-in-law, Syme. With Syme's death, Lister stepped into his place by common consent as the first surgeon in Scotland. He continued to work on his antiseptic methods, carried out laboratory experiments on putrefaction and fermentation, and began his important studies on ligatures. Noting that infections often came from ligatures, he soaked first silk ligatures and later catgut in carbolic acid before employing them and found that this method of treatment prevented putrefaction. He presently became so obsessed with the fear that microbes might fall upon the wound during an operation that he introduced in 1870 the carbolic spray to purify the atmosphere. He clung obstinately to this practice for 17 years but finally admitted that it was superfluous.

Meanwhile on the Continent, Lister's ideas were received with great enthusiasm. After Thiersch's initial support in 1867, Saxtorph of Copenhagen employed the method in his clinic in 1870 and Volkmann of Halle introduced the practice in his clinic. A brilliant surgeon, a man of great literary and artistic ability, a poet as well, and a man who "rather welcomed than avoided a conflict" (Godlee), Volkmann became Lister's most devoted disciple and, by his addresses and papers, did much to introduce antiseptic surgery throughout Germany. Bardeleben and von Bergmann in Berlin, Nussbaum in Munich, and Billroth in Vienna became active champions of Lister. The trip Lister took to Germany in 1875 became a triumphal tour.

In 1877, after an absence of 25 years, Lister returned to his alma mater as professor of clinical surgery at King's College Hospital, London. Fresh from Edinburgh, where he was an idol of the large classes which attended his lectures, he found King's College to be a chilling contrast. The students showed no enthusiasm for their new professor, attendance at his classes became smaller and smaller since the students soon discovered that, if they aired his views in their examinations, conducted by outside examiners, they were likely to fail. "Soon only a few, seldom more than a dozen, came to the lectures, mostly those who had passed in surgery and had no need to think any more about examiners" (Godlee).

Lister occupied the chair of surgery at King's College for 15 years. In 1881, the Seventh International Medical Congress met in London, and the principal addresses were made by Virchow, Pasteur, Huxley and Volkmann. Volkmann, who delivered the address on surgery, said, "England may be proud that it was one of her sons whose name is indissolubly bound up with this greatest advance that surgery has ever made."

Slowly but surely Lister's great eminence was recognized at home as well as abroad. In 1883, he was created a baronet; in 1885, he received the Prussian order, Pour le Mérite; in 1895, he was elected president of the Royal Society; in 1897, he was elevated to the peerage as Lord Lister; and, in 1903, King Edward VII, on the occasion of his coronation, instituted a new order, the Order of Merit, appointing as one of its 12 members Joseph Lord Lister. Lister died in 1912 and, after an impressive funeral service in Westminster Abbey, was buried at his express wish beside his wife in West Hampstead Cemetery.

During Lister's life, an attempt was made to differentiate sharply between antiseptic surgery and aseptic surgery advocated by von Bergmann and thus to minimize the importance of Lister's discovery. Von Bergmann, himself, repudiated such attempts and remarked, "I have been no heaven-storming pathfinder. . . . I have not placed myself in the rank of a Lister. . . . If I have accomplished anything, it has been in the way of critical repetition and improvement." In the last analysis, Lister achieved aseptic surgery by the application of antiseptic methods.

The two revolutionary discoveries in surgery—anesthesia and antisepsis—were made within the span of 20 years. Fate dealt quite differently with the two discoverers. Morton died embittered, discredited by many, and practically penniless. Lister died a peer of the realm, honored by the world.

THE RISE OF BACTERIOLOGY

The dramatic development of antiseptic surgery was simultaneous with the rise of bacteriology. The role of Pasteur in this drama has been mentioned, and, while he unquestionably played one of the major roles, many others were active in creating this new and extremely important science. In medicine, bacteriology dominated the last quarter of the nineteenth century and brought new concepts and mechanisms into medical thinking—physicians thought bacteriologically for the first time in history.

The idea that small animalculae may cause disease is certainly as old as Marcus Terentius Varro (116-27 B.C.). Fracastorius advanced in 1546 the theory of invisible living *semina* which scattered disease, and Kircher saw in 1658 "innumerable small animals" in putrefying meat and claimed that he saw in the blood of plague patients "worms, so small, so fine, so subtle that they elude all discernment by the sense and also are perceived only with a most excellent microscope."

We do not know what Kircher saw with his microscope, but we do know what van Leeuwenhoek saw in 1683, since his letter to the Royal Society contained a sketch of the "little animals," and we recognize among them bacilli and cocci. Leeuwenhoek, however, did not associate these "little animals" with disease, and the subject of bacteriology attracted little attention until the latter half of the nineteenth century.

Meanwhile, Agostino Bassi (1771-1856) carried out some experiments that earned for him in the eyes of some the title of "the founder of the parasitic theory of infection." Bassi, a graduate in law at the University of Pavia, was also interested in natural science and, during his years at the University, in addition to his courses in law, had attended the lectures of Volta the physicist, Scarpa the anatomist, Spallanzani the physiologist, and Rasori the clinician, all of whom made a deep impression on the young student. Bassi, who suffered from continual eye trouble, made several attempts to hold governmental positions but was obliged to retire to his farm near Mairigo, where he lived for 40 years until his death in 1856.

As a scientific farmer, Bassi saw the devastation wrought among silk worms by a disease called in English *muscardine* and in Italian *calcinaccio* because of the white calcareous-appearing patches formed

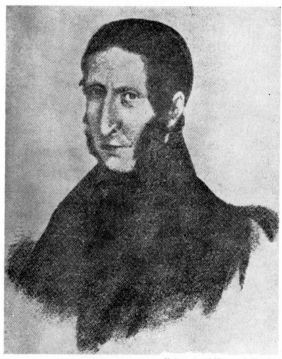

University of Kansas Collection

AGOSTINO BASSI

on the bodies of the worms. In 1835, he published his work, *Del Mal del Segno, Calcinaccio o Moscardino* (The Disease of the Sign, Calcinaccio or Muscardine), in which he showed that the white material, when inoculated into the body of a healthy worm, reproduced the disease. On study with the microscope, he found this white material to be "organic, living and vegetable. It is a plant of the order of a cryptogram, a parasitic fungus." It was later christened the *Botrytis Bassiana*. In his book, Bassi remarks, "Perhaps some of my readers will respond with a smile to my doctrine . . . of living contagions." He described later the methods of preventing the disease by segregation and by treatment of infected places with calcium chloride, potassium nitrate, and other chemicals. In 1844, he published *Sui contagi in generale* (On Contagions in General), in which he asserted, "Smallpox, spotted fever, bubonic plague and syphilis are caused by living parasites, animal or vegetable." The book on muscardine excited much interest among botanists and agriculturists but, apparently, did not impress the medical profession although Schönlein and Henle both referred to it.

In the early years of the century, many zoologists studied the "small animals" in water, vinegar, wine, and other fluids and attempted to classify them. The terms, "monads" (round or oval shape) and "vibrions" (long or short moving rods), soon appeared in the literature. In 1840, Henle called attention to the probability that living parasitic agents caused infectious diseases. In 1849, Pollender, as well as Davaine and Rayer in 1850, saw the anthrax bacillus in the blood of sheep dead from this disease, and Davaine in 1854 saw "monads" in the stools of cholera patients. It remained, however, for Pasteur, a chemist and not a biologist, to excite by his brilliant work a new interest in van Leeuwenhoek's "little animals" and to usher in an exciting period in modern medical history.

LOUIS PASTEUR

Louis Pasteur was born in Dôle, Jura, in 1822, the son of a tanner, who had been an army sergeant during the Napoleonic wars. Soon after his birth, the family moved to Arbois, where he attended school. He was a somewhat slow and methodical youth but early showed considerable talent as an artist. He received his bachelor of letters from the College of Besançon in 1840 and, two years later, his bachelor of science degree. In 1843, he was admitted to the École Normale, heard the lectures of the chemist, Dumas, at the Sorbonne, and was appointed laboratory assistant to A. J. Balard, the chemist. After successfully passing his examinations for the *licence d'agrégation* and for his doctorate in 1848, Pasteur carried out a startling piece of research. It had been known since the investigations of Mitscherlich in 1844 that ordinary commercial racemic or tartaric acid rotated the plane of polarized light to the right, whereas paratartaric acid, when placed in the polariscope, was inactive. Studying the crystals under the microscope, Pasteur found that the crystals of tartaric acid showed faces that were inclined to the right while the crystals of paratartaric acid showed some faces inclined to right and some to the left. Separating the two types, he proved that a solution of "right-faced" crystals rotated polarized light to the right, a solution of "left-faced" crystals rotated the light to the left, and a mixture of the two was inactive. This discovery was reported at the *Académie des Sciences,* and the young man of 26 was highly praised for his remarkable work.

The same year, Pasteur was sent by the government to Dijon as professor of physics in the Lycée and, the following year, was transferred to the academy at Strassburg. In 1854, he was made professor and dean of the new faculty of sciences at Lille, a center for the manufacture of beet-root alcohol. One of the manufacturers, who was having difficulties in his production of alcohol, came to the young dean for assistance. Thus, by chance, Pasteur's interest was turned away from the study of crystals to the investigation of fermentation. In his inaugural address at Lille, he said, "In the fields of observation, chance favors only the prepared minds" *(Dans les champs de l'observation, le hasard ne favorise que les esprits préparés).* He now proceeded to prove the truth of his oft-quoted dictum.

He studied alcoholic fermentation and lactic fermentation in sour milk. In alcoholic fermentation, he saw round globules when the fermentation was healthy, long threads when lactic acid appeared. In 1857, although called back to Paris as director of scientific studies at the École normale, he continued there his studies on alcoholic fermentation. In December of the same year, he stated that the change "of sugar into alcohol and carbonic acid is correlative to a phenomenon of life, an organization of globules." He said further that fermentation is caused by minute organisms and that, when it does not occur, these minute organisms either have not been introduced or find it impossible to live.

Pasteur's investigations revived the old controversy concerning spontaneous generation. His demonstration that both alcoholic and lactic fermentation were produced by minute organisms and were hastened by exposure to the air, brought up the question whether the minute organisms were always present in the air or whether they were spontaneously generated in the solutions. This question Pasteur answered by proving that the microscopic organisms were not spontaneously generated but were introduced by the air. In his well-known experiment, he demonstrated that an infusion, when boiled in a flask which is left open, will putrefy, whereas,

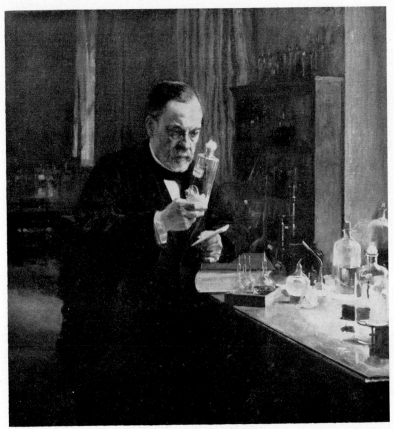

PASTEUR IN HIS LABORATORY
Painting by Edelfelt.

if the neck of the flask is drawn out to a fine point, the solution will remain pure because the air will "drop its dusts and germs that it carries, at the opening of the neck or in the first curves." This was the crucial experiment that suggested antisepsis to Lister.

In 1864, Pasteur was asked to study a disease which was ruining the wine industry of Jura, making the wine sour and unpalatable. He found that wines were spoiled by parasitic growths and that these could be destroyed by heating the wine for a few moments at a temperature of 50 to 60 degrees C. This process has since been extended to other fields and has perpetuated his name with the term, "pasteurization."

An epidemic began to destroy silk worms in enormous numbers in 1865 and bid fair to ruin the silk industry. This disease, called *pébrine* because the worms developed black spots like pepper (*pébré*) grains, raged not only in France but also in Italy, Spain and Austria. Microscopical study of the eggs convinced Pasteur that certain glistening oval bodies, or corpuscles, were the cause of *pébrine,* and he showed that the disease could be stamped out by using only healthy eggs, those proved by microscopic study to be free of corpuscles, for the breeding of silk worms. Diseased eggs, he emphasized, should be destroyed. In this investigation, he also found diseased silk worms that showed no corpuscles but large numbers of "vibrions." These worms he realized were suffering from a different disease, *flacherie,* a very contagious intestinal disease of the worms, resembling cholera. The disease was caused by feeding the worms with damp mulberry leaves, in which he found innumerable "vibrions." He demonstrated that this disease could be prevented by proper feeding. These studies saved the silk industry in France, which in the course of 10 years had already suffered a loss of 2,000,000 francs from *pébrine* alone. While in the midst of this work in 1868, Pasteur suffered a cerebral hemorrhage with a complete left hemiplegia but, after an invalidism of three months, returned to his investigations.

The war of 1870 aroused such intense bitterness in Pasteur that he returned the honorary diploma of doctor of medicine sent him in 1868 by the University of Bonn. "Influenced by patriotic motives" and realizing that "Germany was incontestably superior to France in the manufacture of beer," as his biographer and son-in-law Vallery-Radot states, Pasteur "conceived the thought of making France a successful rival." He studied the manufacture of beer in a number of French breweries and then went to London, where he investigated the large British establishments. He presently stated, "Every marked alteration in the quality of the beer coincides with the development of microorganisms foreign to the nature of true beer yeast." He showed this could be prevented, as in the case of wine, by heating the beer to a temperature of 50 to 60 degrees C. This "pasteurized" beer was much superior to previous French beer, but whether it made French beer the equal of German beer is perhaps a matter of individual taste.

In 1877, after having revolutionized the manufacture of wine and beer and after having firmly established the germ theory and saved the silk industry of France, Pasteur turned his attention to splenic fever, or anthrax, a scourge which was decimating the flocks of sheep, sometimes killing as many as 50 per cent of the flocks. After three years, this work was interrupted by studies on chicken cholera that had appeared in an epidemic form and was destroying a large number of fowls. He soon isolated the offending microbe and found that old cultures not only lost their virulence but, when injected into hens, protected them from a second inoculation with a fresh and virulent culture. He now returned to the study of anthrax and, employing similar methods, announced two years later that animals injected with a culture of the anthrax bacillus, attenuated by growing the organisms at 42 degrees C., were protected from the fatal results of a later injection of a virulent culture.

This announcement was received with great skepticism, and, to test Pasteur's claims, the Melun Agricultural Society placed 60 sheep at Pasteur's disposal. The news of the proposed experiment attracted much attention, and a large crowd of physicians, veterinarians, journalists and farmers gathered at Melun on May 31, 1881, to witness Pasteur's crucial experiment. Twenty-four sheep which had previously been vaccinated with attenuated cultures of the anthrax bacillus and an equal number of unvaccinated sheep were injected with virulent anthrax cultures. Two days later, all the vaccinated sheep remained well, while 22 of the unvaccinated sheep were dead and the other two were dying. The experiment had been a spectacular success; "the whole of France burst out into an explosion of enthusiasm" (Vallery-Radot). Pasteur christened his method "vaccination" in homage to Jenner.

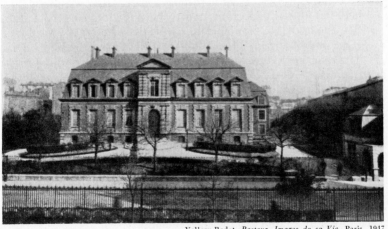

Vallery-Radot, *Pasteur, Images de sa Vie*, Paris, 1947

PASTEUR INSTITUTE

While still working on the problem of anthrax, Pasteur began another series of experiments which led to the most startling and dramatic discovery of his entire career, a career already filled to overflowing, it seemed, with astonishing discoveries. In 1880, when a veterinary surgeon brought to his laboratory two dogs suffering from rabies, Pasteur began his studies on this disease.

His first experiments were with the transmission of the disease. It was well known that rabies was transmitted by the saliva of a rabid dog, but Pasteur, convinced from the appearance of the animals that the virus must be present also in the nervous system, inoculated healthy dogs with bits of the medulla oblongata from a rabid animal and found that the dogs soon developed rabies. "Since this unknown being is living," thought Pasteur, "we must cultivate it; failing an artificial medium, let us try the brain of living rabbits." As soon as a rabbit died of rabies, a bit of the medulla was removed and inoculated directly into the brain of a healthy rabbit, and the process repeated when the inoculated rabbit succumbed. An inoculation succeeded inoculation, the period of incubation was steadily reduced until, after 100 successive inoculations, it was reduced to seven days. Inoculations past this point produced no reduction in the incubation period, which remained fixed at seven days. This virus was subsequently referred to as the fixed virus. Pasteur could now predict the day of death in an inoculated animal.

After having learned how to increase the virulence of the virus, he now sought to attenuate its virulence, as he had done in chicken cholera and anthrax. After numerous experiments, he found that a bit of rabid medulla, after having been desiccated for 14 days, lost its virulence. He then performed the experiment of inoculating dogs the first day with bits of medulla which had been dried for 14 days, the next day a 13 day fragment, continuing this process until, on the 15th day, the dog received a bit of fresh rabic material. These dogs, when inoculated with fresh rabic material, did not develop the disease.

Pasteur continued these experiments and demonstrated before a commission appointed by the Minister of Public Instruction that, by his method, he could protect healthy dogs from the bite of a rabid animal. He had had, however, no opportunity to test his method on a human being. On July 6, 1885, he had this opportunity when Joseph Meister, a little Alsatian boy, aged nine, was brought to Pasteur's laboratory by his mother, who related that her son had been bitten by a rabid dog two days previously.

Pasteur's emotions were deeply stirred at the sight of the boy, who had lost 14 wounds and was so weak he could scarcely stand. Even then hesitant to employ his method on the little patient, he first consulted Dr. Vulpian and Dr. Grancher. When they urged him to apply the antirabic vaccination, the boy was immediately injected with material from a 14-day desiccated rabic cord. The injections were continued daily, Pasteur going through a succession of hopes, fears and anguish. His mental agitation was such that he could not work or even sleep. On July 16, he inoculated the boy with some material only one day old, material which would surely produce hydrophobia in rabbits after only seven days' incubation. The boy continued well; the treatment was a success. Pasteur, worn out by the long vigil, retired to the country to rest. On August 3, he wrote to his son, "Very good news last night of the bitten lad. . . . It will be 31 days tomorrow since he was bitten." On October 26, Pasteur described the treatment of Joseph Meister before the *Académie des Sciences* and added that three months and three days had passed and the child remained perfectly well. Soon patients who had been bitten by rabid dogs came from far and wide to receive the treatment.

The news of Pasteur's successful treatment spread like wild-fire. The *Académie des Sciences* recommended that an establishment be founded in Paris for the prevention of rabies and that it be called the *Institut Pasteur*. A wave of enthusiasm and generosity spread from one end of France to the other and to other countries. Presently, the sum of 2,500,000 francs had been raised for this purpose, the list of contributors containing such notable personages as the Czar of Russia, the Emperor of Brazil, and the Sultan of Turkey. The completed buildings of the Pasteur Institute were dedicated at a simple ceremony in 1888. Ill and weary at this time, Pasteur himself was never able to take up active work in the new laboratories. In 1892, on the occasion of his seventieth birthday, a great international celebration was held in Paris. He visited the Institute for the last time in June, 1895, and, in September of that year, died quietly, one hand clasping a crucifix, the other the hand of his wife.

During his lifetime, Pasteur received all the honors that France could bestow—membership in the *Académie des Sciences* (1862), the *Académie de Médecine* (1873), the *Académie Française* (1862), the Grand Cross of the Legion of Honor (1880). During his Paris period, he was successively director of scientific studies at the École normale (1857-1863), professor of geology and chemistry at the École des beaux-arts (1863-1867), professor of chemistry at the Sorbonne (1867-1889), and director of the Institut Pasteur. Most of his great discoveries were first described at either the *Académie des Sciences* or the *Académie de Médecine* and published in their transactions. Four important monographs—*Études sur le vin*, 1866; *Études sur le vinaigre*, 1868; *Études sur la maladie des vers à soie*, 1870; and *Études sur la bière*, 1876—appeared during his lifetime.

Pasteur's eminence in science was the result of a remarkable imagination tinged with an uncanny intuition, both producing great achievements because of his indomitable patience, persistence and industry. Theories interested him only when capable of translation into facts. He has been justly described as the man who proved the germ theory of disease, but his chief interest in bacteriology was not that of a "pure" scientist but as a "practical" one whose aim was to eradicate or control the diseases due to germs. His practical methods of controlling silkworm disease, anthrax, chicken cholera, and the diseases of wine and beer brought immense financial gain to France. These economic benefits he conferred upon his native land were, however, overshadowed by his greater contribution to humanity.

Pasteur was a very devout Catholic, but, as a scientist, he claimed absolute liberty of research. "Science," he said, "should not concern itself in any way with the philosophical consequences of its discoveries." He considered it a waste of time to seek an explanation for primary causes or the mystery of the universe. He believed that the domain of religion and science "are distinct, and woe to him who tries to let them trespass on each other in the so imperfect state of human knowledge."

ROBERT KOCH

In 1843, the same year that young Louis Pasteur entered the École Normale at Paris, Robert Koch, the son of a mining engineer, was born in Klausthal, Hanover. Twenty-one years the junior of Pasteur, Koch, in his early years, did not seem destined for a brilliant career, as did his older rival. Koch graduated at Göttingen in 1866, having been deeply influenced by one of his teachers, Jacob Henle, whose theory of contagion has already been mentioned. Following graduation, he served as an army surgeon in the war of 1870, after which he settled in Wollstein as a district physician (*Kreisphysicus*), varying the monotony of country practice with microscopic studies in the tradition of Henle. During the years when Pasteur was making important discoveries regarding the diseases of the silkworm and of beer, Koch was busy with the uninspiring routine of a country practice.

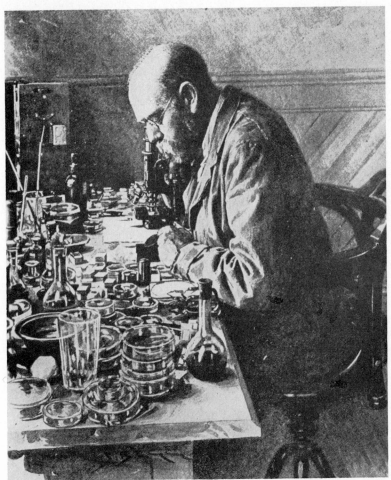

Osler, *Evolution of Modern Medicine*, New Haven, 1921

ROBERT KOCH

In 1876, Robert Koch, aged 33, wrote to Professor Ferdinand Cohn, professor of botany at the University of Breslau, asking for permission to demonstrate this work on anthrax, stating, "After many vain attempts, I have finally been successful in discovering the process of development of the bacillus anthracis." Cohn invited the country doctor to present his work, and Koch gave a three-day demonstration of his culture methods and results to a group of well-known scientists, including Cohn, Weigert, Traube and Cohnheim. He demonstrated to his astonished spectators pure cultures of the anthrax bacillus, the development of spores from the bacilli with the later transformation of spores back to bacilli and proved that pure cultures of the anthrax bacillus would cause the disease when injected into animals. He also solved the riddle that had troubled Cohn—the fact that blood from animals dead of anthrax could produce the disease although no bacilli were present in the blood —by showing that spores in the blood would cause the disease.

Cohn was deeply impressed by the work of this doctor done entirely on his own initiative and with no university connections. He immediately published Koch's paper in his *Beiträge zur Biologie der Planzen* under the title, *Die Ätiologie der Milzbrandkrankheit begründet auf die Entwicklungsgeschichte des Bacillus Anthracis* (The etiology of anthrax based on the development of the anthrax bacillus). The news of Koch's discovery spread to France. Paul Bert countered that it was possible to destroy the anthrax bacillus in the blood by treating it with compressed oxygen, so, since the blood would still produce the disease, he concluded, "Bacteridia are therefore neither the cause nor the necessary effect of spelnic fever." Pasteur, however, who was just beginning his studies on splenic fever, or anthrax, repeated Koch's work and confirmed it in every detail, seeing the spores Koch had described.

After his demonstration, Koch returned to his country practice at Wollstein and continued his bacteriological work in an improvised laboratory in his home. The following year (1877), he published in Cohn's *Beiträge* a paper describing his methods of fixing and drying bacterial films on cover-slips, staining them with aniline dyes and photographing them for study and comparison—techniques of fundamental importance in bacteriology. The article contains three plates with 24 remarkable microphotographs. In 1878, he published his important monograph on wound infections, *Untersuchungen über die Aetiologie der Wundinfektionskrankheiten*. By employing the techniques he himself had worked out, he was able to describe the bacteria of six different varieties of wound infections, each bacterium characteristic in its appearance, retaining the same appearance after several transfers on culture medium or passage through animals. In addition to the bacteriological studies, he described in detail the pathological findings.

Still a country doctor and now 35 years old, Koch had within two years through the achievements recorded in these three papers advanced to the first rank in medical science. Through the influence of Cohn, he was appointed to a position in the Imperial Health

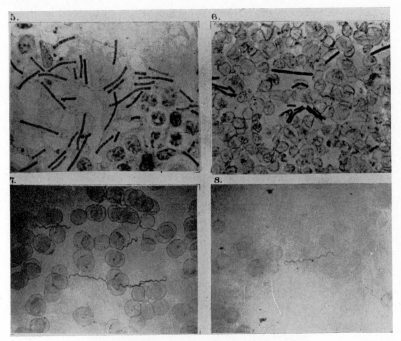

KOCH'S MICROPHOTOGRAPHS OF BACTERIA

Four microphotographs from Koch's paper, *Untersuchungen über Bacterien,* published in 1877. Note the excellence of these photographs made by Koch himself while still Kreisphysikus in Wollstein.

Office *(Kaiserliches Gesundheitsamt)* in 1880 and moved to Berlin, where Löffler and Gaffky became his assistants. Here, in 1881, he worked out a new method of obtaining pure cultures of bacteria by using a meat infusion mixed with warm gelatin, which hardened after being poured upon glass plates. He demonstrated this method at King's College during the International Medical Congress held in London the same year. While the Congress was dominated by three outstanding personalities—Lister, Virchow and Pasteur—Pasteur was deeply impressed by young Koch's discovery and, after the demonstration, shook Koch's hand, exclaiming, "C'est un grand progrès!" And it proved to be. By some, it has been considered Koch's greatest contribution to medical science since it enabled the bacteriologist to obtain pure cultures of microorganisms.

Employing this new method, together with the staining methods he had previously devised, Koch, in 1882, discovered the tubercle bacillus, the most spectacular achievement of his career. The existence of such an organism had long been postulated and had seemed a certainty since Villemin had shown that tuberculous sputum and the fluid of tubercular cavities, when injected into rabbits, produced tuberculosis. Koch's demonstration of the tubercle bacillus wrote the final chapter in the history of the cause of this age old disease.

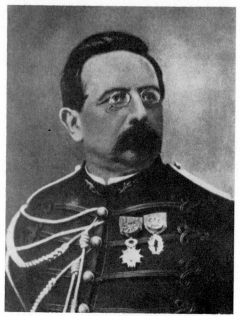

Les Médecins Célèbres, Paris, 1947

JEAN ANTOINE VILLEMIN

Villemin was the undisputed demonstrator of the contagiousness of tuberculosis. (Portrait in the *Musée* de Vâl de Grace.)

As Rieux wrote in 1927, the three fundamental advances in the history of tuberculosis were made by three men—"Laennec, who proclaimed its unity; Villemin, who demonstrated it was due to a virus; Koch, who discovered and identified its pathogenic agent."

The paper describing Koch's discovery also contains a statement of what have since become known as "Koch's postulates." The specificity of a microorganism and its relation to a disease are not demonstrated until the following conditions are fulfilled: (1) the microorganism is present and demonstrable in every case of the disease;

(2) it must be cultivated in pure culture; (3) inoculation of the culture must produce the disease in susceptible animals; and (4) it must be recovered from such animals and grown in pure culture. *These postulates are the pillars upon which the whole structure of modern bacteriology rests.*

In 1883, Koch, while carrying out investigations in Egypt and India as head of the German Cholera Commission, discovered the cholera vibrio and proved the transmission of cholera by water, food and clothing. He also discovered at this time the microorganism of Egyptian ophthalmia, the Koch-Weeks bacillus.

It was in 1890 that he discovered tuberculin, which he hoped would be a remedy for tuberculosis. While Koch himself was very conservative in his claims, the discovery was hailed as a cure for tuberculosis. The great hopes so raised, however, were later doomed to disappointment. This disappointment has been somewhat mitigated by the demonstration of the great value of tuberculin in diagnosis.

Koch was appointed professor of hygiene and bacteriology in the University of Berlin in 1885 and director of the new Institute of Infectious Diseases in Berlin in 1891. He held the latter position until 1904, when he resigned in favor of his pupil Gaffky. In 1893, he wrote an important paper on water-borne diseases, pointing out that they could be prevented by proper filtration. Three years later at the request of the British Government, he went to South Africa to study Rinderpest (cattle plague). He did not discover the etiologic agent of this disease, which is still unknown, but did work out a successful method of vaccination for its prevention. While in Africa, he also studied Texas fever, blackwater fever, malaria, surra and plague. He revisited Africa in 1906 to study sleeping sickness and, at that time, introduced atoxyl into its treatment.

Koch was now a famous savant whose name was known around the world. In Japan, a shrine was erected in his honor. Although he received the Nobel prize in 1905, was elected to the Prussian *Akademie der Wissenschaften,* and was given the title of *Excellenz,* the latter years of his life were unhappy. He became infatuated with a young actress, divorced his wife, and married the young woman, to the intense indignation of the entire German nation. He died of heart disease in 1910 at the age of 67.

Koch was one of the greatest bacteriologists of history. His scientific horizon was not so broad as Pasteur's but, for meticulous, accurate and exact bacteriological studies, Koch was without a peer. It may be doubted whether Pasteur in most of his research ever worked with pure cultures of microorganisms, whereas Koch not only worked with pure cultures but also demonstrated how this perfection was to be acquired and stressed the fundamental scientific principle that microorganisms must be studied in pure culture to determine their etiologic and pathogenic role. When Koch began his work, the bacterial origin of only two diseases had been established with any degree of probability—anthrax and relapsing fever. Armauer Hansen of Bergen, Norway, had seen the lepra bacillus and was studying its relationship to leprosy (1871-1874), but his work was neither widely known nor accepted.

The work of Koch gave bacteriology an impetus it had never known before. In his laboratories in Berlin, he was soon surrounded by a group of eager young students actively engaged in the study of bacteriology and making important discoveries. This investigative ferment spread rapidly throughout Germany to distant lands. Many important bacteriological discoveries were made elsewhere, but, in a true sense, all of these investigators were pupils of Koch, who had not only provided the initial stimulus but had developed the methods necessary for successful research in this field.

The list of important diseases, the etiology of which was demonstrated by the discovery of the specific microorganism responsible, is a long and impressive one. The achievement of bacteriology during this period is one of the chief glories of nineteenth century medicine. Neisser, in 1879, discovered the gonococcus; Eberth, in 1880, discovered the typhoid bacillus; the pneumococcus, previously observed by Pasteur and Sternberg, was shown to be the cause of pneumonia by Fraenkel in 1884; the bacillus of glanders was demonstrated by Löffler in 1882-1886; the streptococcus of erysipelas by Fehleisen in 1883; the diphtheria bacillus by Klebs in 1883; the bacillus of tetanus by Nicholaier in 1884; the meningococcus by Weichselbaum in 1887; the *Micrococcus melitensis* by Bruce in 1887; the gas bacillus by Welch and Nuttall in 1892; the plague bacillus by Kitasato and Yersin, working independently, in 1894—and this by no means exhausts the list. In addition to these bacterial diseases, Evans, in 1880, demonstrated that surra, a disease of horses in India, was due to an unusual type of parasite—a trypanosome—a discovery that was followed by the work of Bruce, who found trypanosomes in the blood of cattle in Africa suffering from nagana.

Koch, who inaugurated the era of bacteriological research, had, as we have seen, a most important precursor in Louis Pasteur. Another precursor, not so well known to posterity, was a fellow countryman, Edwin Klebs, who made many important and lasting contributions to bacteriology. Klebs was born in Königsberg, East Prussia, in 1834. He studied first at Königsberg, where Rathke and Helmholtz were teaching, and then at Würzburg, where he came under the influence of Kölliker and Virchow. He was so impressed with Virchow that he followed him to Berlin, where he took his medical

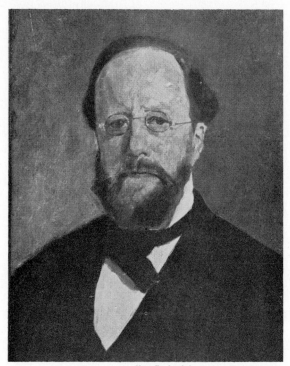

New England Journal of Medicine, 1935

EDWIN KLEBS

Portrait by H. Treuenfels, 1879.

degree in 1856, writing a dissertation on tuberculosis, a disease the study of which remained his greatest interest throughout his life.

After graduation, he became a *Privatdozent* at Königsberg and, in 1861, returned to Berlin as assistant to Virchow. After five years, he went to Bern as professor of pathology, then to Würzburg in 1871, to Prague in 1873, and to Zürich in 1882. After 11 years, he left Zürich for Karlsruhe, came to Asheville, North Carolina, as director of the laboratory in a private sanitarium for tuberculosis, and, in 1896, became professor of pathology in Rush Medical College, Chicago. In 1900, he returned to Europe, working successively in Hanover, Berlin, Laussane and Bern. He died in 1913.

The restless, nomadic instincts of Klebs, characterized by his frequent change of residence, is reflected in his scientific activities. He made many capital discoveries, but, becoming impatient, wandered off to other fields before he had impressed on others the value of his initial discovery and before he himself had pursued the discovery to its logical conclusion. Whereas Virchow adjusted his thinking from morphological concepts with great difficulty and viewed with suspicion the new theories of immunity as a reversion to the old humoral pathology, Klebs early recognized the importance of bacteriology. Klebs's reputation as a pathologist, particularly after the publication of his excellent *Handbuch des pathologischen Anatomie,* 1869-1876, was so great that he won most pathologists over to his viewpoint.

Studying the pathology of gunshot wounds in 1871, Klebs saw bacteria of different forms in almost every case. This investigation preceded that of Koch but was not, however, so meticulously carried out. Klebs came to the conclusion that these different forms were varieties of the same organism, to which he gave the name of *microsporon septicum.* The same year, working on anthrax, he devised a filter impervious to bacteria and worked with the filtrates, showing that they were toxic but could not infect animals with anthrax. These significant facts were the starting point for the later work of von Behring, Roux and Yersin on toxins and antitoxins. In 1872, Klebs employed as culture media sturgeon's glue—the first use of solid media in bacteriology. In 1878, he successfully inoculated monkeys with syphilis, although credit is commonly assigned to Metchnikoff's experiments in 1905, and he saw the typhoid bacillus before Eberth (1881) and the diphtheria bacillus before Löffler (1883). In 1884, he published, with Fritzsche, the first description of a case of acromegaly with autopsy.

One of the reasons for Klebs's failure to receive the credit that seems his due was stated by Klebs himself, according to one of his students: "I was the first to see and partially describe many pathogenic bacteria, but I had no success with those methods which yielded conclusive evidence."

Vallery-Radot, in his *Life of Pasteur,* writes that Pasteur was intensely interested in diphtheria and "had hopes that he would yet live to see the defeat of the foe so dreaded by mothers." He writes, perhaps a bit grudgingly, "A German by the name of Klebs discovered the bacillus of diphtheria in 1883 by studying the characteristic membranes; it was afterwards isolated by Löffler, another German."

Roux and Yersin, working in the Pasteur Institute, showed that the effects produced by the diphtheria bacillus were due to the toxin which it produced, a discovery which greatly interested the failing Pasteur. The following year, Behring and Kitasato, working in Koch's Institute, announced the discovery of tetanus antitoxin on December 3, 1890. One week after this joint publication, Behring alone published a paper on immunization against diphtheria. "Priority claims have been made by or on behalf of Hericourt and Richet (1888), and Babes and Lepp (1889), but history must assign unchallenged to Behring and Kitasato the discovery of antitoxic immunity" (Bullock). Roux, at the Pasteur Institute, began the production of diphtheria antitoxin, treated children suffering from diphtheria in the Children's Hospital with the new preparation, and immediately reduced the mortality from 51 per cent to 24 per cent. In rapid succession, reports appeared in large numbers confirming the value of diphtheria antitoxin. "Pasteur, who was then at Arbois, followed every detail with passionate interest" (Vallery-Radot).

THE PREDOMINANCE OF GERMAN MEDICINE

Medical science had now received two powerful impacts within the space of less than 25 years. Virchow had discovered that diseases are due to diseased cells; Koch had demonstrated the bacterial origin of many diseases and given the investigator the techniques necessary to prove a bacterial origin. The stimulus imparted by these two men, transmitted to an extraordinary number of gifted young chemists, physicists, anatomists, pathologists and physiologists, soon raised Germany to the front rank in medicine. This ferment, which had been apparent for several years, was greatly accelerated by the outcome of the Franco-German War of 1870. Following this war, victorious Germany embarked upon a building program for her universities and hospitals, which program made them at once an object of admiration and envy to their contemporaries in other lands. With this went a prodigality in support and maintenance that had been previously unknown. Pasteur wrote in 1867,

Some nations have felt the wholesome breath of truth. During the past thirty years, Germany has been covered with large and rich laboratories and every day sees new ones born. Berlin and Bonn have constructed two palaces, worth four million francs, both designed for chemical studies.

Pasteur continued in this strain, castigating the French Government for its penurious policy in regard to science. "Pasteur," says

his biographer, Vallery-Radot, "had the greatest admiration foɩ
the German system: popular instruction liberally provided for and,
in addition, an intellectually independent higher instruction." This,
however, was before the War of 1870, which transformed Pasteur into
an enemy of all things German. After 1870, although Pasteur made
no more comparisons between Germany and France to the advantage
of the former, the disparity between the liberality of science of the
two nations became even more marked. The new German Empire
lavished large sums on their universities and hospitals; France did
not follow her example, so Germany presently became the leader in
medicine and science and held this position until World War I.

The powerful stimulus to German scientific medicine, stemming
from the pioneer work of Liebig, Johannes Müller, Virchow and
Koch, initiated one of the most productive periods in the history
of medicine. Microscopic anatomy, pathological anatomy, normal
and pathological physiology, pharmacology and bacteriology, cultivated with such prodigious intensity, yielded an amazingly rich
harvest. Clinical medicine and surgery, the heirs of the great mass
of new knowledge, made corresponding advances. With Berlin as
its center, Germany became a vast network of scientific activity, a
network which included all the universities and technical institutes.
Many of the smaller universities developed into centers of scientific
activity, the peer of those which had developed in the capital itself,
and, in many of these smaller universities, renowned investigators
carried out work unequaled elsewhere in the empire. Not infre-
quently, the professors, for various reasons, moved from one university to another, and the students invariably changed with the se-
mesters, as they sought one teacher in a certain subject, another
teacher in another subject. This free interchange, in which the
Swiss universities also participated, was stimulating to both teacher
and student.

The list of great teachers and investigators in Germany at this
period is a very long one and includes some of the greatest names
in modern medical history. In anatomy, the names of Rudolf Albert
Kölliker of Würzburg, the creator of systematic histology, and of
Wilhelm His of Leipzig, the pioneer in histogenesis, are outstanding. In pathology, Julius Cohnheim of Breslau and Leipzig, the
most brilliant of Virchow's pupils; Carl Weigert, assistant of Cohnheim, who first stained bacteria and introduced aniline dyes into
the study of microscopic anatomy and pathology; Friedrich Daniel
von Recklinghausen, pathologist of Strassburg, who described three
diseases bearing his name; and Johannes Orth, Virchow's successor

in Berlin, all earned enduring fame in this field. In physiology, E. F. W. Pflüger of Bonn solved many complex problems of metabolism; Willy Kühne elucidated many physiological problems and discovered trypsin; and Hugo Kronecker at Leipzig, Berlin and Bern made notable contributions to the physiology of the heart, circulation and respiration. In Munich, Max von Pettenkofer and Carl von Voit in their "Respiration Chamber" founded the modern study of metabolism and worked out the caloric values of foods. Here also Pettenkofer established the first modern hygienic institute. In Strassburg, Felix Hoppe-Seyler made great advances in physiological chemistry, and Oswald Schmiedeberg established pharmacology as an important branch of medicine and trained a new generation of pharmacologists.

Clinical medicine was represented by a veritable galaxy of prominent names. Friedrich Theodor von Frerichs, the successor of Schönlein in Berlin, was one of the founders of scientific medical teaching. Ludwig Traube, von Frerich's successor, was an able clinician and

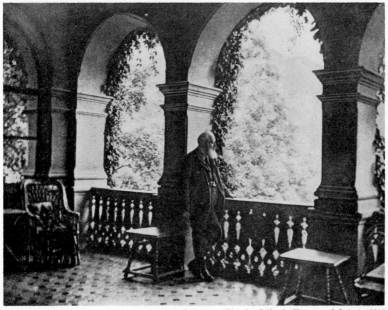

Briefe von Theodor Billroth, Hannover & Leipzig, 1895

THEODOR BILLROTH

Photograph with the notation, "St. Gilgen, September, 1892," and the quotation from Hebbel, "Diess ist ein Herbsttag wie ich keinen sah."

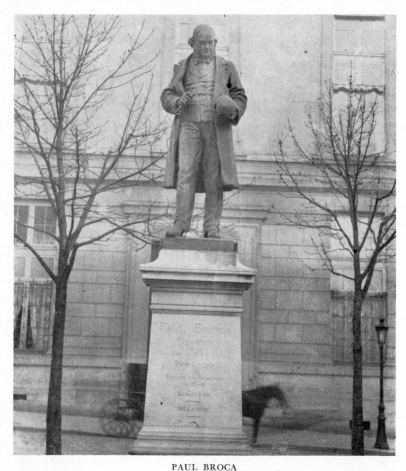

PAUL BROCA

Statue which stood on the Boulevard St. Germain before World War II.

one of the founders of experimental pathology. Karl Wunderlich of
Leipzig studied the relation of body heat to disease and was the
founder of modern clinical thermometry. Adolf Kussmaul, professor
in four different universities, made important contributions to many
phases of clinical medicine. In Strassburg, Naunyn's clinic became
the mecca for students of diabetes, and here Oskar Minkowsky produced diabetes by extirpation of the pancreas and demonstrated the
role of B-oxybutyric acid in diabetic acidosis. Heinrich Quincke,
professor at Kiel, introduced lumbar puncture as a diagnostic and
therapeutic procedure.

In surgery, the achievements were impressive. Karl Thiersch of Leipzig, Friedrich von Esmarch of Kiel, Richard von Volkmann of Halle, Ernest von Bergmann of Berlin, Gustav Simon of Heidelberg and Johann von Mikulicz-Radecki of Breslau made surgical history. In Berlin, Albrecht von Graefe founded scientific ophthalmology.

German-speaking Vienna also contributed to the glory of German medicine. Ernst Wilhelm von Brücke, a transplanted Berliner, was a remarkable all around physiologist and anatomist; Willy Kühne, a native of Hamburg, studied for the first time the split products of gastric digestion; and Hermann Nothnagel, born in Brandenburg, was a popular teacher who has earned lasting fame by his encyclopedic *Handbuch*. But the best known of all was the gifted Theodor Billroth, another North German, one of the greatest surgeons of all time, whose originality of mind was equalled by his skill and boldness in surgical operations.

France, although she had lost the leadership in medicine to her younger rival across the Rhine, continued to produce men worthy of her best tradition. Armand Duchenne made fundamental studies on nervous diseases; Paul Broca investigated the cerebral localization of motor functions and placed brain surgery on a scientific basis. Jean Martin Charcot, perhaps the greatest and certainly one of the most dramatic and interesting teachers of his time, created the greatest clinic in Europe for the study of nervous diseases. "Modern neurology," says Garrison, "is mainly of French extraction and derives from Duchenne of Boulogne through Charcot and his pupils."

French scientific activity was further stimulated by the work of the group at the Pasteur Institute. Roux, upon whom the mantle of Pasteur had fallen, proved to be an extremely capable and brilliant investigator. In 1888, Metchnikoff, a young Russian biologist who had discovered the new and important phenomena of phagocytosis came to Paris and joined the staff of the Institute.

In Great Britain, where clinical practice was still the goal of most physicians and where the separate fields of anatomy, physiology and pathology were not cultivated with the same intensity as in Germany, there were nevertheless many physicians who made important contributions to medical science. Among them were William Bowman, pathologist and ophthalmologist; J. H. Bennett, pathologist and microscopist; William S. Kirkes, who made important studies on thrombosis and embolism; Samuel Wilks, pathologist and medical historian; Hughlings Jackson, pioneer neurologist; William Broadbent, who achieved fame, particularly as a cardiologist; and

Thomas Lauder Brunton, who introduced pharmacological methods into Great Britain and taught the value of nitrates in angina pectoris. During this period, Patrick Manson returned from China to initiate the study of tropical diseases, and Michael Foster founded the Cambridge school of physiologists, whose contributions made Cambridge a leader in this field.

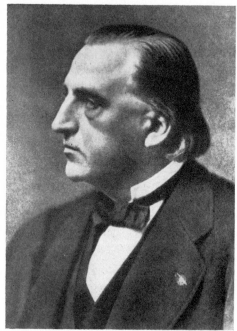

Les Médecins Célèbres, Paris, 1947

JEAN MARTIN CHARCOT

THE INFLUENCE OF GERMAN MEDICINE ON AMERICA

"The universities of Germany," wrote Osler in 1890, "are her chief glory, and the greatest boon she can give us in the New World is to return our young men infected with the spirit of earnestness and with the love of thoroughness which characterizes the work done in them." Many young physicians went to Germany for their further education and on their return home brought with them the spirit of earnestness and thoroughness that Osler had praised.

Henry P. Bowditch, after study with Claude Bernard in Paris

and with Carl Ludwig in Leipzig, returned to Boston and established at Harvard in 1871 the first well equipped laboratory of physiology in America. After two years' study in Vienna with Rokitansky and Skoda and with Virchow in Berlin, Reginald Fitz returned to Boston and became professor of pathology at Harvard. Later, turning to clinical medicine, he became one of the outstand-

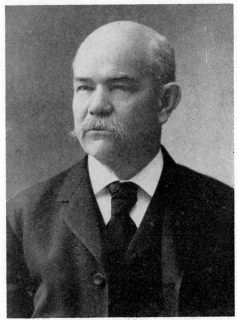

Library, Jackson Co. (Mo.) Medical Society

REGINALD FITZ

ing physicians of his time. In 1886, he pointed out the importance of diseases of the appendix and focused the attention of the profession upon this common and hitherto neglected cause of disease and death. It was one of the great achievements of nineteenth century medicine. The same year Krönlein of Zürich performed the first appendectomy for appendicitis.

Nowhere, however, was the deep impress of German medicine felt so strongly as at the new school of medicine which arose in Baltimore during the closing years of the nineteenth century. The establishment of the Johns Hopkins medical school marks the beginning of a new era in American medicine.

JOHNS HOPKINS

When Johns Hopkins, shrewd and thrifty Quaker merchant and banker, reached the age of 72, he was possessed of the largest fortune of his time in Baltimore. He regarded his fortune of some $7,000,000 as a trust to be used for the benefit of his fellowmen and divided it into two equal portions, one half for the founding of a university, the other half for the establishment of a hospital. In 1867, bills were introduced into the Maryland General Assembly authorizing the formation of two corporations, the Johns Hopkins University and the Johns Hopkins Hospital. Both bills were duly passed, and the charters were granted. Johns Hopkins University was formally opened in 1876; Johns Hopkins Hospital in 1889; and the School of Medicine in 1893.

Johns Hopkins himself selected the site for the hospital, bought the land, and presented it to the trustees of the hospital. He died in 1873, and, a year later, the trustees he had appointed chose Daniel Coit Gilman, then president of the University of California, to head the new Johns Hopkins University. Gilman's brilliant achievements as president of the new university wrote a new chapter in the history of higher education in America. Universities in America up to this time had been mainly overgrown colleges. Gilman planned a university in which emphasis should be on graduate study, an institution composed of professors of great distinction,

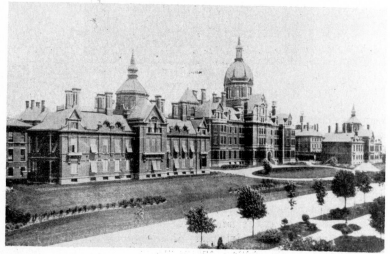

JOHNS HOPKINS HOSPITAL, 1889

where unusual facilities should be available for superior students. He assembled a group of outstanding scholars so that, when the university was opened in 1876, the faculty contained such notables as B. L. Gildersleeve in Greek, J. J. Sylvester in mathematics, Ira Remsen in chemistry, H. Newell Martin in biology, W. K. Brooks in zoology, and H. A. Rowland in physics. In a short period of time, these men, under the inspiring leadership of Gilman, had made the name of Johns Hopkins University well known throughout the educational world.

Gilman next turned his great talents to the establishment of the Johns Hopkins Hospital and medical school, which he wished to make as distinctive in their fields as the university itself had become. In this work, he was ably assisted by H. Newell Martin, professor of biology in the university, and John Shaw Billings of the Surgeon-General's Office in Washington, who gave lectures at the universiy on the history of medicine, medical education, and medical jurisprudence. Billings influenced deeply the plans for the organization of the new medical school and was the chief adviser to the hospital trustees during the period of construction. His judgment in regard to the selection of the new faculty had also great influence with Gilman.

In 1876, Billings went to Europe in the interest of the Johns Hopkins Hospital. In Leipzig, he visited Ludwig's laboratory, where he met a young American doctor, William H. Welch, who was actively at work there. Billings was much impressed by Welch and remarked to Francis T. King, the chairman of the hospital board, who had accompanied him on the trip, "That young man should be, in my opinion, one of the first men to be secured when the time comes to begin the medical school."

Welch, who had received his doctor's degree from the College of Physicians and Surgeons of New York in 1875, spent nearly two years in Germany working with Ludwig in Leipzig and with Cohnheim in Breslau. On his return to New York, he began to practice medicine but was more interested in a small laboratory of pathology in the Bellevue Hospital, where he conducted courses in pathology and bacteriology.

In 1884, President Gilman, after receiving most favorable reports from Billings and Cohnheim, appointed William H. Welch professor of pathology. Welch moved to Baltimore to assume his duties, but his appearance on the new stage was, as Chesney remarks, "more like a prologue than the first act of a play" since the medical school

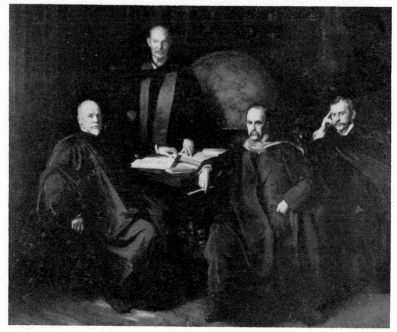

THE FOUR DOCTORS

This portrait by John Singer Sargent is one of his masterpieces. Sitting
from left to right are Welch, Osler and Kelly, standing Halsted.

did not open until nine years later. Welch began a series of lectures
for physicians soon after he arrived in Baltimore, even before the
pathological laboratory was built. With the completion of this laboratory, he established courses in pathology and bacteriology for
physicians and also offered facilities for research in these fields.
Among his distinguished pupils of this period were Walter Reed,
James Carroll, Simon Flexner, and Reid Hunt.

William Osler, professor of clinical medicine in the University of
Pennsylvania, was appointed in 1888 Physician-in-chief to the Johns
Hopkins Hospital and professor of medicine in the university.
Welch had known Osler for several years, having met him while he
was still in Montreal. "I was captivated," wrote Welch, "and I think
that he was my choice for the Hopkins from the time I first became
connected with it."

The well-known Sargent portrait of the "Four Doctors" portrays
Welch and Osler in the foreground. "It is entirely fitting," Chesney
comments, "for Welch and Osler were unquestionably the two most

commanding figures in the Hospital in those early days." As Chesney, however, notes, the other two men in the portrait, Halsted and Kelly, also made notable contributions to the progress of the new hospital and medical school as well as to American medicine.

William Stewart Halsted, a native of New York, graduated at the New York College of Physicians and Surgeons in 1877 and, after two years of study in Vienna, Würzburg, Leipzig and Halle, returned to New York, where he soon acquired an active surgical practice, serving on the staffs of six widely separated hospitals. In 1881, he introduced the procedure of re-infusion of aerated blood and devised the well-known "cigarette" drain for wounds. In 1885, he discovered the principle of conduction, or block anesthesia with cocaine, performing some of his operations, as he states, "in a large tent which I built on the grounds of Bellevue Hospital, having found it impossible to carry out antiseptic precautions in the general amphitheatre of Bellevue, where the numerous anti-Lister surgeons dominated and predominated." In the course of his experiments, many performed on himself, he became temporarily addicted to cocaine, a habit which he overcame completely but which for a time wrecked his health and forced his retirement from practice. Two years later, fully recovered, he went to Welch's laboratory in Baltimore, where he worked on problems relating to the healing of wounds and the function of the thyroid gland. In 1889, he was appointed associate professor of surgery and, the following year, professor of surgery, a position he held for 32 years.

The fourth of the doctors in Sargent's picture was Howard Atwood Kelly, a graduate of the University of Pennsylvania. At the time of his appointment as professor of gynecology and obstetrics in Johns Hopkins, he was only 31 years of age and only seven years out of medical school, but already professor of obstetrics at the University of Pennsylvania. His later achievements in gynecology and obstetrics proved him a peer of the three other brilliant men with whom he was associated.

When the medical school was opened in 1893, other promising young men joined the original four doctors. Franklin P. Mall, age 31, a graduate of Michigan, who had worked in Leipzig with the anatomist His and the physiologist Ludwig, was appointed professor of anatomy. John J. Abel, a native of Ohio, who had studied seven years in Germany and had received his medical degree at Strassburg in 1888, was appointed professor of pharmacology. William H. Howell, an old pupil of H. Newell Martin, was called to the chair of physiology.

Two characteristics of the new faculty were noteworthy. The first was the age of the professors. At the time they were appointed to their chairs, Kelly and Mall were 31, Howell 33, Abel 36, Halsted 38; while of the older men, Welch and Osler were both 45. The second characteristic was the fact that all of them, except Howell, had studied extensively in Germany.

The new medical school, following the ideas of Gilman that it should be a graduate school, required that all students who were admitted should have a bachelor's degree, a good reading knowledge of French and German, and must have finished prescribed courses in physics, chemistry and biology. These high entrance requirements caused much shaking of heads among the doctors of America and called forth the oft-quoted remark from Osler that he was lucky to be a professor in the new medical school because he never could have gained entrance as a student. Women were admitted on the same terms as men, another new departure in medical education. The members of the faculty by their scientific contributions soon made the new school the unquestioned medical center of the country.

Welch continued to be the inspiring teacher and thinker, a powerful influence in moulding the course of American medical education and in initiating and encouraging research in all fields of medicine. Osler succeeded in his great ambition: "To build up a great clinic on Teutonic lines, not on those previously followed here and in England, but on lines which have proved so successful on the Continent and which have placed the scientific medicine of Germany in the forefront of the world." How well he succeeded is described by Welch:

Osler created a medical clinic of a new order, at least for this country. He brought the senior students into the wards of the hospital not simply to look on at demonstrations, not simply to accompany the physician on his rounds in the wards, but as a part of the actual machinery of the hospital. . . . He was familiar with the organization of medical clinics in Germany, France and England; he took the best, and I think he established a type of organization which marked a great advance in medical education.

In addition to many papers and addresses, Osler wrote the greatest textbook of medicine in his time. His *Principles and Practice of Medicine*, which appeared in 1892, sold 23,000 copies in its first edition, went through eight editions during his lifetime, and was translated into French, German, Spanish and Chinese. The publisher announced with the publication of the sixth edition that 105,000 copies of the book had been sold. Frederick T. Gates, financial adviser to John D. Rockefeller, read this book during his summer

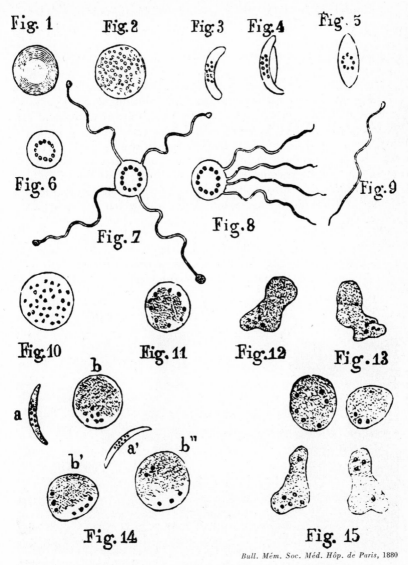

Fig. 1 Fig. 2 Fig. 3 Fig. 4 Fig. 5

Fig. 6 Fig. 7 Fig. 8 Fig. 9

Fig. 10 Fig. 11 Fig. 12 Fig. 13

Fig. 14 Fig. 15

Bull. Mém. Soc. Méd. Hôp. de Paris, 1880

ILLUSTRATIONS OF MALARIAL PARASITES IN LAVERAN'S
COMMUNICATION

vacation of 1897 and, deeply impressed with the importance of medical research, persuaded Mr. Rockefeller to establish an institute for medical research.

Osler was a man of unusual charm and geniality, an interesting and inspiring teacher, a person of wide cultural interests, and a graceful and witty writer. From his earliest years an enthusiastic student of medical history and an avid collector of old books, he contributed many noteworthy articles on historical topics and collected one of the best private medical libraries of modern times. He had an unusual capacity for friendships, enjoyed a wide acquaintance among the medical profession, and his departure from Baltimore in 1905 to become Regius Professor of Medicine at Oxford called forth wide spread expressions of regret and unprecedented demonstrations of the esteem and affection in which he was held.

W. S. Halsted was, in personality, a marked contrast to Welch and Osler. He was not, like Welch, a brilliant speaker whose extemporaneous talks had the polish and accuracy of a carefully prepared address, and he lacked the infectious geniality and the spon-

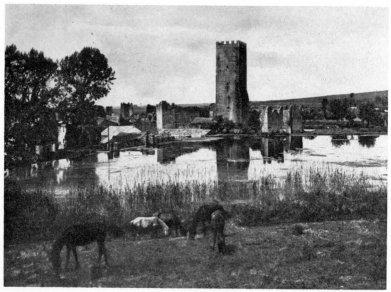

Photo Alinari

THE RUINS OF NINFA

A dramatic victim of malaria is the deserted city of Ninfa. In 1150, it was a thriving, well-populated community. By mid-eighteenth century, malaria had driven away Ninfa's last inhabitant.

taneous wit of Osler. He was a somewhat "remote, austere, Olympian figure" (Chesney), and his bedside teaching, as the undergraduates said, began as a dialogue, which was over the heads of the students, between the professor and his resident and, then getting beyond the depth of the resident, became a monologue with Halsted carrying on alone. The nicknames bestowed by the students on the three men were unconsciously revealing: Welch was "Popsy," Osler "The Chief," and Halsted "The Professor."

Halsted had a great distaste for publicity and an aversion to dramatic and spectacular surgery. A profound student of pathology and physiology, he tested surgical procedures in the experimental laboratory before employing them in the operating room. He stressed gentleness and absolute aseptic technique in the handling of tissues and never sacrificed safety for speed. He was deeply devoted to the progress of surgery and quite uninterested in questions of priority. He never referred to his great discovery of block anesthesia made in 1885, and the recognition of his claims to priority was literally forced upon him 37 years later when the American National Dental Association awarded him a gold medal for his achievement. He was one of the greatest scientific surgeons of his day, and his institution of surgical residencies in Johns Hopkins marks the beginning of a new era in American surgery.

Howard A. Kelly, aggressive and dynamic, a fluent speaker and a skillful operator, developed a clinic which equaled that of his colleagues. His boldness and skill in operating, his powers of observation, his ability to think and write clearly placed him in the forefront of American gynecologists and, according to many, the leader. A forceful and ready speaker and a very devout churchman, Kelly was, during his entire career, a vigorous campaigner for reform in civic government, in public health, and in personal morals. An enthusiastic collector of old books and deeply interested in medical history, he made many contributions to this field. He was a deep student of fungi and had a large collection of mushrooms.

All the other young men who established the new medical school became noted in their fields. Franklin P. Mall, the new professor of anatomy, carried out investigations in embryology which are among the most significant of their time. John J. Abel, the pharmacologist, isolated epinephrin and bufagin, did pioneer work on phthaleins, devised vividiffusion, and made important studies on pituitary extracts. He was an indefatigable worker throughout his life, crystallized insulin at the age of 69, and, the last year of his life when 81 years of age, made important studies on the properties of tetanus toxin. William H. Howell rapidly rose to a place of leadership in American physiology, made fundamental observations on the coagulation of the blood, discovered heparin and cephalin, and wrote the outstanding textbook on physiology, which passed through 14 editions during his lifetime and from which most American students learned their physiology for 40 years.

The list of the men who taught or studied at Johns Hopkins during its formative years is a long and impressive one. Among the pathologists, it includes such names as Councilman, MacCallum, Le Count, Winternitz and Whipple; among bacteriologists, George M. Sternberg, Simon Flexner, Alexander Abbott, P. H. Hiss, Richard P. Strong, Walter Reed, James Carroll, W. W. Ford, and G. H. P. Nuttall; among anatomists, W. H. Lewis, Florence R. Sabin, Herbert M. Evans, and L. H. Weed; in physiology, J. A. E. Eyster, P. M. Dawson, and D. R. Hooker; in clinical medicine, W. S. Thayer, L. F. Barker, Thomas McCrae, T. B. Futcher, Henry Christian, Joseph Pratt, Allen Krause, George Blumer, John Howland, Henry M. Thomas, W. T. Longcope, and Wilbur Davidson; in surgery, Harvey Cushing, J. M. T. Finney, Hugh Young, Joseph Bloodgood, Dean Lewis, Mont Reid, Walter Dandy, William Sharpe, H. C. Naffziger, George Heuer, and Willis Gatch; in gynecology, Thomas S. Cullen and John T. Sampson; in obstetrics, J. Whitridge Williams; in pharmacology, Reid Hunt, Paul Lamson, L. G. Rowntree, E. K. Marshall, and H. K. Geiling. All of these men achieved fame and distinction. They left an indelible impress on American medicine.

The Johns Hopkins group contributed to the advance of scientific medicine by their medical achievements. The medical school had a potent influence in elevating the standards of medical education. The Johns Hopkins Hospital with its system of residencies, medical, surgical, gynecological and obstetrical, introduced a new era in professional training in America.

FURTHER SCIENTIFIC ACHIEVEMENTS

In the latter years of the nineteenth century, several noteworthy discoveries were made which took their place beside the astounding advances already recorded.

MALARIA

In 1880, Alphonse Laveran, a French Army physician stationed at Constantine, was engaged in the study of malaria. He noted at autopsy the constant presence of pigment granules, especially in the liver and in the cerebral blood vessels, and began an intensive study of the pigment in the blood vessels and in the blood. He wrote:

> In 1880, at the military hospital of Constantine, I discovered on the edges of the round pigmented bodies in the blood of a patient with malaria filiform elements resembling flagella which moved about with great vivacity, displacing the neighboring red cells: from that time I had no doubts on the parasitic nature of these bodies which I had discovered in malarial blood.

Laveran sent a memoir describing his discovery to the Paris *Académie des Sciences*. This was read and published the same year but was received with great skepticism. However, he continued his investigations and found that these bodies were invariably present when the blood was examined during the chill before the administration of quinine. In 1882, he went to Rome, where he again found the same parasites in the blood of malarial patients and demonstrated them to Baccelli, Bastianelli, Celli, Grassi, Marchiafava, and other Italian scientists. Golgi, in 1886, showed that the attack of fever commences at the moment the merozoites are liberated and pointed out the difference in the appearance of the tertian and quartan parasites. In 1889, Celli and Marchiafava differentiated the malaria parasites into the three types recognized today—tertian, quartan, and aestivo autumnal. Celli later formed a society for combatting malaria and suceeded in stamping out the disease in the Roman Compagna, a hot bed of malaria since the days of the ancient Roman republic. All of this work was accomplished by the study of fresh preparations. Dimitri Romanowsky of St. Petersburg devised in 1891 a stain which stained the parasites and has since been of great value in the study of malaria.

The skepticism regarding Laveran's discovery continued, however, for several years. Gradually, as techniques improved, the truth of his claims was established. Osler observed in the first edition of his *Principles and Practice of Medicine,* 1892: "So far as I know, not a single observer, who has had the necessary training and the material at his command, has failed to demonstrate the existence of these parasites." In a later passage, Osler adds: "We do not know how the parasite enters, or how or in what form it leaves the body; how or where it is propagated, under what outside conditions it develops, whether free or in some aquatic plant or animal."

Five years were to elapse after Osler wrote these words before the answer was found. In 1883, Albert F. A. King had already published a paper in which he gave 19 reasons for believing that malaria is transmitted by the mosquito, although he was apparently unfamiliar with Laveran's great discovery. Laveran, himself, became convinced in 1884 that the disease was transmitted by mosquitoes and stressed the fact that mosquitoes were extremely numerous in areas where malaria was prevalent. Meanwhile, Sir Patrick Manson, who had demonstrated while in China in 1879 that filariasis is transmitted by the bite of a mosquito and that the life cycle of the *filaria Bancrofti* takes place in the mosquito, returned to England and became interested in the subject of malarial transmission by mosquitoes.

In 1894, Ronald Ross, a surgeon in the Indian Medical Service, returned for a leave and saw Manson in London. Ross had been studying malaria in India 13 years but had made little headway and had never even seen the malarial parasite. Manson demonstrated to him at the Charing Cross Hospital the parasites in the blood of a patient who was suffering from malaria and also expounded the mosquito theory to him. On his return to India, Ross continued his work with new enthusiasm, aided by better technique and a better microscope of his own invention. In 1895, he demonstrated the parasites in the stomach of an anopheles mosquito which had fed on a malarial patient. This was the same year that W. G. MacCallum of Johns Hopkins showed that the so-called flagella were really sexual forms of the parasite. In 1898, Ross demonstrated the parasites in the salivary glands of the anopheles mosquito.

Manson was delighted and most enthusiastic over Ross's success. As a final clinching proof, Manson received in 1900 from Dr. Sambon in Italy some mosquitoes which had fed on a malarial patient and were presumably infected. Manson's son, Thurburn, allowed the mosquitoes to bite him and, two weeks later, came down with malaria. Grassi and Bignami had previously succeeded in transmitting malaria by the bite of an infected mosquito, but their experiments, carried out in a malarious country, were not so conclusive as Manson's experiments in London, which was free from malaria. At the same time as Manson's experiments, Doctors Sambon and Low, with a friend Terzi, lived three months during the malarial season in one of the most malarious districts in the Roman Campagna in a hut screened against mosquitoes, never leaving the hut until an hour after sunrise and always returning indoors an hour before sunset. They remained free of the disease although their hut was located in the deadliest place in the region and the fluctuating population, consisting mainly of migratory farm laborers, suffered severely from malaria during that period.

The importance of these discoveries is difficult to exaggerate. Malaria has been one of the greatest killers of history. While never appearing with the dramatic suddenness of an outbreak of bubonic plaque or of yellow fever, striking a community, destroying thousands in a few days or weeks, and then moving to fresh victims, malaria comes in quietly and unobstrusively but settles down as a permanent inhabitant, exacting its daily toll year by year and, as time rolls on, century by century. From the days of Aristophanes until the period of the conquistadores of Peru in the seventeenth century, the disease exacted a huge toll of life on four continents with no remedy available. Laveran had now made it possible to dif-

ferentiate malaria from a group of fevers with which it had long been confused; Ross had proved that it was transmitted by the mosquito, the destruction of which must be accomplished if the disease were ever to be controlled or eradicated. Malaria still exacts a heavy toll, but the mortality from this disease has definitely declined since the work of Laveran and Ross.

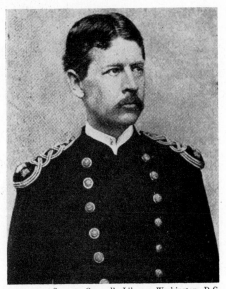

Surgeon General's Library, Washington, D.C.

WALTER REED

YELLOW FEVER

The mode of transmission of yellow fever was demonstrated less than five years later. Yellow fever had been present on the American continent since the time of Columbus. As early as 1493, an epidemic appeared in Santo Domingo. From that time, the disease appeared in epidemic form in various American cities, one of the most destructive outbreaks being the epidemic of 1793 in Philadelphia, where, in four months, 4,041 deaths were recorded, Philadelphia then having a population of 40,000. In 1870, a Napoleonic army, which had landed in the West Indies, was almost completely destroyed by yellow fever.

In 1881, Carlos Findlay, a Cuban physician, at the International Sanitary Conference held in Washington, expressed his belief that yellow fever was transmitted by the bite of a mosquito. He published an article in the *American Journal of the Medical Sciences*, 1886, describing his experiments on five men who were subjected to the bites of mosquitoes which had bitten patients suffering from yellow fever. In all of the subjects, yellow fever developed. Findlay's experiments, however, either were ignored or failed to impress most investigators.

In 1900, following the Spanish-American War, an outbreak of yellow fever appeared in Havana. The army sent the well-known Yellow Fever Commission, consisting of Walter Reed, James Carroll,

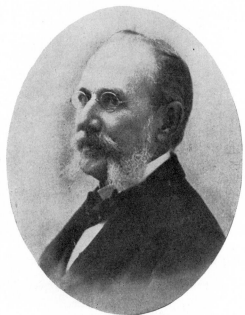

Surgeon General's Library, Washington, D.C.

CARLOS J. FINLAY

Jesse Lazear, and Arístides Agramonte, to study the disease. In Havana, they worked in close collaboration with Major W. C. Gorgas, who was the sanitary chief of Havana, and with Carlos Findlay, whose insistence on the mosquito theory they listened to with much skepticism but agreed to test.

The commission soon proved that yellow fever was transmitted by the bite of a mosquito, known then as the *Culex fasciatus,* later as the *Stegomyia fasciata,* and now called the *Aëdes aegypti.* They showed further that the disease was not transmitted by contact or other means. In the course of their experiments, Carroll submitted to the bite of an infected mosquito, developed yellow fever, but recovered. Lazear was bitten accidentally by an infected mosquito and died of yellow fever. Gorgas now initiated a thorough campaign of mosquito extermination. In three months, yellow fever was eradicated, and Havana, for the first time in 150 years, was free of the disease. Four years later, Gorgas was placed in charge of sanitation during the construction of the Panama Canal. Here he was largely responsible for the successful completion of this project, at which De Lesseps had previously failed. De Lesseps and the French had not lacked engineering skill, but the high mortality of their workers from yellow fever and malaria had doomed their efforts to failure.

DISCOVERY OF THE X-RAYS

The closing years of the century saw a great discovery in physics, a discovery which was to be of incalculable value to medical science —the discovery of the x-rays. This discovery was another vindication of Pasteur's statement that "in the field of observation, chance favors only the prepared mind." Its discoverer was Wilhelm Conrad Röntgen, a well-known physicist and, at the time, professor of physics and director of the Physical Institute at the University of Würzburg.

On November 8, 1895, Röntgen, while working at a late hour in a dark laboratory, noted that, when an electric current was passed through a Hittorf-Crookes tube, which was covered with black paper, some crystals of barium platinocyanide, which lay on the table, began to fluoresce. Further investigation revealed that a screen of the same material showed fluorescence when a current was passed through the tube and that opaque objects placed in front of the screen produced varying degrees of intensity in the glow on the screen. He then placed his hand in front of the screen and saw upon the screen the dense shadows of the bones within the outlines of the flesh. The next step was obviously to replace the screen with a photographic plate and thus obtain a permanent picture.

Röntgen's first publication on the subject was a preliminary report to the Würzburg Physical-Medical Society, which was received by the secretary on December 28, 1895, and bore the title, *Ueber eine neue Art von Strahlen*. Few discoveries in the history of science have created a greater sensation in scientific or lay circles. The medical applications of the new rays, which Röntgen called the x-rays, were obvious. Three months after Röntgen's announcement, the *Journal of the American Medical Association* noted:

The surgeons of Vienna and Berlin believe that the Roentgen photograph is destined to render inestimable services to surgery. . . . Half an hour is the shortest exposure possible, and most require one hour. The electric apparatus required is so expensive, $100.00 and upward, that few surgeons can use it yet in their private practice.

Two years after Röntgen's discovery, the new rays were employed by surgeons in the Greek-Turkish War of 1897 and, the following year, by American army surgeons in the Spanish-American War, the official report, remarkable for its understatement, noting, "The use

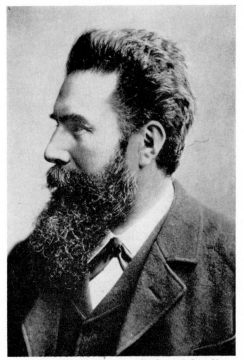

Kindness of Otto Glasser

WILHELM CONRAD RÖNTGEN

of the Röntgen ray has marked a distinct advance in military surgery." At first limited largely to the diagnoses of surgical conditions, such as fractures and bullet wounds, later improvements soon showed its great value in the study of the heart, lungs, and gastro-intestinal tract, also its great value as a therapeutic agent.

As we look back over the medical achievements of the nineteenth century, they are very impressive. The discovery of *auscultation* removed diagnosis, particularly in pulmonary and cardiac diseases, from the realms of speculation to the field of demonstrated fact. The later introduction of the x-ray gave a precision to diagnosis, which would have delighted Laennec, Skoda, and their numerous disciples, who did not live to see these later spectacular advances. Virchow, with his *cellular theory,* introduced a new concept into medical thinking, which shed light upon every phase of disease and destroyed the erroneous humoral theory, which had dominated medicine for more than 2,000 years. *Bacteriology,* through the discoveries of Pasteur, Koch, and their pupils, introduced a new era in medicine, demonstrated the cause of many diseases, which for centuries had seemed insoluble mysteries, and introduced new methods for the prevention, control and cure of diseases which had exacted an enormous toll of life since the beginnings of history.

The advances in surgery were equally spectacular. The discovery of *ether anesthesia* by Morton permitted both surgeon and patient to regard with equanimity operations which had previously caused excruciating pain to the patient and made even the most cold-blooded surgeon shudder. The development of *antiseptic and aseptic surgery* by Lister and his disciples made operations hitherto attended by a high mortality now relatively safe procedures. The later spectacular discoveries in bacteriology were as great a boon to surgery as to medicine.

REVOLUTION IN NURSING

During the latter half of the century, nursing, that indispensable adjunct to the successful treatment of medical and surgical conditions, underwent a veritable revolution, particularly in English-speaking countries. This was the achievement of Florence Nightingale (1820-1910), a young woman of wealth and education, who, appalled by the poor nursing conditions in England, resolved to devote her life to the reform of nursing. After study at the Institute of Protestant Deaconesses at Kaiserswerth, Germany, where she took the regular training courses for nurses, she studied in the hospitals of London, Edinburgh and Paris and, in 1853, became superintendent of the Hospital for Invalid Gentlewomen in London.

In 1854, England was profoundly stirred by the reports of the sufferings of the sick and wounded in the British Army during the Crimean War. Miss Nightingale set out with a staff of 38 nurses and took charge of the huge unsanitary barracks hospital at Scutari. Here she found a filthy hospital, swarming with vermin and lacking the most simple items of medical care as well as even primitive sanitary arrangements. She soon had more than 10,000 patients under her

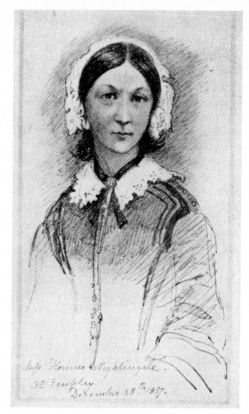

FLORENCE NIGHTINGALE IN 1857
Pencil drawing by Sir George Scharf in the
National Portrait Gallery.

care and, with almost superhuman energy, succeeded, in spite of
constant obstruction from the military authorities, in cleaning up
the hospital and instituting sanitary measures. The death rate in the
hospital, which was 42 per cent in February, 1855, fell to two per
cent in June of the same year.

Miss Nightingale's achievements in the Crimea made her a national heroine. After the conclusion of the Crimean War, the British
Government sent a man-of-war to bring her home, and London made
preparations for a triumphal reception, but Miss Nightingale returned quietly on a French ship, crossed the channel, and was in her
country home before the news of her whereabouts was known. With

50,000 pounds raised by public subscription, she founded a school of nursing at St. Thomas' Hospital, which became the model for subsequent training schools in England and in America. She was the founder of modern nursing. In 1907 at the age of 87, she received the Order of Merit, three years before her death.

HENRI DUNANT AND THE RED CROSS

Three years after the publication of Florence Nightingale's report on the sufferings of the British soldiers in the Crimea, J. Henri Dunant, a wealthy Swiss banker and philanthropist, while traveling in northern Italy, witnessed one of the bloodiest battles of modern times, the Battle of Solferino. This sanguinary encounter on June 24, 1859, between the Austrian army and the combined Italian and French forces lasted but 15 hours; but, at the end of the holocaust, more than 40,000 of the 300,000 troops engaged lay dead, dying, or wounded on the field of battle with practically no facilities for the care of the suffering.

Dunant was so moved and shattered by the horrors he had seen that he poured out his feelings in a book which described the terrible sights he had witnessed. *Un Souvenir de Solférino* was published in

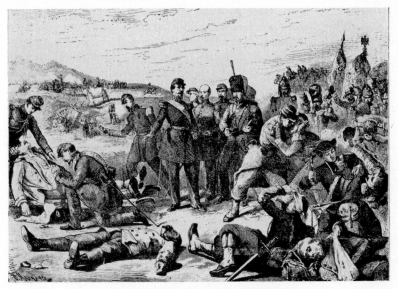

AFTER THE BATTLE OF SOLFERINO
Painting by T. Veron in the chapel of Vâl de Grace.

1862. In this small book, he wrote a shocking account of the wounded left to perish on the battlefield without medical care and proposed a world conference to found and organize in all civilized countries permanent societies of volunteers which, in time of war, would render succor to the wounded without distinction of nationality.

Dunant's book created a sensation and reached much wider fields through German, Italian and Swedish translations. Victor Hugo was deeply moved by it; the brothers Goncourt described it "as a thousand times more beautiful than Homer"; and Ernst Renan wrote the author, "You have created the greatest work of the century." Prince Frederick Karl of Prussia, Grand Master of the Order of St. John of Jerusalem, pledged his support to such an international organization as suggested by Dunant; the King of Saxony and Napoleon III, who himself had witnessed the Battle of Solferino, both promised all possible assistance.

The appeal of Dunant was soon translated into action. In 1863, a congress attended by 36 delegates from 14 nations assembled in Geneva and drew up a series of proposals. The following year, a second international conference, known now as the Geneva Convention, attended by 26 delegates from 16 governments, signed a treaty or agreement, embodying in its 10 articles the principles of the Red Cross. The essential principles of the articles were: the wounded were to be respected; military hospitals were to be treated as neutral territory; the personnel and the property of the medical services were to be protected; and the symbol of this protection was to be a white flag bearing a red cross.

Dunant, who had spent most of his fortune in founding the Red Cross, became bankrupt in 1867 and disappeared. During the War of 1870, he emerged from the slums of Paris, where he had been living as a pauper, with the demand that Article Five of the Convention, "The inhabitants of a country who administer aid to the wounded shall be free and unmolested," to be respected. Then again in 1875, he disappeared from view.

For 15 years, Dunant's whereabout were unknown. He became a legend, while the organization he had founded swept over the world and established branches in every civilized country. In 1890, Dunant, aged 62, was found in a hospice for old men in Heiden, Switzerland, suffering from delusions. Five years later, he was a patient at the Hospice in Heiden, where he was interviewed by a Swiss journalist, who found him "a deserted and poor but not a broken and embittered man . . . demanding nothing of the world for himself." In 1901, Dunant, with Frederic Passy, received the first award of the Nobel Peace Prize and, with characteristic generosity, gave his portion to charity. He died in 1910 at the age of 82. Dunant's name remains virtually unknown to the countless victims of war and disaster who owe their lives to the organization which he founded. The Red Cross is without question one of the great humanitarian achievements of all time.

MENDEL'S LAW

In 1865, the year that Lister employed carbolic acid in a compound fracture and Villemin demonstrated the infectiousness of tuberculosis and six years after Darwin published his *Origin of the Species,* an Augustinian monk, Gregor Johann Mendel, abbot of Brünn, in Moravia, announced the results of his experiments on hybridization in peas and formulated what has since been known as Mendel's Law. Unlike the publications of Darwin, Lister and Villemin, Mendel's paper, published in the *Verhandlungen der Naturforchers Vereins in Brünn,* remained unnoticed for 35 years. Mendel, working with the common pea, described the prevailing character, which appeared in the experiment of hybridization, as the dominant character, that which was suppressed as the recessive. When two peas were bred which contained both dominant and recessive factors, one-half of the progeny bred true to the parental characters (hybrids), whereas the other half was divided equally between offspring showing only the dominant and those showing only the recessive characters. In subsequent generations, self fertilized, the hybrid offspring bred as before while the dominants and recessives bred true to their kinds.

Mendel's law has had a wide application in the study of biology, of eugenics, and of heredity, including the hereditary characteristics of certain diseases. It has profoundly modified the earlier Darwinian theories that the external factor of environmental stress in the struggle for existence gave rise to new species.

RELATIONS BETWEEN THE MEDICAL PROFESSION AND THE PUBLIC

The relations between the medical profession and the public underwent marked changes during the nineteenth century. Richard H. Shryock, in his excellent book, *The Development of Modern Medicine,* has one chapter on "Public Confidence Lost" and a later chapter on "Public Confidence Regained," which very accurately describe the two phases of change in the attitude of the public.

During the eighteenth century, the line of cleavage between the learned professions—law, theology and medicine—and the general public was more sharply drawn than in the nineteenth. Law was a highly complex affair, understood only by those learned in this specialty, and the decisions of its experts were final. Theology was something sacred, studied by a select group whose conclusions were handed down to the faithful, who accepted them in the main as the revelations from a higher power. Medicine again was a very complex affair, the mysteries of which were understood by the select few who spoke with authority on the great problems of disease and death and whose words to the suffering were almost oracular. In the fields of both theology and medicine, there were rival sects, to be sure, but each sect had its own leaders who exercised great authority among its respective followers. Dissenters from the established sects of religion and medicine appeared from time to time, the religious dissenters forming a new religion and the medical dissenters forming a new system of medicine.

Vincent Priessnitz (1799-1851), a Silesian peasant, was run over by a wagon and severely injured. The surgeon, who was summoned, declared the patient would be an invalid for life. Priessnitz, however, by keeping wet compresses on his chest for a year and drinking large quantities of water, recovered completely. He then, at the age of 18, instituted his water cure for disease, a treatment which soon found many adherents among the high and the low, the rich and the poor.

In America, Samuel Thomson (1769-1843), who, like Priessnitz, had never studied medicine, cured with steam inhalations and lobelia one of his children who was suffering from scarlet fever and had been given up by a physician. Soon afterwards, he became a traveling herb doctor and worked out a medical theory of his own. He believed that metals and minerals are obtained from the earth and, being heavy, have a tendency to draw one down and, therefore, should not be employed; plants, on the contrary, grow upward and tend to elevate anyone who ingests them, and, therefore, herb medicines alone were indicated in disease. He used only plant remedies, chiefly lobelia. He later patented his system of practice and granted for a consideration exclusive rights for certain areas and sold many copies of his *New Guide to Health,* which outlined his new system. Thomsonianism, as it came to be called, had numerous lay followers and many zealous professional champions, the latter founding two medical schools in Ohio to teach the doctrines of Thomson.

Another American product and, in the light of subsequent history, quite an influential one, was Mary Baker Eddy, whose theories stem back to Quimby and beyond him to magnetism and mesmerism. When she founded "Christian Science," it was not a religion but a healing cult. She states quite frankly in her *Retrospection and Intraspection,*

My immediate recovery from the effects of an injury caused by an accident, an injury that neither medicine nor surgery could reach, was the falling apple that led me to the discovery how to be well myself, and how to make others so.

Christian Science, according to Mrs. Eddy, is "divine metaphysics," "the scientific system of divine healing," "the law of God, the law of good, interpreting and demonstrating the divine Principle and rule of universal harmony." "This religion teaches its adherents to forsake and overcome every form of error or evil on the basis of its unreality" (Smith). What is called in the common vernacular, "disease," is in reality an error and is unreal.

Osteopathy, another American "discovery," was formally organized by A. T. Still, who established the American School of Osteopathy at Kirksville, Missouri, in 1892. Still, whose formal education was exceedingly limited and who had been a free lance practitioner after attending medical lectures in Kansas City, became convinced of the futility of drugs and, as early as 1874, formulated his new system of healing, which was based largely on "structural derangement." "Osteopathy," according to Hulburt, one of its advocates, "is a system of health founded on the theory that the living body is a vital machine which will make the remedies necessary to protect itself against disease as long as it is in correct mechanical adjustment."

In the course of the years, osteopathy apparently wandered far from its original precepts. Osteopathic physicians presently employed the drugs so vehemently denounced by its founder, quite as liberally as members of the regular medical profession. They found that the body did not make the necessary remedies in sufficient amounts, so began the use of vaccines and antitoxins, and, learning by experience that mechanical adjustments were of little value in such conditions as appendicitis and cholelithiasis, they resorted to surgical operations and other procedures which were scarcely included in the "adjustments" that Still regarded as completely sufficient for the healing of disease.

The advances in physical science during the eighteenth and nineteenth century profoundly influenced the theological concepts of
life. The promulgation of the Darwinian theory compelled the
intelligent clergy to alter their concepts of the origin of man and
made untenable the teaching that Adam was the first man and that
sin came into the world through the eating of an apple. The social
and economic upheavals following the French Revolution brought
about a new evaluation of the rights and duties of men, expressed by
revolutionary changes in the legal codes. The elevation of the
level of education and its extension to all classes increased the numbers of those who no longer accepted the pronouncements of priests
and physicians as revelations either inspired or produced by a superior intellect.

The period between 1830 and 1850, during which medicine made
phenomenal advances, was not one which inspired the public with
great confidence. They saw a new generation of physicians disputing
the commonly accepted doctrine that all fevers were a single disease
and attacking vigorously the value of an age-old conviction that
bleeding was a panacea for all diseases. Further, they saw a group
spearheaded by the brilliant Skoda abandoning bleeding, opposing
the drastic purging with calomel and other purgatives, and fighting
against the employment of emetics, two unpleasant methods of treatment, which the public had come to accept as necessary evils in order
to regain health. They heard the same school of "Therapeutic Nihil-
ism" proclaim the uselessness of many therapeutic measures in vogue
and that, in many diseases, the patients would recover sooner if left
alone instead of being bled, purged, and treated with emetics. We
now recognize that these Vienna pioneers had to clear away a vast
amount of rubbish and rubble before a solid foundation for medicine could be laid, but the suffering sick saw no cheer in these new
pronouncements. "Hence the paradox," as Shryock writes, "that the
most hopeful period in the history of medicine was the one in which
the public looked to medicine with the least hope."

The public, feeling it was deserted by the medical profession,
turned in increasing numbers to quacks, patent medicines, food
faddists, and new healing sects. Honest physicians admitted that they
could cure few diseases; their rivals claimed that they could cure all
ills. The sale of "consumption cures" increased by leaps and bounds.
American newspapers were filled with advertisements of patent medicines, and many fortunes were made by their exploiters. In England,
the same situation developed. Morrison, of the "London College
of Health," took in 80,000 pounds annually from the sale of his

purgative pills, and Beecham's pills, "a shilling a box worth a guinea," netted their manufacturer a fortune and a baronetcy. In France, the laws forbade the sale and advertising of patent medicines, but the laws were a dead letter. In Germany, strict laws were passed against quacks and patent medicines, but, as these laws soon created a group of people who were widely regarded as martyrs striving only to serve humanity, the laws were, on the advice of Virchow, repealed, and quackery flourished as never before. A large number of new schools of healing appeared.

With the new birth of bacteriology, confidence in the medical profession rose. Among the great achievements of these pioneers, nothing perhaps stirred the imagination of the public as much as Pasteur's conquest of rabies—although this disease is relatively rare. The demonstration of the healing properties of diphtheria and of tetanus antitoxins also made a deep impression. When Röntgen, at the turn of the century, demonstrated to an incredulous public that it was possible to see the outlines of bones and his successors began making pictures of the heart and lungs, public confidence grew apace.

ADVANCES IN PUBLIC HEALTH AND HEALTH LEGISLATION

The nineteenth century witnessed also a renewed interest in public health and an increasing conviction that the health of the people was a concern of the state. The idea was by no means entirely new. In antiquity, we find in both Greece and Rome public physicians, whose salaries were paid by the state and whose services were accessible to the poorer classes who were unable to pay for medical care. In the Middle Ages and later in the cities of the fifteenth, sixteenth and seventeenth centuries, city physicians were appointed who were charged with the treatment of poor patients and with the maintenance of the local health. With the advent of the industrial revolution, it became more and more apparent that these old methods, hallowed by centuries of tradition, were inadequate to insure a healthy population. With the rapid growth of new cities, it became quite necessary, if the inhabitants were to survive, to make these cities safe and healthful places in which to live. While these problems were most acute in the cities, yet they were present also in the villages and hamlets.

When Johann Peter Frank finished in 1813 the last volume of his *Medicinische Polizey*, his great work apparently had no influence upon his generation. Thirty-four years later, Virchow, investigating the typhus epidemic in Silesia, became interested in the problems of public health and used his powerful and trenchant pen in its behalf. Virchow pointed out that the health of the people is a concern of the state, that social and economic conditions have a powerful influence on health and disease, and that the state itself must take measures, both social and medical, to promote health and combat disease. "History has shown more than once," declared Virchow, "how the fates of the greatest empires were decided by the health of their peoples or of their armies." Justinian, in his Twelve Tables, had set down his memorable dictum—*Salus populi suprema lex*. History had shown that the safety of the people rested not only on their protection from civil and military enemies but also on their protection from disease, often due in large measure to inseparably linked economic and hygienic conditions.

The development of bacteriology, the demonstration of the bacterial and parasitic cause of many diseases pointed the way to their control or eventual elimination. The demonstration that typhoid fever was the result, in great measure, of a contaminated water supply, that cholera commonly was caused by infected food, that many epidemics were caused by infected milk, that tuberculosis was disseminated by dried sputum, that malaria and yellow fever were carried by mosquitoes, that sleeping sickness was transmitted by the bite of a fly, and that the common house fly was a carrier of typhoid and other diseases—all these discoveries called for the application of measures that were obviously outside and beyond the field of private medical practice. The ancient principle of prevention of diseases now acquired a new meaning and a new force since the means of prevention were clearly understood. The old teachings of Johann Peter Frank in his *Medicinische Polizey* acquired a new meaning as well as a belated recognition.

The further study of these problems stressed anew the prevalence of disease among the poor. Virchow pointed out the importance of statistics, as Rosen has emphasized, in the relationship between social conditions and medical problems. "Medical statistics will be our standard of measurement: we will weigh life for life and see where the dead lie thicker, among the workers or among the privileged" (Virchow). The accuracy of morbidity and mortality statistics constantly improved, and the government became interested in public health and sanitation as never before both from the standpoint of humanitarianism and of economic gain.

Max von Pettenkofer, the director of the first hygienic institute,

established in Munich, summarized the growing trend in a notable
address on "The Value of Health to a City":

It has become the fashion to think that the health conditions of a city
are determined exclusively by good sewage, abundant water supply, and
good toilets. . . . [In applying these measures,] we solve not even one-third
of our problems. . . .

Our health is also determined, to a large extent, by nutrition: not only
by the quality of our food but also by its quantity. . . .

Housing conditions are also extremely important. . . .

Political and social conditions are also influential upon the health and
mortality of a population.

"It was left for the nineteenth century," Rosen points out, "to
develop the idea of medicine as a social science, and eventually to
formulate with greater precision and clarity the concept of social
medicine."

In Germany, the work of Pettenkofer and of other pioneers was
influential in the establishment of pure water supplies for cities and
towns and in 'the passage of regulations for food inspection to insure
the people healthful food. Some of the enthusiastic bacteriologists,
like Behring, saw in bacteriology the solution of the problems of
public health.

The rise of capitalism following the industrial revolution increased the insecurity of the working classes. Labor became a com-
modity on the market, wages fluctuated as did the price of commodi-
ties. During economic crises, large numbers of workers lost their
jobs and became public charges. When illness struck, the problem
was further aggravated, and society seemed totally unable to cope
with it. Unrest and dissatisfaction were widespread, and, in Germany, the Social-Democratic party grew rapidly in numbers and in
influence.

Bismarck, who had welded the 30-odd German states into a powerful empire under the leadership of Prussia, saw in this political development a menace to his new creation. A member of the Prussian
landed aristocracy, he had a feudal paternalistic attitude towards the
workers and distrusted the growing power of the bankers and in-
dustrialists. As early as 1849, he said in an address, "The social insecurity of the worker is the real cause of their being a peril to the
state." When he became Chancellor of the German Empire, he expressed the view that the socialist claims should be allowed in as far
as possible within the framework of the existing political institutions
of the country.

Bismarck's first proposal for compulsory social insurance was presented to the Reichstag in 1881. It was supported by the Conservatives but defeated by a coalition of the Liberals, who resented government interference in the field of insurance and by the Social-Democrats, who distrusted Bismarck and looked upon him as an enemy of their class. The following year, he returned to the fray, and his bill, with certain modifications, was again introduced. The Liberals attacked him as a socialist, and the Social-Democrats denounced the bill as "poor relief" and "beggars' insurance," but he was finally successful by adroit maneuvering and by making concessions to various groups, and his bill for sickness insurance passed the Reichstag in 1884. Three years later, in 1887, he proposed a further extension of social security legislation by introducing a bill for old age and invalidity insurance. Again, he was opposed by the Liberals and Social-Democrats but once more triumphed, and the bill passed in 1889 with a majority of 20 votes.

This new legislation of Bismarck did not destroy the Social-Democratic party. On the contrary, it grew in numbers with each successive election. It did, however, apparently check the party in its "present aberration," and it killed the revolutionary policy of the Social-Democrats. In time, they became the strongest supporters of the legislation originally introduced by Bismarck, the Iron Chancellor.

Thus, Germany, under the leadership of the arch-conservative Bismarck, became the pioneer in sickness, disability, unemployment, and old age insurance. Her example was soon followed by many other nations. It was a politico-medical event of the first magnitude.

Biographical Addenda

THE NINETEENTH CENTURY—THE SECOND HALF

1799-1870—James S. Syme was the most celebrated Scottish surgeon of his time. He was born in Edinburgh and studied with his cousin, James Liston, who conducted a private anatomical school. Here Syme later became Liston's prosector. In 1821, he was appointed house surgeon to the Royal Infirmary; in 1823, fellow of the Royal College of Surgeons; and, the same year, carried out the first hip exarticulation performed in Great Britain. In 1833, he was elected professor of clinical surgery at the University of Edinburgh and, in 1834, following the departure of Liston, surgeon to the Royal Infirmary. After the death of Liston, he was called to London as professor of clinical surgery in University College Hospital, but did not like London, and presently returned to Edinburgh, where he again occupied his old chair.

Syme made many contributions to surgical literature and gained a great reputation as a bold, resourceful, careful and skillful surgeon. Joseph Lister became his house surgeon in 1854 and subsequently married Syme's daughter. Syme was a champion of Lister's antiseptic method and wrote an early article on the subject. Gurlt, the noted historian of surgery, described him "as beyond question, belonging with the first surgeons of the modern period."

1800-1890—Sir Edwin Chadwick, the father of modern sanitary science in England, was born near Manchester and was educated for the bar. In 1832, the Royal Commission on Poor Laws appointed him an investigator, and, the following year, he was appointed a member, holding this position until 1846. His report on *The Sanitary Condition of the Labouring Population,* 1842, pointed out the necessity for improving the water supply, drainage and sewage disposal of the large cities. He stressed the results of public neglect and urged that public health was the concern of the state.

1801-1858—Johannes Müller.

1801-1867—Armand Trousseau.

1801-1881—Maximilien Paul Émile Littré is noted as a lexicographer, philologist, and medical historian. He was born in Paris and received an excellent classical education, becoming proficient in Latin, Greek, Sanskrit and Arabic as well as in English and German. He studied medicine, completed the necessary studies, but never practiced. He was one of the editors with Bouillaud and Andral of the *Journal hebdomadaire de médecine* and editor of the paper, *National,* and the magazine, *L'Expérience.* His great translation of Hippocrates was the labor of nearly 30 years, the first volume appearing in 1839 and the tenth volume in 1861. It remains the best, the most scholarly, and the most comprehensive translation. His second great achievement, the

Dictionnaire de la langue française, appeared in four volumes, 1863-1874, and remains a monument to his erudition and his accuracy as a scholar. He also translated Homer, Pliny, Goethe and Schiller.

1802-1880—William Sharpey was born in Arbroath, Scotland, and graduated at Edinburgh in 1823. He practiced for several years and then went to the Continent, where he studied at Pavia, Berlin, Heidelberg, Paris and Vienna. In 1831, he was appointed professor of anatomy in Edinburgh and, in 1836, became professor of anatomy and physiology in University College, London, holding this position until his retirement in 1874.

Sharpey was one of the founders of modern physiology in England and numbered among his pupils Joseph Lister, Michael Foster, and Burdon Sanderson.

1803-1873—Justus von Liebig.

1804-1881—Matthias Jakob Schleiden.

1805-1881—Josef Skoda.

1804-1892—Sir Richard Owen.

1806-1865—Joseph François Magendie.

1806-1875—Guillaume Benjamin Armand Duchenne, a native of Boulogne, studied medicine in Paris and, after graduating in 1831, returned to Boulogne, where he practiced for 11 years. In 1836, he became interested in electricity as a therapeutic measure and, eight years later, went to Paris because he saw there a greater opportunity to study patients. He lived in Paris from 1842 until his death in 1875 without ever seeking a teaching or hospital appointment, either of which he felt would take too much time from his investigations. Instead, he visited all the hospitals, studying their cases of nervous diseases and acquiring an extraordinary experience and skill in diagnosis. He has been rightly called "the creator of electro diagnosis and electro therapy." He was the first to describe accurately and delineate bulbar paralysis, progressive muscular atrophy, and pseudo hypertrophic paralysis. He also made important fundamental studies on many diseases of the nervous system, particularly tabes dorsalis.

1807-1873—Auguste Nélaton was born in Paris, where he graduated in 1836. In 1851. He became professor of surgery and was later in 1867 surgeon to Napoleon III. He was an excellent teacher and a skillful operator and was highly respected for his sound judgment, based on great experience. He introduced a flexible rubber catheter, a probe for bullets with a porcelain tip, which he employed on General Garibaldi. His chief work was his *Éléments de pathologie chirurgicale* in five volumes, published in Paris, 1844-1860.

1808-1877—Sir William Fergusson, a native of Scotland, studied at Edinburgh, and practiced there until 1840, when he went to London as professor of surgery in King's College. He was the author of *A System of Practical Surgery*, London, 1842, which ran through five editions, was published later in Philadelphia, and was translated into German. He employed but few instruments in his operations and was described by his contemporaries as having "the eagle's eye, the lion's heart, and the lady's hand." He was surgeon to Prince Albert and to Queen Victoria.

1809-1882—Charles Robert Darwin.

1809-1854—Sir William James Erasmus Wilson was born in London of Scotch parents, studied at St. Bartholomew's Hospital under Abernethy, and became a member of the Royal College of Surgeons in 1831. He was later prosector to Richard Quain at the University College, and, while there, published *Practical and Surgical Anatomy*, 1838. In 1840, he was appointed lecturer on anatomy and physiology at Middlesex Hospital, and, the same year, his *Anatomist's Vademecum* was published, a work which passed through 11 English editions and eight American editions and was translated into German. Becoming interested in diseases of the skin, Wilson published two notable works—*Diseases of the Skin*, 1842; and *Healthy Skin*, 1847. In 1869, he became professor of dermatology at the Royal College of Surgeons, endowing the chair himself. In 1881, he founded and endowed a chair of dermatology at the University of Aberdeen in memory of his father. Wilson was much interested in Egyptology, wrote a book on *Egypt of the Past* in 1881, and was instrumental in bringing the obelisk known as "Cleopatra's Needle" to London.

1809-1896—Friedrich Gustav Jakob Henle.

1810-1882—Theodor Schwann.

1810-1892—Jean-Louis-Armand Quatrefages de Bréau, the well-known French anthropologist, studied medicine at Strassburg, practiced there for a time, then taught biology at Toulouse, and went to Paris in 1850 as professor at the Lycée Napoleon. He wrote treatises on comparative anatomy, biology of the lower animals, ethnology, and kindred subjects. His pamphlet, *La race prussienne*, published in Paris in 1879, claimed that the Prussians were not a Germanic race but a barbaric, destructive Mongol race. "This stirred Virchow's patriotism to the extent of instigating a colossal public census of the color of the hair and eyes in 6,000,000 German school-children, the solemn official character of which frightened some of the children out of their wits" (Garrison).

1810-1894—Joseph Hyrtl.

1810-1896—Marie Philibert Constant Sappey, born in Cerdon near Bourg, studied at Paris, where he received his doctor's degree in 1843. He became professor of anatomy at Paris in 1868 and was one of the leading anatomists of the nineteenth century, his work on the anatomy of the lymphatic system being especially noteworthy. His outstanding works were *Traité d'anatomie descriptive*, 1847-1863 and 1867-1874; and *Anatomie, physiologie, pathologie des vaisseaux lymphatiques*, Paris, 1874, both illustrated with excellent plates.

1811-1884—Heinrich Haeser was born in Rome of German parents, received his early education in Weimar, where his father was a director of music, and studied medicine at Jena, receiving there his doctor's degree in 1834. He became a *Privatdozent* in Jena and, in 1840, started the publication of a new medical journal, the *Archiv für die gesammte Medicin.* He was an active opponent of *Naturphilosophie* and assisted in its downfall at Jena. In 1845, the first edition of his history of medicine, *Lehrbuch der Geschichte der Medicin und der Volkskrankheiten,* was published at Jena. He went to Leipzig in 1840 to carry on the editorial work of his medical journal, was called to Greifswald in 1846 as professor, and to Breslau in 1862. The third edition of his history of medicine appeared in three volumes in 1875. This work is a masterpiece of erudition, accuracy and scholarship and remains today a most valuable reference work on the history of medicine.

1811-1888—Thomas Blizard Curling, at the age of 21, was appointed assistant surgeon to the London Hospital, holding this position until 1826, when he became surgeon. He was active in this post until his resignation after 20 years of service. Curling pointed out in 1842 that severe burns of the skin often produced duodenal ulcers. In his paper on "Two Cases of Absence of the Thyroid Body," published in the *Medical Chirurgical Transactions* in 1850, he gave an early excellent description of cretinism.

1811-1870—Sir James Young Simpson.

1812-1875—John Hughes Bennett was born in London and studied medicine in Edinburgh, where he received his M.D. degree in 1837. He then studied two years in France and two years in Germany, after which he returned to Edinburgh, where he gave lectures on histology and conducted a private course in microscopy. He was a candidate in 1842 for the chair of general pathology but was unsuccessful. The same year, he was appointed physician to the Royal Dispensary and, in 1848, was elected professor of the Institutes of Medicine. In 1855, he was a candidate for the chair of the Practice of Physic at Edinburgh but was not chosen. He resigned his professorship in 1874 and, the following year, received the LL.D. degree from Edinburgh. He died following an operation for stone.

Bennett was an excellent teacher, clear, incisive, at times eloquent, but, because of his frequent sarcasms and his great frankness in expressing his opinions, was never very popular with his colleagues. He was instrumental in introducing into Britain cod liver oil for the treatment of tuberculosis and protested against the depleting methods in vogue for the treatment of pneumonia. He was quite an active writer and was the author of more than 100 papers. In 1845, he published in the *Edinburgh Medical and Surgical Journal* a paper on "A Case of Hypertrophy of the Spleen and Liver in which Death took place from Suppuration of the Blood," a case of leukemia, which, however, he interpreted incorrectly. Virchow, the same year, described a similar case, interpreted it correctly, and gave it the name of leukemia.

1814-1878—Claude Bernard.

1814-1894—William Alexander Greenhill, medical historian, edited Sydenham's works and the writings of Sir Thomas Browne and translated Rhazes's *On Small Pox and Measles* from the original Arabic.

1814-1899—Sir James Paget.

1815-1878—Crawford W. Long.

1815-1848—Horace Wells.

1815-1877—Karl Reinhold August Wunderlich was born in Sulz-on-the-Neckar and studied medicine at Tübingen, where he received his doctor's degree in 1838. After graduation, he joined the faculty as a *Privatdozent*, became full professor in 1846, but left Tübingen to become professor at Leipzig and director of the medical clinic. Wunderlich was the originator of modern clinical thermometry, the foundation of which he laid in his treatise on the relation of body heat to disease, *Das Verhalten der Eigenwärme in Krankheiten*, Leipzig, 1868. He also wrote an excellent history of medicine, *Geschichte der Medicin*, Stuttgart, 1859.

1816-1872—Charles Victor Daremberg, one of the greatest French medical historians, was born in Dijon and received his M.D. at Paris in 1841. He became librarian of the *Académie de Médecine* in 1846 and of the Mazarin Library in 1849. In 1864, he inaugurated a course on the history of medicine at the Collège de France. Seven years later, he was appointed professor of the history of medicine in the faculty of Paris. He was an excellent classical scholar, a man of broad education and interests, and as Haeser noted, "in the beginning of his career, Daremberg searched through most of the European libraries in order to improve by examination of the manuscripts the texts of the medical authors of antiquity." Daremberg published translations of Caelius Aurelianus, Ruphos of Ephesus, Galen, Oreibasios, the Four Masters, selections from Homer, Celsus's *De Medicina* and wrote an outstanding history of medicine, *Histoire des Sciences Médicales*, Paris, 1870.

1816-1880—Ferdinand von Hebra.

1816-1890—Sir William Gull

1816-1892—Sir William Bowman was born in Nantwich and, after serving five years as a resident pupil at the General Hospital in Birmingham, became a student at King's College, London, studying especially anatomy and physiology. In 1841 and 1842, he contributed to the Royal Society papers on the minute structure and movements of muscles, as the result of which he was elected a Fellow. In 1842, he contributed another paper, "On the Structure and Use of the Malpighian Bodies of the Kidney," in which he described "Bowman's capsule."

In 1840, Bowman, when 24 years of age, was appointed surgeon to King's College Hospital. Six years later, he joined the staff of the Royal London Ophthalmic Hospital and presently became the leading ophthalmic surgeon in London.

1816-1895—Carl Ludwig.

1817-1894—Charles Édouard Brown-Séquard.

1817-1905—Rudolf Albert Kölliker was born in Zürich and studied medicine in Zürich, Bonn, Berlin and Heidelberg, where he received his M.D. in 1843. He was Henle's prosector in Zürich from 1843 to

1845, became professor of physiology and anatomy at Zürich in 1845, and went to Würzburg in 1847 as professor, remaining there until his retirement in 1897. Kölliker was one of the greatest biologists of his time. His famous work, *Handbuch der Gewebelehre*, Leipzig, 1852, is a landmark in the history of anatomy and biology, the first sytematic book on histology. It went through six editions and was translated into English, French and Italian. Kölliker "knew more by direct personal observation of the microscopic structure of animals than any one else who has ever lived" (Minot). His *Entwicklungsgeschichte* was the first book on comparative embryology.

1817-1894—August Hirsch, a native of Danzig, received his M.D. from Berlin in 1843 and then practiced at Danzig. In 1863, he was called to Berlin as professor of medicine. He wrote extensively on the epidemiology of infectious diseases, and, in 1859-1864, his great work, *Handbuch der historisch-geographischen Pathologie,* was published, which, in 1883, was translated into English and published by the New Sydenham Society with the title, *Handbook of historic-geographic Pathology.* This exhaustive work, containing more than 14,000 references, continues to be a standard work for students of tropical medicine and hygiene. He was an editor of the *Biographisches Lexikon* of physicians and wrote a noteworthy history of ophthalmology, which formed Volume VII of von Graefe and Saemisch's *Handbook der Augenheilkunde,* 1877.

1818-1865—Ignaz Philipp Semmelweis.

1818-1876—Ludwig Traube was born in Ratibor, Silesia, studied in Breslau under Purkinje and in Berlin under Johannes Müller and Schönlein. He received his doctor's degree in Berlin in 1840 and then studied in Vienna under Rokitansky and Škoda. He returned to Berlin, gave courses in auscultation and percussion, and later turned to experimental pathology, studying especially the changes following section of the vagus nerves, the changes produced by suffocation, the effects of digitalis, and the relationship between heart disease and kidney disease. His *Gesammelte Beiträge zur experimentallen Pathologie,* published in 1871-1878, gave him a wide reputation. He became Schönlein's assistant in 1849 and professor in 1857, and he first called attention to the well-known phenomenon, the *plusus alternans,* in 1872. He was greatly esteemed as a physician, teacher and man.

1818-1901—Max von Pettenkofer was born in Lichtenberg, Bavaria, and studied medicine at the University of Munich, where he received his doctor's degree in 1843. While a student, he became deeply interested in chemistry and made two important chemical discoveries—one, the detection of arsenic by the Marsch apparatus; and, the second, a method of separating arsenic from antimony. After graduation, he studied chemistry further in Würzburg, where he devised the well-known Pettenkofer test for bile in the urine—the production of a purplish crimson when a few drops are added to a solution of sugar and sulphuric acid. Shortly afterwards, he discovered in the urine a new nitrogenous substance, which later investigations proved to be creatinin.

In 1845, Pettenkofer returned to Munich, where he obtained a position in the royal mint. While holding this position, he discovered a new method of assaying silver and gold, proved definitely that saliva contains sulphocyanic acid, and worked out a method of producing haematinon, a substance used in the manufacture of the red antique glass at Pompeii. In 1847, he was appointed associate professor of medical chemistry in the University of Munich.

His first investigations in his new position were on the chemistry of cement, followed by his discovery of a successful method of obtaining suitable illuminating gas from wood. In 1853, he was made professor of medical chemistry; in 1855, he was given a suite of rooms in the Physiological Institute; and, in 1878, a Hygienic Institute of his own. From the beginning of his professorship in 1853, he devoted his energies and great talents to the study of hygiene in all its aspects—air, clothing, ventilation, heating, lighting, soil, water, food, excreta, the life of man in all his surroundings, and even the disposition of his body after death. He was the undisputed founder of experimental hygiene.

The name of Pettenkofer is associated especially with his work on metabolism and cholera. His studies on respiration, metabolism, nutrition, and food values, which were carried out with his pupil, Carl von Voit, and which extended over a period of 20 years in the famous "Respiration Chamber," the gift of King Maximilian II, marks an epoch in modern medicine and dietetics. They were the first studies of metabolism in health and disease and the first accurate studies of the caloric values of a large number of foodstuffs. "Imagine our sensations," Voit wrote, "as the picture of the remarkable processes of life unrolled before our eyes and a mass of new facts became known to us."

Pettenkofer's *Boden* theory of cholera aroused a long and bitter controversy. While admitting that Koch's comma bacillus was the specific germ of the disease, Pettenkofer held that it alone cannot cause the disease without susceptibility of the individual, favorable local conditions and the proper seasonal conditions. The immunity of certain localities to cholera, according to him, was due to the condition of the soil and to the ground water level, and he stated that the highest cholera incidence occurs simultaneously with the lowest rainfall. To prove his point, he drank in 1892 when 74 years of age a culture of virulent cholera bacilli, but experienced no ill effects beyond "a light diarrhoea with an enormous proliferation of the bacilli in the stools."

Pettenkofer's *Boden* theory is no longer tenable, but it stimulated an enormous amount of experimental work. His other contributions to the subject of public health were numerous and important. Hume lists 228 articles or monographs in Pettenkofer's bibliography. He trained many pupils whose contributions were important and of permanent value. At the age of 83, in bad health, his wife, two sons and a daughter dead, he ended his own life.

1818-1896—Emil du Bois-Reymond.

1818-1897—Sir Thomas Spencer Wells.

1819-1868—William Thomas Green Morton.

1819-1885—Friedrich Theodor von Frerichs was born at Aurich, in Hanover, received his degree at Göttingen in 1841, and, returning to his home town, soon achieved a great reputation as an ophthalmologist. From ophthalmology, however, he turned to medicine and became later one of the founders of experimental pathology. He went to Göttingen as associate professor in 1848, then to Kiel in 1850, where he laid the foundation of his reputation with his monograph on Bright's disease, a clinical and pathological study. In 1852, he was appointed professor at Breslau and remained there seven years, during which time he discovered leucin and tyrosin in the urine of patients with acute yellow atrophy (1855) and published his *Klinik der Leberkrankheiten*, 1858. This work contains a notable chapter on melanemia, in which Frerichs, according to Laveran, describes the malarial parasite but failed to appreciate its significance.

In 1850, Frerichs was called to Berlin as successor to Schönlein. He came to Berlin at the height of his reputation but soon seemed to undergo, according to his pupil Naunyn, a certain intellectual deterioration, intensified by his quarrels with Traube, his colleague at the Charité, and by the aggres-sive hostility of Virchow. He did little productive work for several years, but his clinics and lectures were still models of accuracy and conciseness. In 1876, he again began his investigations, and in 1884 his *Ueber den Diabetes* appeared, a scholarly treatise, worthy of his fame. All of his pupils praised Frerichs as a remarkable clinician and an outstanding teacher. Among his pupils were some of the best known physicians of modern times, including Ehrlich, Naunyn, Leyden, and von Mering. He stressed the relationship between experimental pathology, including chemistry, and clinical medicine and was one of the founders of scientific clinical teaching in Germany.

1819-1892—Ernst Wilhelm von Brücke was born in Berlin and studied medicine at Berlin and Heidelberg, receiving his degree in 1842. He was assistant to Johannes Müller in Berlin, was called to Königsberg as associate professor of physiology in 1848, and went the following year to Vienna, where he worked for more than 40 years, becoming one of the celebrities of the New Vienna School. In 1879, he was rector of the University of Vienna, the first Protestant to hold this post since the founding of the university, and, the same year, was raised to rank of nobility.

Brücke was a remarkable all-round physiologist and anatomist. He investigated vision, phonetics, cardiac physiology, digestion, glyco-suria, and muscle movements and wrote a noteworthy book on artistic anatomy.

1820-1910—Eduard Henoch was

born in Berlin, received his medical degree at the University of Berlin in 1843, and established in 1860 a clinic for children in Berlin. He was a pioneer in German pediatrics and described "Henoch's purpura" in 1874.

1821-1894—Hermann Helmholtz.

1821-1902—Rudolf Virchow.

1822-1895—Louis Pasteur.

1822-1884—Gregor Mendel was born in Heinzendorf, Moravia, and entered the Augustinian order as a novice in the cloister at Alt-Brünn in 1843. He later attended the University of Vienna for two years and then returned to Brünn, where he taught in the town school for 14 years. During this period he carried out in the garden of the monastery his famous experiments on hybridization in peas and founded the Brünn Society of Natural Science (*Naturforscher Verein in Brünn*). His famous paper, *Versuche über Planzenhybriden,* was published in the transactions of the *Verein* for 1866, where it remained buried and unnoticed for 35 years, until after Hugo de Vries, in 1900, had made the same discovery. Mendel's law, which has had a tremendous influence on medical and biological thinking, postulates that, in the generation of hybrids, one-half of the progeny will breed true to the parental characters, whereas the other half will be equally divided between offspring possessing only the dominant or the recessive characters. Mendel became abbot of the monastery in 1868 and, because of his duties in this position, was unable to continue his scientific investigations.

1822-1902—Adolf Kussmaul, one of the outstanding German clinicians of his day, was born near Karlsruhe, studied at Heidelberg, and, on the completion of his studies, entered the army, serving for two years as an army surgeon. He then practiced as a country physician, but, deciding to embark upon an academic career, he matriculated at Würzburg, attracted there by the growing reputation of Rudolf Virchow. He received his doctor's degree in 1855 and was later professor of medicine at Heidelberg, Erlangen, Freiburg and Strassburg. He was the first to describe periarteritis nodosa and progressive bulbar paralysis, to diagnose mesenteric thrombosis, to attempt esophagoscopy and gastroscopy, to practice gastric lavage for dilatation of the stomach; and was one of the first physicians to employ thoracentesis. He described the peculiar type of respiration associated with diabetic acidosis—"Kussmaul's air-hunger." His *Recollections (Jugenderinnerungen eines alten Arztes),* published in 1899, is an interesting and fascinating autobiography.

1823-1864—William Senhouse Kirkes was born in Holker, Lancashire, and studied at St. Bartholomew's Hospital in London and then at Berlin, where he received his M.D. in 1846. He was appointed assistant physician to St. Bartholomew's Hospital in 1854 and physician in 1864. His *Handbook of Physiology,* first published in 1848, went through five editions and was one of the best texts of its time. His article on "The Detachment of Fibrinous Deposits from the Interior of the Heart," published in the *Medico-Chirurgical*

Transactions for 1852, was an early and important contribution to the subject of embolism.

1822-1895—Karl Thiersch was born in Munich, where he received his doctor's degree in 1843. He served as an army surgeon in the war with Denmark in 1850. He was prosector in pathological anatomy in Munich for six years, was called to Erlangen as professor of surgery in 1854, and went to Leipzig in 1867 as professor, holding this position until his death. He served as a consulting surgeon during the Franco-German War of 1870 and, on his return to Leipzig, became a vigorous champion of Lister's antiseptic method and the first prominent Continental surgeon to introduce this practice into his clinic. He made important studies on epithelial cancer (1865), phosphorus necrosis of the jaws (1867), and the healing of wounds (1867), and he is especially remembered for the Thiersch skin graft, which he introduced in 1874.

1823-1908—Johann Friedrich August von Esmarch was born in Tönning, Schleswig-Holstein, studied at Kiel and Göttingen, and, in 1854, became professor of surgery at Kiel. He was a great military surgeon and served in the campaigns of 1848-1850, 1864-1866, and 1870-1871. He is remembered chiefly for his introduction of the first-aid bandage on the battle field (1869-1870) and for the well-known "Esmarch bandage" (1873).

1824-1876—Gustav Simon, native of Darmstadt, professor of surgery at Rostock (1861) and Heidelberg (1867), performed the first excision of the kidney in Europe in 1869 and splenectomy in 1857.

1824-1881—Paul Broca was born in Sainte-Foy-la-Grande, in the Gironde, received his bachelor's degree in the College of his native city at the early age of 16, and then began the study of medicine in Paris. He received his doctor's degree in 1849, became professor *agrégé* in 1856, and served successively as surgeon to St. Antoine, La Pitié, Hôpital des Cliniques, and Hôpital Necker. He early devoted himself to an intensive study of pathology and wrote an excellent treatise on cancer (1852) and on aneurysms (1856). In 1863 appeared the first volume of his *Traité des tumeurs*.

Broca was the founder of modern brain surgery and, in 1861, localized the center of articulate speech in the third left frontal convolution. This discovery, although disputed, led to a systematic mapping out of various areas of the brain on the basis of their function, a work of fundamental importance in the development of brain surgery. He was the first surgeon to operate upon an abscess of the brain, the site of which he determined on the basis of his studies on the localization of function. He also achieved a great reputation as an anthropologist, devised the modern methods of measuring the skull and of determining the ratio between the dimensions of the skull and those of the brain, and invented new instruments for these studies. He was the creator of the modern science of craniology.

In addition to these outstanding

services to surgery and anthropology, Broca made important contributions to the field of public health, to infant mortality, to the study of the birth rate in France, and to the organization of sanitation in the French Army. He was created a senator in 1880 and died a few months later. His career was epitomized in the eulogy of Trélat: "Forty years of work without respite, 40 years of dignity, of generosity, of exalted patriotism, of devotion to all noble causes: that is the life of Broca."

1824-1911—Samuel Wilks was born in Camberwell, a borough of London, studied at University College, and received his M.D. degree from the University of London in 1850. He was appointed physician to Guy's Hospital in 1856 and was connected with Guy's the rest of his life. He introduced the term, "enteric fever," was one of the earliest to study the visceral lesions of syphilis (1857-1863), and studied osteitis deformans (1868), bacterial endocarditis (1868), acromegaly (1869), alcoholic paraplegia (1868), and subcutaneous tuberculosis (1862). His writings "really gave the diseases called after Bright, Addison, and Hodgkin their place in English medicine" (Garrison). His *Lectures on Pathological Anatomy*, 1859, and his *Lectures on the Diseases of the Nervous System*, 1878-1883, were standard works in their time. The former contains the earliest clear description of chronic ulcerative colitis.

As a loyal son of Guy's, Wilks wrote, with the collaboration of G. T. Bettany, *A Biographical History of Guy's Hospital*, which was published in 1892 and is an interesting and charming account of the hospital and of its distinguished men. His *Biographical Reminiscences*, 1911, is a fascinating autobiographical study. Wilks was not only a great physician but also a man of great kindliness and rare charm. He was described by Osler as one of the handsomest men in London.

1825-1899—Ernst Julius Gurlt was born in Berlin, where he studied medicine and graduated in 1848. He was subsequently *Privatdozent* and professor of surgery at Berlin. He took part in the wars of 1848, 1864, 1866 and 1870, was the author of numerous articles on military surgery, and wrote books on fractures and on operative surgery. He was one of the most learned surgeons of his period, and his *Geschichte der Chirurgie*, 1898, a history of surgery down through the Renaissance period, remains unrivaled for its "scholarship, exhaustive treatment, and accurate bibliography" (Garrison). It is without question the greatest history of surgery, a lasting monument to its author.

1825-1895—Thomas Henry Huxley.

1825-1893—Jean Martin Charcot, one of the greatest French teachers and clinicians, was born in Paris and, as a youth, had difficulty in deciding whether he wished to be a physician or an artist. He finally chose medicine and graduated at Paris, presenting a thesis on chronic arthritis. In 1862, he became physician to the Salpêtrière, where he lectured regularly on chronic diseases, on diseases of the aged, and especially on diseases of the nervous system. He became professor of pathological anatomy in 1872 and conducted the courses in pathology at the medical school, in addition to his clinical lectures and demonstrations. In 1882, he was appointed to the newly established position of professor of nervous diseases and created the greatest neurological clinic of modern times, attracting students from all over the world.

The public clinics of Charcot were not only instructive but very dramatic. The patients were presented in a small theatre equipped with a stage, foot-lights, and other lighting accessories so that the lights could be thrown on the patients from various angles. After presenting the patient and demonstrating the clinical findings, Charcot then dismissed the patient and threw on a screen a picture of the pathological findings in the disease. The somewhat theatrical techniques of his presentation invariably made a deep impression upon the throngs that attended his clinics.

Charcot, however, was more than a showman, he was a great neurologist. He studied the pathological lesions in locomotor ataxia and described gastric crises and the trophic joint affections (Charcot's joint) in this disease. He differentiated the Aran-Duchenne progressive muscular atrophy from amyotrophic lateral sclerosis and separated paralysis agitans from multiple sclerosis. He regarded hysteria as a neurosis produced by suggestion, believed that hypnosis was a condition similar to, if not identical with, hysteria, and was very skeptical of hypnosis as a therapeutic measure.

Charcot was not only a great neurologist but a first class clinician and pathologist. He wrote excellent articles on diseases of the liver, kidneys, bile ducts, pneumonia, gout, rheumatism, endocarditis and tuberculosis. He carried out important investigations on localization in cerebral disease and on the lesions of the cortical motor centers in man. He described with Bouchard in 1866 military aneurysms of the cerebral arteries and pointed out their importance as a cause of cerebral hemorrhage. In 1853, he described with Robin "lozenge shaped" crystals in the spleen and blood of a patient who had died of leukemia, later described by Leyden in the sputum of asthmatics and since known as Charcot-Leyden crystals.

1827-1894—Emanuel Fredrik Hagbarth Winge, born in Fredriksvaern, Norway, was first a practicing physician, then a ship's surgeon. After two years in Berlin, Prague, Vienna and Paris, he was appointed assistant in the medical clinic at Christiania, in 1866 was appointed professor of pathology, and in 1869 was made professor of internal medicine. Winge made several contributions of solid worth to pathology and internal medicine and, in 1869, described a case of endocarditis with thrombosis, demonstrating microorganisms in the endocardial lesions and also in the thrombi. This was the first positive proof of the bacterial origin of ulcerative endocarditis.

1825-1901—Pierre Carl Potain was

born in Paris and studied medicine in his native city, receiving the degree of M.D. in 1853. His doctor's dissertation, *Quelques recherches sur les bruits vasculaires anormaux qui suivent les hémorrhagies,* indicated his early interest in cardiac conditions. In 1856, he became chief of the clinic of Bouillaud and, in 1861, was appointed professor *agrégé.* During the war of 1870, he was asked to take charge of an ambulance but declined and instead served as an infantryman, participating in several battles. While Potain was a young physician, Trousseau predicted he would become the first clinician of Paris, a prediction which was gradually fulfilled. In 1882, Potain became physician to the Charité, where he was active until his retirement in 1900.

Potain was a great clinician and a remarkably keen observer. He wrote little but lavished great care on what he wrote. He was the author of *Clinique médicale de la Charité,* 1894. He was the first to study gallop rhythm, wrote an exhaustive treatise on functional heart murmurs, invented a sphygmomanometer which was used for a generation, and devised the well-known Potain aspirator.

1825-1895—Ernest Felix Immanuel Hoppe-Seyler, the greatest physiological chemist between Liebig and Emil Fischer, was born in Freiburg, Saxony, and took his medical degree at Berlin in 1850. He was successively prosector in Greifswald (1854-1856), assistant at the Pathological Institute at Berlin under Virchow (1856-1864), professor of applied chemistry at Tübingen (1861-1872), and professor of physiological chemistry at Strassburg from 1872 until his death.

Hoppe-Seyler's first important paper was on the physics of percussion (1854), in which he classified the percussion note according to its physical characteristics. His later publications were in the field of physiological chemistry. He was the first to obtain crystalline hemoglobin and to describe the spectum of oxyhemoglobin (1862). He worked out the chemical formulas of hemin, hematin, hematoporphyrin (1863); discovered hemochromogen and methemoglobin (1864); and proved that hemoglobin is loosely bound to oxygen but cannot be readily separated from carbon monoxide. He described bubbles in the blood following a sudden drop in atmospheric pressure; isolated lecithin; and studied the chemistry of milk, pus, cartilage, and the products of fermentation. He introduced the term, "proteid."

1826-1897—Paul Louis Duroziez was born in Paris, where he received his doctor's degree in 1853. He was never professor at the medical school and never had a service in any of the great hospitals of Paris, and, although he had no hospital service of his own, the doors of all the hospitals were open to him. He was a general practitioner, a remarkably keen observer, and a simple and gentle man who was universally respected by the physicians of Paris. He was elected president of the *Société de Médecine* in 1882 and was created Chevalier of the Legion of Honor in 1895. His *Traité Clinique des Maladies du Coeur,* which appeared in 1891, earned for its author the Itard Prize of the Academy of Medicine and the Montjou Prize of the Institut de France. Duroziez is best remembered for his description of "pure" mitral stenosis (Duroziez's disease) and for his account of the double femoral murmurs in aortic insufficiency (Duroziez's sign).

1827-1892—Jean Antoine Villemin, who demonstrated the contagiousness of tuberculosis, was a French army surgeon who was born at Prey in the Vosges and studied medicine at Strassburg and later at the army medical school of Val-de-Grâce. In 1863, he was appointed professor at Val-de-Grâce, where he worked until his retirement. His great work, *Études sur la Tuberculose,* which appeared in 1868, contains an account of his careful experiments in which he proved that sputum from a tuberculous person, fluid from a tuberculous cavity, and material from scrofulous glands produced, when injected subcutaneously or into the trachea, tuberculosis in rabbits.

1827-1912—Lord Lister (Joseph).

1828-1870—Albrecht von Graefe, the creator of modern ophthalmology, was born in Berlin, the son of Carl Ferdinand von Graefe, an eminent military surgeon. He studied medicine at Berlin, where he received his degree in 1847. He then studied at Prague, where he came under the influence of Ferdinand Arlt, professor of ophthalmology, and decided to become an ophthalmologist. After further study in Paris, Vienna and London, he returned to Berlin in 1850 and began practice as an eye specialist. The discovery of the ophthalmoscope by Helmholtz in 1851 aroused great enthusiasm in von Graefe, who exclaimed, "Helmholtz has opened up a new world to us."

Von Graefe was the first ophthalmologist to employ the ophthalmoscope. He diagnosed sudden loss of vision from embolism of the retinal artery (1859), pointed out the importance of optic retinitis in diagnosis, and differentiated functional from organic loss of vision. He introduced the operation of iridectomy in the treatment of iritis, iridochoroiditis and glaucoma, employed linear extraction in the operation for cataract, and noted the lid lay in exophthalmic goitre (von Graefe's sign). He founded the *Archiv für Ophthalmologie* in 1857, in which he described most of his important discoveries and which was a journal that led its field for more than half a century. His *Handbuch der gesammten Augenheilkunde,* in which Saemisch was associated as an editor, appeared in seven volumes in 1874-1880.

Von Graefe became associate professor of ophthalmology at Berlin in 1857, professor in 1866 and directed the most active and productive clinic of ophthalmology of its time. He was a man of a refined, spiritual type, endowed with great personal charm as well as with remarkable intelligence and unbounded energy. Doctors came to him from all over the world seeking instruction, and patients in large numbers in search of relief. He died at the early age of 42.

1828-1898—Ferdinand Julius Cohn was born in Breslau, studied natural science in Breslau and Berlin, became associate professor of botany in Breslau in 1859 and full professor in 1870. He established the university institute of plant physiology in 1866 and, in 1875, founded the *Beiträge zur Biologie der Planzen*, in which was published much of the pioneer work in bacteriology. He recognized the importance of Koch's early work on the anthrax bacillus, which Koch demonstrated in his laboratory and the report of which Cohn published in his *Beiträge*. Cohn was the recognized authority in the field of bacteriology during its early history, published many important papers, and proposed in 1875 the first practical classification of bacteria, dividing them into four groups—Sphaero bacteria (cocci), rod shaped bacteria (bacilli), Desmo bacteria (thread-like bacteria), and Spiro bacteria (spirilli and spirochaete).

1829-1896—George Harley was born in Haddington, England, and studied medicine at Edinburgh, where he received his doctor's degree in 1850. After graduation, he went to Paris, where he worked with Magendie and Claude Bernard for two years and then went to Germany, where he spent two additional years, working with Liebig, Virchow, Kölliker and Bunsen. On his return to England, he was appointed lecturer in physiology at University College, London, in 1856, professor of legal medicine in 1859, and physician to the University College Hospital in 1860. In 1865, he was elected Fellow of the Royal Society.

Harley wrote important papers and monographs on diabetes, on diseases of the suprarenal glands, on jaundice, and on the urine, discovered the urinary pigment, urohematin, and proved that it contained iron. He was one of the first to describe and study paroxysmal hemoglobinuria, which he found disappeared after mercurial treatment.

1828-1913—Sir Jonathan Hutchinson, a native of Selby, in Yorkshire, studied first at the York School of Medicine and Surgery, later studied at St. Bartholomew's Hospital in London, and received the degree of M.R.C.S. in 1850. He was surgeon to the London Hospital from 1859 until 1883 and professor of surgery in the Royal College of Surgeons from 1879 to 1883. He was an extremely versatile man, an eminent general surgeon, ophthalmologist, dermatologist, syphilologist, pathologist and neurologist as well as a man of remarkably broad culture and learning. He edited the *Archives of Surgery* from 1889 to 1899, writing all the contributions himself, and also edited a popular encyclopedia of knowledge, again writing all the articles. He described "Hutchinson's teeth" in congenital syphilis, "Hutchinson's triad" (interstitial keratitis, notched teeth, and labyrinthine disease) in syphilis, "Hutchinson's facies" in ophthalmoplegia, and "Hutchinson's mask" in tabes. He was a great student of syphilis and, during his lifetime saw more than one million cases.

1829-1902—Hugo Wilhelm von Ziemssen was born in Griefswald, received his M.D. degree in 1853, was professor of medicine at Erlangen in 1863 and at Munich in 1874. He was the author of many articles and editor of the authoritative *Handbuch der speciellen Pathologie und Therapie,* which appeared in 17 volumes in 1875-1885.

1829-1910—Eduard Friedrich Wilhelm Pflüger was born in Hanau and studied in Marburg and Berlin, where he was a pupil of Johannes Müller and of du Bois-Reymond. He received his doctor's degree in 1853 in Berlin, became *Privatdozent* there in 1858, and, in 1859, succeeded Helmholtz as professor of physiology at Bonn, holding this chair the rest of his life.

Pflüger was one of the master physiologists of his time and founded in 1868 the famous *Archiv für die gesamte Physiologie* (Pflüger's Archiv), in which much of his best work and that of his pupils appeared. He made many fundamental discoveries in the physiology of respiration and metabolism, proving that the seat of respiration is in the tissues and not in the blood. This thesis he established by his monographs on gasometry of the blood (1866), on the cause of dyspnea (1868), on oxidation processes in the body (1872), and on heat production and oxidation (1878). He also showed that proteid metabolism could not take place until proteids are built up into protoplasm and that all the nitrogen produced by the breaking down of proteids appears in the urine and feces. He was the founder of experimental embryology and invented a number of new physiological instruments, such as his gas-pump, lung catheter, aerotonometer and pneumonometer.

1829-1894—Christian Albert Theodor Billroth, one of the greatest surgeons of his time, was born on the Island of Ruegen, the son of a minister who died and left a widow with five children, Theodor, the eldest, being five years old at the time of his father's death. Young Billroth wished to become a musician but, on the insistence of his mother, began his medical studies at Greifswald. From there, he went to Göttingen, thence to Berlin, where he received his M.D. degree in 1852. He served first as assistant in the surgical clinic of Langenbeck, became *Privatdozent in* 1856, and, four years later, went to Zürich as professor of surgery. In 1867, he went to Vienna as professor of surgery, serving in this position for 25 years and making his clinic the most renowned surgical clinic of its time.

Billroth's early work while in Berlin was mostly in the field of pathology and was so excellent that, during the time he was assistant in the surgical clinic of Langenbeck, he was called to Greifswald as professor of pathological anatomy, but declined the call. His first publications in the field of surgical pathology culminated in his excellent *Die allgemeine chirurgische Pathologie und Therapie,* which was published in 1863, went through 11 editions, and was translated into English, French, Italian, Spanish, Hungarian, Polish, Russian, Serbian, Croatian and Japanese. He was early interested in the study of wound infections and, after preliminary studies, began in 1868 a systematic series of bacteriological investigations. He grasped at once the causal relationship between bacteria and wound infection and described one generic group the "cocco-bacteria septica," which he held responsible for wound infections (*Untersuchungen über die Vegetationsformen von Coccobacteria septica,* Berlin, 1874).

In operative surgery, Billroth is remembered particularly as a pioneer in surgery of the gastro-intestinal tract. In 1872, he carried out the first resection of the esophagus and, in 1881, the first resection of the pylorus for cancer, and he devised a number of operations still known by his name. He also carried out the first excision of the larynx. He was an early champion of Lister's antiseptic methods, which made his brilliant surgical achievements possible.

Billroth was a man with a charming and genial personality, had a marked artistic bent, and was devoted to music, being himself an excellent pianist. He was a life-long friend of Johannes Brahms, the composer, and, when he received a call to Berlin as professor of surgery, declined, giving as his reason that he could not persuade Brahms to leave Vienna. His *Briefe,* first published in 1896, went through nine editions.

1830-1889—Richard von Volkmann was born in Leipzig, the son of Alfred Wilhelm Volkmann, a well-known physiologist, at that time *Privatdozent* in Leipzig, later professor in Halle. Richard von Volkmann graduated at Berlin in 1854 and, in 1867, became professor and director of the surgical clinic at Halle, remaining there until his retirement. He served as a consulting surgeon in the war of 1870 and was

one of the earliest and most influential champions of Lister's methods. He was the first surgeon to excise the rectum for carcinoma, described ischaemic contractures (Volkmann's contractures), and originated the splint and spoon, since known by his name. He founded in 1870 the well-known *Sammlung Klinischer Vorträge,* "which contains some of the most valuable monographs of recent times" (Garrison). He possessed unusually literary ability, and his poems and charming stories, written under the pen-name of Richard Leander, have won for him a lasting place in the history of German literature.

1830-1914—Silas Weir Mitchell, the leading American neurologist of his time, was born in Philadelphia the son of the well-known physician, John Kearsley Mitchell. Weir Mitchell graduated at Jefferson Medical College in 1850 and, after studying in Paris under Claude Bernard, returned to Philadelphia. During the Civil War, he studied nerve injuries in Turner's Lane Hospital in Philadelphia, and, in 1872 appeared his important book, *Injuries to Nerves and their Consequences.* In this work, he described for the first time ascending neuritis and its treatment by cold and splints, the psychology of amputations, reflex paralysis, and many other pathological states. He was the first to describe causalgia (1864), erythromalalgia (1872), and post paraplegic chorea (1874). In 1863, he discovered with Morehouse the laryngeal chiasma and, from 1863-1869, carried out important observations on the coordinating function of the cerebellum. In 1875, he introduced the treatment of nervous diseases by prolonged rest in bed, aided by a full diet, massage, and electrical treatment—a method since known as the "Rest Treatment" or "Weir Mitchell Treatment." This method was immediately adopted all over the world and made its originator famous. He described the treatment in his monograph, *Fat and Blood,* 1877, which was immediately successful and was translated into French, German, Italian, Spanish and Russian.

Weir Mitchell carried out important investigations on the toxicity of arrow poison and snake venom and studied the physiological effects of amyl nitrite, atropin and opium. He was a pioneer in the exact study of pharmacology.

He also had unusual gifts as a poet and prose writer. His novels, *Hugh Wynne,* 1897, and *The Adventures of François,* 1898, were both phenomenally successful. Sir Lauder Brunton called Weir Mitchell "the most accomplished and versatile physician of his time."

1831-1908—Karl von Voit was born in Amberg and studied medicine in Munich, where he received his doctor's degree in 1854. He was later successively *Privatdozent* for physiology, then associate professor, and professor in 1863. Voit was a pupil and colleague of Pettenkofer and assisted him in his epochal work on respiration and metabolism, later taking over himself the greater part of the investigation.

1831-1904—Wilhelm His was born in Basel, Switzerland, the scion of a very distinguished Swiss family, and studied medicine in Berlin, Würzburg, Bern, Vienna and Paris, having as his teachers Johannes Müller,

Remak, Virchow and Kölliker. He received his medical degree in 1854, was appointed three years later professor of anatomy and physiology in Basel, and was called in 1872 to Leipzig as professor of anatomy. "As Bichat dealt with the coarser aspects of tissues, Henle and Kölliker with their microscopic appearances in health, Virchow with the same in disease, so the name of His will always be associated with the science of their origins (histogenesis)" (Garrison). His invented a microtome and, using serial sections and the wax method of Born, drew the sections on wax plates, then, placing them together, demonstrated morphological relations in three dimensions. His famous *Anatomie menschlicher Embryonen,* 1880-1885, was the first accurate and exhaustive study of the development of the human embryo. In 1886, he demonstrated by embryological investigations that the axis cylinder arose from the nerve cell.

1832-1913—William Howship Dickinson was born in Brighton and received the degree of M.B. at Cambridge in 1850. Returning to London, he was successively assistant physician, physician, and consulting physician to St. George's Hospital. In 1865, he published in *The Lancet* an early account of paroxysmal hemoglobinuria.

1832-1910—Ernst von Leyden was born in Danzig and was a pupil of Schönlein and of Traube. On the death of Frerichs in 1885, he became his successor at Berlin and soon acquired a great reputation. He was the author of monographs on tabes dorsalis, on the respiration in fever, on poliomyelitis and was especially active in the establishment of sanitaria for the treatment of tuberculosis.

1833-1910—Friedrich Daniel von Recklinghausen was born in Gütersloh, Westphalia, and received his medical degree at Berlin in 1855. He was assistant in the pathological institute under Virchow for six years, then became professor of pathology at Königsberg, then at Würzburg, and, in 1872, was called to Strassburg, where he was very active as a teacher and an investigator until his death 38 years later. He described three diseases which bear his name—*neurofibromatosis generalis* (von Recklinghausen's disease), *osteitis fibrosa cystica* (associated with a parathyroid tumor), and the lesser known *arthritis deformans neoplastica.*

1833-1900—Jacob M. Da Costa, one of the ablest teachers of his time, was born on the Island of St. Thomas, West Indies, of Spanish and Portuguese extraction. As a boy, he was educated in Europe, mainly at Dresden, and, at an early age, gained a complete mastery of French and German, as well as becoming fluent in Spanish, Portuguese, Italian and Dutch. After graduation at Jefferson Medical College in 1852 at the age of 19, he spent 18 months at Paris and Vienna, returning to Philadelphia in 1853. In 1864, he was appointed lecturer in medicine at Jefferson Medical College, and in the same year appeared his *Medical Diagnosis,* which passed through nine editions during his life-time and was translated into German, Italian and Russian. In 1872, he was elected professor of the theory and practice of medicine at Jefferson and held this position until his retirement in 1891. During the Civil War, he served at a military hospital in Philadelphia and saw among the soldiers many cases of "irritable heart," which he mentioned in his *Medical Diagnosis* and later described more fully in an article published in 1871 in the *American Journal of Medical Science.*

Da Costa was a renowned clinician and teacher. His public clinics were events in the medical life of Philadelphia.

1833-1915—Carlos Findlay was born in Camagüey, Cuba, the son of a Scotch father and a French mother. He received his early education in France and later entered the Jefferson Medical College in Philadelphia, where he graduated in 1855. On his return to Cuba, he became a general practitioner in Havana and, after many years of study, became convinced that yellow fever was transmitted by the bite of the Stegomyia mosquito. He advocated this theory at a meeting of the International Sanitary Conference in Washington in 1881 and published five years later in the *American Journal of Medical Sciences* an article describing the experimental transmission of yellow fever by the bite of infected mosquitoes. When the American Yellow Fever Commission went to Havana in 1900, Findlay convinced the members, although they were at first skeptical, of the correctness of his theory.

1834-1897—Rudolf Peter Heinrich Heidenhain was born in Marienwerder and studied medicine at Königsberg, Halle and Berlin, receiving his degree at Berlin in 1854.

In 1859, he was appointed professor of physiology and histology at the University of Breslau, where he remained until his death.

Heidenhain was one of the outstanding physiologists of his century, and many of his students became later prominent physiologists. He made notable investigations on gastric and urinary secretion and on the formation of lymph. Discovered by and named after him were Heidenhain's cells, Heidenhain's rods, Heidenhain's stain, and Heidenhain's law—that glandular secretion always involves changes in structure of the gland.

1834-1911—Hermann Senator was born in Gnesen, Polish Prussia, and studied under Johannes Müller, Schönlein and Traube in Berlin, where he received his degree in 1857. He spent his entire professional life in Berlin, where he became associate professor in 1875 and, in 1888, was given a separate clinic and placed in charge of the polyclinic of the University. His reputation rests on his work on fever (1873), diabetes (1879), albuminuria (1882), and on his monograph on kidney disease (1896).

1834-1911—John Hughlings Jackson was born in York and studied medicine first in his native city and then at St. Bartholomew's Hospital in London. He received his M.D. degree at the University of St. Andrew's, Scotland, and was appointed assistant physician at the London Hospital. He was one of the leading British neurologists of his time, did much to establish the value of the ophthalmoscope in the diagnosis of cerebral disease, made important

studies on aphasia in 1864 and described unilateral convulsions, or "Jacksonian epilepsy," in 1875.

1834-1881—Maurice Raynaud, the son of a distinguished university professor, studied medicine at Paris, receiving his medical degree in 1862 and submitting as a thesis a monograph, *Sur l'asphyxie locale et la gangrène symétrique des extremités,* in which he described the syndrome since known as Raynaud's disease. He became *agrégé* in 1866, was made officer of the Legion of Honor in 1811 and member of the *Académie de Médecine* in 1879. He taught with great success but died suddenly at the age of 47.

Raynaud was deeply interested in the history of medicine and was the author of a charming and scholarly book, *Les médecins au temps de Molière,* 1862.

1835-1907—Sir William Broadbent, born in Huddersfield, Yorkshire, studied medicine first at Manchester and received his M.B. at London University in 1858. He obtained a post at St. Mary's Hospital the following year and was connected with the hospital and its medical school for 40 years. He was elected a Fellow of the Royal Society in 1896 and created a baronet in 1893.

Broadbent was an excellent clinician, a forceful teacher, and one of the leading consultants in London. He was the author of *The Pulse,* 1890, and *Heart Disease,* 1897, and is remembered for his description of "Broadbent's sign" in adhesive pericarditis.

1835-1935—Griffith Evans was born in Towyn, England, studied at the Royal Veterinary College in London, and, in 1860, entered the British Army as a veterinary surgeon. He was stationed for a time in Montreal, Canada, where he entered the medical school of McGill University and received the M.D. degree in 1864. In 1877, he was sent to India and, in 1880, investigated a disease of horses and camels called surra. He found the causative agent to be a trypanosome, since called the *Trypanosoma Evansi*. This was the first demonstration of a disease due to a pathogenic trypanosome. Evans returned to England in 1885 and, from 1892 until 1912, lectured on veterinary medicine at University College, Bangor, Wales.

1836-1907—Sir Michael Foster was born in Huntington, the son of a surgeon. He studied at University College, and, after further study in Paris, returned to University College, where he taught physiology. On Huxley's recommendation, he was appointed praelector of physiology at the University of Cambridge in 1870 and became professor of physiology when that position was created in 1883. He was the founder of the Cambridge School of Physiology and numbered among his pupils such distinguished scientists as Balfour, Liversidge, Marshall, Sidgwick, Ray, Gaskell, Langley, Sherrington, Henry Head, Adami, and Newell Martin. "He made an epoch in teaching which was only excelled by Ludwig's" (Garrison). Most of Foster's original work was one on the heart and circulation. He was the author with Balfour of the *Elements of Embryology*, 1874, which, for more than a quarter of a century, was a widely used text, and in 1876 appeared his *Text-Book of Physiol-*

ogy, which passed through seven editions and was translated into German, Italian and Russian. His *Lectures on the History of Physiology*, 1901, is a most readable book and remains the standard work on the subject.

1836-1907—Ernst von Bergmann was born in Riga, Latvia, and studied at Dorpat, Vienna and Berlin, receiving his doctor's degree at Berlin in 1860. He served as an army surgeon during the wars of 1866 and 1870 in the German armies and, in 1871, was appointed professor of surgery at Dorpat. In the Russo-Turkish War of 1877-1878, he served as a consulting surgeon to the Russian Army. In 1878, he was appointed professor of surgery at Würzburg, and, in 1882, he went to Berlin as professor of surgery.

Von Bergmann was recognized as one of the great surgeons of his time. He advanced cranial surgery by his memoir on head injuries, *Die Lehre von den Kopfverletzungen*, 1877, and made important contributions on surgery of the joints, on surgical pathology, on fat embolism, and on ligations. He was an early advocate of Lister's methods, introduced steam sterilization in surgery (1886), and began to employ in 1891 asepsis in surgery.

1837-1900—Willy Kühne was born in Hamburg, studied in Göttingen, Jena, Berlin, Paris and Vienna, having as teachers such noted men as Woehler, Weber, Henle, Virchow, Claude Bernard, Ludwig, Brücke, and du Bois-Reymond. He received his medical degree at Berlin in 1862, was assistant in Virchow's pathological institute, went to Amsterdam as professor of physiology in 1868, and then went to Heidelberg, where he was professor of physiology from 1871 until his retirement in 1899. He carried out important investigations on the end organs of motor nerves, on hemoglobin, on pancreatic digestion, discovering trypsin, and on rhodopsin, or visual purple, and, with his pupil, Chittenden of New Haven, isolated many new split products of proteins.

1837-1905—Samuel Siegfried Karl von Basch was born in Prague and studied medicine in Prague and in Vienna, where he received his degree in 1862. He worked in the physiological laboratory of von Brücke in Vienna for many years and was assistant in the medical clinic from 1861 to 1865. In 1865, he went to Mexico, where he became personal physician to the unfortunate emperor Maximilian. Returning to Vienna after Maximilian's death, he became *Privatdozent* for experimental pathology in 1870 and professor in 1877. He made many interesting contributions to physiology and, in 1880, devised the first practical instrument for the estimation of the blood pressure in patients.

1838-1896—Jules Edouard Nicaise was born in Pont-à-Binson and studied at Rheims and later at Paris, where he received his doctor's degree in 1866. After serving as surgeon to several hospitals, he was appointed surgeon to the Laennec Hospital in 1880 and held this position until his death. He was a very prolific writer, publishing more than 300 articles, mainly on surgical subjects. He is remembered especially for his excellent editions of the works of Guy de Chauliac (1891), Henri de Mondeville (1893), and Pierre Franco (1895), which are accompanied by extensive commentaries.

1838-1921—Oswald Schmiedeberg, one of the greatest of modern pharmacologists, was born in Laidsen, Courland, and received his doctor's degree at Dorpat in 1866, where he was appointed professor of materia medica in 1871. The following year, he went to Strassburg as professor and worked here until the end of the first World War, carrying out a large amount of important and fundamental work in pharmacology. His colleague, Naunyn, wrote of him: "Schmiedeberg lived only in his institute. He was, at that time, at the height of his activity as a teacher; all the pharmacologists of the world came to him in Strassburg for their training." His *Grundriss der Arzneimittellehre,* later called *Grundriss der Pharmakologie,* appeared first in 1883, went through seven editions, and was translated into Dutch and English. It remains a standard treatise on pharmacology and contains many of his original observations.

1838-1913—John Shaw Billings was born in Indiana and studied medicine at the Medical College of Ohio, graduating in 1860. During the Civil War, he was medical director of the Army of the Potomac and, after the war, went to the Surgeon-General's Office in Washington, where he worked for 30 years. He was the founder of the Surgeon-General's Library and, in 1880, issued, with the assistance of Robert Fletcher, the first volume of the *Index Medicus,* the most exhaustive medical bibliography ever undertaken. Billings was an able operative surgeon and an authority on military medicine, hygiene, sanitary engineering, statistics, and hospital construction. He wrote the "best history of surgery that has been published in English" (Garrison) (in F. . Dennis's *System of Surgery,* New York, 1895) and was widely known as the planner of the Johns Hopkins Hospital. He left Washington to become administrator of the New York Public Library, which he designed and brought to a high state of efficiency.

1838-1915—George Miller Sternberg was born in Hartwick, New York, graduated in 1860 at the College of Physicians and Surgeons of New York City, and began practice in Elizabeth City, New York. At the outbreak of the Civil War, he became an army surgeon and, after the war, remained in the army, becoming Surgeon-General in 1893. A pioneer in bacteriology, he discovered the pneumococcus in 1880, advanced a theory of phagocytosis in 1881, and demonstrated the plasmodium of malaria in 1885, for the first time in the United States. He was an authority on sanitation and disinfection and the founder of the Army Medical School in Washington. His valuable and popular *Manual of Bacteriology,* 1892, later republished as *Textbook of Bacteriology,* was the first work of its kind by an American author.

1839-1884—Julius Friedrich Cohnheim was born in Demmin, Pomerania, and received his medical degree at Berlin in 1861. He served in the war of 1864 and, the same year, became assistant to Virchow in Berlin. He was subsequently professor of pathology at Kiel (1868-1872), Breslau (1872-1878) and Leipzig (1878-1884).

The most eminent of Virchow's pupils, Cohnheim made important studies on sugar forming ferments (1863), introduced the method of freezing tissue for microscopic study, and employed silver and gold salts for the staining of nerve endings. His monograph on inflammation, *Neue Untersuchungen über die Entzündung,* Berlin, 1873, revolutionized pathology, showing that the essential feature of inflammation is the passage of leukocytes through the walls of the capillaries and that pus cells are white blood cells which have wandered from the blood vessels. This work was a clear refutation of Virchow's teaching that diapedesis does not occur. He witnessed Robert Koch's historic demonstration in 1876 of the life cycle of the anthrax bacillus and predicted that Koch would become the first bacteriologist of his time. The following year, Cohnheim successfully inoculated tuberculosis into the anterior chamber of the eye of a rabbit.

Cohnheim was a resourceful investigator and an inspiring teacher. Among his pupils were Heidenhain, Ehrlich, Neisser, Weigert, and the Americans Welch and Councilman. He was long a sufferer from gout, the complications of which cut short his brilliant career at the age of 45.

1839-1914—Hugo Kronecker was born in Liegnitz, Silesia, studied medicine at Heidelberg, Berlin and

Pisa, and was a pupil of Helmholtz, Wundt, Traube, Kühne and Ludwig. He received his doctor's degree at Berlin in 1863, was *Privatdozent,* then associate professor at Leipzig and Berlin, and, in 1885, went to Bern as professor of physiology. Kronecker and his pupils carried out important researches on fatigue and recovery of striped muscle (1871) and on the mechanism of deglutition (1880) and demonstrated that heart muscle cannot be tetanized (1874) and that the heart beat is "all or none." He studied the role of inorganic salts in the heart beat, the physiology of mountain-sickness, reflex action, animal heat, and innervation of respiration, assisted von Basch in studies on blood pressure in man, and invented the phrenograph, thermoesthesiometer, and the graduated induction coil.

1839-1925—Bernard Naunyn, the son of the burgomaster of Berlin, was born in Berlin and studied first in Bonn, then in Berlin, where he received his doctor's degree in 1862. The first clinic conducted by Frerich made a deep impression on Naunyn, who later wrote, "After the first lecture of Frerich, my goal stood clearly before my eyes . . . that my life belonged to internal medicine." He remained in Berlin as Frerichs' assistant for seven years, went to Dorpat as professor in 1869, to Bern in 1871, became professor at Königsberg in 1872, and succeeded Kussmaul at Strassburg in 1888, remaining there until his retirement in 1904, meanwhile declining a call to Vienna in 1894.

Naunyn's "rigorous Prussian temperament" excited at first considerable opposition in the newly acquired province of Alsace, but, in the end, his remarkable abilities as a teacher and organizer, his obvious integrity, his love of truth, and his wide culture gained the admiration and respect of his colleagues, patients, and fellow townsmen. In Strassburg, he succeeded in persuading the authorities to construct a splendid new building for his clinic, which became one of the outstanding medical clinics of the new German Empire. He devoted his life to the study of diseases of the liver and of diabetes, his most outstanding contributions being his work on gall-stones, *Klinik der Cholelithiasis,* Leipzig, 1892, and his monograph on diabetes, *Der Diabetes mellitus,* Vienna, 1898. Many foreign students came to his Strassburg Clinic to study his methods of treating diabetes. Among them were Petrèn of Sweden, Cushny of Scotland, later in Ann Arbor, and Joslin of Boston. Joslin, he relates, "remained really little longer than three weeks; but, with the large material at my disposal and with his great zeal, he was able in this short time to become familiar with my views and maxims. Then, with a 24-hour stop in Paris, he went directly back to Boston."

At Naunyn's suggestion, his assistants, von Mering and Minkowsky, removed the pancreas from a dog and produced diabetes in the animal. His assistant in Königsberg, Stadelmann, discovered β-oxybutyric acid while studying acidosis under his direction. Naunyn introduced the term, "acidosis," to describe the metabolic condition of acid formation in diabetes and made careful studies of this condition. His autobiography, *Erinnerungen, Gedanken, und Meinungen,* published in 1925, is one of the most interesting books in this field.

1839-1911—Georges Dieulafoy, born in Toulouse, received his medical degree at Paris in 1869 and became professor in 1886 and, 10 years later, chief of the medical service at l'Hôtel-Dieu. A pupil of Trousseau, he first attracted his master's attention by supplying him with a correct quotation from Ovid. He was a good classical scholar and a man of wide culture. A natural orator with all the fervor of a native of southern France, a born actor and mimic, he held clinics that were dramatic and fascinating as well as instructive and impressive. His *Manuel de pathologie interne,* first published in 1880, went through 16 editions during his life-time, a testimonial of its great popularity as a text on internal medicine.

1840-1910—Joseph Frank Payne was born in Camberwell and received his medical degree at Oxford in 1867. After postgraduate work in Paris, Berlin and Vienna, he returned to London, where he was appointed assistant physician to St. Thomas' Hospital in 1871 and physician in 1887. In 1888, he published a *Manuel of Pathology,* a subject in which he had a deep interest. A scholar and a student of medical history, he wrote a *Life of Linacre* in 1881, *Life of Sydenham* in 1900, and several authoritative articles on English medicine in Anglo-Saxon times.

1840-1921—Wilhelm Erb, one of the greatest neurologists of his time, was born in Winneweiler and received his medical degree at Heidelberg. He became *Privatdozent* for medicine at Heidelberg in 1865 and associate professor in 1869 and, in 1880, went to Leipzig as full professor. In 1883, he returned to Heidelberg as professor, holding this position until his retirement in 1907.

One of the first to employ electricity as a diagnostic aid in neurology, Erb demonstrated in 1874 the increased irritability of motor nerves in tetany. He described palsy of the brachial plexus (Erb-Duchenne palsy) in 1873 and spastic spinal paralysis (Erb-Charcot disease) in 1875. In 1875, he pointed out the absence of the knee kick in tabes dorsalis; in 1878, described myasthenia gravis with bulbar symptoms; and, in 1884, gave the first clear description of progressive muscular dystrophy. During his years at Heidelberg, his clinic became outstanding for the investigation of nervous diseases. In his *Die Aetiologie der Tabes,* 1892, he maintained that this disease was caused by syphilis.

1841-1914—Alfred Freeman Africanus King was born in Oxfordshire, England, and came to America when 20 years of age. He received his M.D. degree at the University of Pennsylvania and settled in Washington, D.C. Being present in the theatre, he attended President Lincoln immediately after his assassination. He devoted himself to the practice of obstetrics and wrote a *Manual of Obstetrics,* 1882, which went through 11 editions. In 1882, he wrote a paper, published in *Popular Science Monthly* for September, 1883, in which he gave 19 reasons for believing that malaria is transmitted by the bite of a mosquito.

1840-1911—Henry Pickering Bowditch was born in Boston, studied at Harvard College, and, at the outbreak of the Civil War, enlisted in the Union Army, serving four years and being advanced to the grade of major. He received his M.D. degree from Harvard in 1868 and then proceeded abroad, where he remained two years studying with Claude Bernard in Paris and Carl Ludwig in Leipzig. On his return to Boston, he became assistant professor of physiology and established one of the first physiological laboratories in America. He invented many types of physiological apparatus in common use and was one of the founders of the *American Journal of Physiology*. He made many important contributions to physiology, including studies on cardiac irritability, innervation of blood vessels, respiration, and the digestion of fat.

1841-1898—Joseph O'Dwyer, a native of Cleveland, Ohio, and surgeon to the Foundling Hospital in 1884, perfected and made practical the method of intubation of the larynx as a substitute for tracheotomy. This procedure was first carried out by Bouchut in 1856-1858 and by Trousseau in Paris in 1859.

1841-1905—Hermann Nothnagel, a pupil of Traube and Virchow in Berlin, was born in Alt-Lietzgöricke, in Brandenburg, became professor at Freiburg in 1872, at Jena in 1874, and was called to the chair of internal medicine at Vienna in 1882,

where he remained until his death. He was an excellent teacher and an impressive lecturer. He is remembered especially for the encyclopedic system of medicine, *Handbuch der speziellen Pathologie und Therapie,* 1894-1905, which he edited, a storehouse of information and an enduring monument to German scholarship.

1842-1922—Heinrich Quincke was born in Frankfur a.O. and received his degree at Berlin in 1863, remaining as Frerichs' assistant for six years. He was subsequently professor at Bern in 1873 and was called to Kiel in 1878, where he remained until his retirement in 1908. He was the first to study carefully the capillary pulse in aortic insufficiency, described a new disease —angioneurotic edema, or Quincke's disease—was the first to note poikilocytosis in pernicious anemia, and introduced lumbar puncture as a diagnostic and therapeutic measure.

1843-1910—Robert Koch.

1843-1913—Reginald Fitz was born in Chelsea, Massachusetts, and received his M.D. at Harvard in 1843. After two years of study in Europe, chiefly with Rokitansky and Skoda in Vienna and with Virchow in Berlin, he returned to Boston and, in 1879, was appointed professor of pathological anatomy at Harvard. Later, his interests centered more in clinical medicine, and, in 1892, he became professor of medicine, holding this chair until his retirement in 1908.

At the first meeting of the Association of American Physicians in 1886, Fitz read a paper on "Perforating Inflammation of the Vermiform Appendix," which clearly described the early symptoms and signs of this disease. The paper aroused the attention of the entire medical profession in a disease which is very common and hitherto neglected—acute appendicitis. In 1889, Fitz wrote a paper on "Acute pancreatitis," published in the *Boston Medical and Surgical Journal,* which clearly outlined this disease and pointed out its diagnostic criteria.

1844-1916—Thomas Lauder Brunton, a native of Roxburghshire, Scotland, received his M.D. at Edinburgh in 1868 and then studied with Brücke in Vienna, Kühne in Heidelberg, and Ludwig in Leipzig. Returning to England, he settled in London, where he became assistant physician to St. Bartholomew's Hospital in 1875 and physician in 1897, teaching materia medica in the medical school. He became the leading exponent of the application of pharmacologic findings to the practice of medicine and made important observations on the action of digitalis. He introduced amyl nitrite in the treatment of angina pectoris, after demonstrating that the rise of blood pressure which occurs in angina pectoris is relieved by the vaso-dilating action of amyl nitrite ("On the use of nitrite of amyl in angina pectoris," *Lancet,* 1867). He was the author of *A Text-Book of Pharmacology, Therapeutics and Materia Medica,* 1885, and wrote a large number of monographs and articles on pharmacologic and physiological subjects.

1844-1922—Sir Patrick Manson, "Father of Tropical Medicine in Great Britain," was born in Cromlet Hill, Aberdeenshire, Scotland, and received his doctor's degree in 1866 at Aberdeen. He went to the Far East the same year, spent five years on the island of Formosa, then in Amoy, China, where he remained four years. He returned to England in 1875 and, while in London, noted an article on filaria, which attracted his attention. On his return to China the same year, he began to study filariasis in Amoy and demonstrated the life cycle of the *filaria Bancrofti* in the mosquito. The same year, he discovered the eggs of a hitherto unknown worm, the lung fluke, *Paragonimus,* in the bloody sputum of a patient with hemoptysis. In 1883, he moved to Hong Kong, where he was active in medical circles and soon had an enormous practice.

In 1889, Manson retired and bought an estate in Scotland, but, the same year, lost most of his fortune through the depreciation in Chinese currency, and, seeing the pressing necessity of earning a living, went to London to practice. He became physician to the Seamen's Hospital and began lecturing on tropical medicine first at Livingstone College, then at Charing Cross Hospital and St. George's Hospital. Meanwhile, he carried out experiments in his home with mice, rats, birds and mosquitoes, and he became convinced that mosquitoes transmitted malaria just as they did filariasis but was unable to prove it as there was no endemic malaria in London. He passed the idea on to a new doctor from India—Ronald

Ross. Manson was instrumental in founding the London School of Tropical Medicine.

1844-1926—Camillo Golgi was born in Corteno and received his medical education at Pavia, where he was appointed professor of histology in 1876 and professor of pathology in 1881. He made many important studies in pathology but is remembered best for his method of staining nervous tissue with his silver nitrate stain, a method which he applied with great success to the study of the finer anatomy of the nervous system. He also did pioneer work on malaria, showing in 1886 that the paroxysm begins at the moment the merozoites are liberated and demonstrating the differences in the morphology of the tertian and quartan parasites. Golgi received the Nobel prize in 1906.

1845-1904—Carl Weigert was born in Munsterberg, Silesia, and received his medical degree in Berlin in 1866. After serving as clinical assistant to Waldeyer in Berlin, he went to Breslau as Cohnheim's assistant in pathology and followed Cohnheim to Leipzig in 1878. Weigert was made associate professor in 1879, but went to Frankfurt in 1885 as director of the Pathological Institute, and was active in this position until his death. Weigert introduced aniline dyes in the study of bacteria, and his staining methods made progress in bacteriology possible. He also introduced many new staining methods in the study of tissue and made important pathological studies of smallpox and chronic neritis.

1845-1915—Sir William Richard

Gowers, one of the founders of modern neurology, was born in London and received his medical education at University College, taking his M.D. degree in 1870. He was appointed assistant physician to University College Hospital in 1872, physician in 1883, and consulting physician in 1888. He was early interested in the anatomical pathology and diseases of the spinal cord. In his *Diagnosis of Diseases of the Spinal Cord*, published in 1880, he described the tract in the spinal cord since known by his name. His *Manual of Diseases of the Nervous System*, in two volumes, was published in 1886, went through three editions and was translated into German and Italian. Gowers was an accomplished artist, drawing many illustrations for his scientific articles and books. He also devised a hemoglobinometer, which was widely used for many years.

1845-1916—Ilia (Elie) Metchnikoff was born in the province of Kharkoff and studied zoology and natural sciences at Kharkoff University, where he received his degree. He was docent at Odessa, lecturer on zoology at St. Petersburg, and, from 1873 to 1882, was professor of zoology at Odessa, but resigned because of dissatisfaction with the repressive policies of the government. Henceforth, he held no university positions. In 1883, he went to Messina, attracted by its rich marine fauna, and noted in an experiment that a splinter, when introduced into the body of a transparent starfish larva, soon drew to it large number of cells, which presently surrounded it. "That experiment formed the basis of the phagocyte theory, to the development of which I devoted the next 25 years of my life." Passing through Messina, Virchow saw Metchnikoff's experiments, was much impressed, and encouraged him to continue his work. The first report of Metchnikoff appeared in the *Arbeiten des zoologischen Instituts zu Wien*, 1883. He pursued his investigations further and noted that the *daphnia*, a small transparent fresh-water crustacean, when attacked by a parasitic fungus, sends out cells which attack the spores of the fungus. If the spores are destroyed, the *daphnia* recovers. Metchnikoff now applied this principle to infectious diseases due to bacteria, calling the protecting cells "phagocytes," a name suggested to him by the Vienna scientists when he asked for a Greek term meaning "devouring cells."

Metchnikoff returned to Odessa in 1886 as director of the bacteriological station, but, two years later, went to Paris and became a worker at the Pasteur Institute. He later made important contributions in the field of embryology, comparative anatomy, and anthropology, but his greatest contribution was the discovery and study of phagocytosis.

While on a visit to the Balkans, Metchnikoff was much impressed by the apparent longevity of Bulgarian peasants, which he attributed to their generous consumption of yoghurt or curdled milk. He attained considerable notoriety through his advocacy of yoghurt, but subsequent investigations indicated that "old" Bulgarian peasants were not so old as they appeared and that their supposed longevity was largely a myth.

1845-1922—Charles Leon Alphonse Laveran, the son of a distinguished army physician, was born in Paris and studied medicine at Paris and Strassburg, graduating at Strassburg in 1867. He decided to follow the same career as his father, so entered the army. He served in the Franco-German War of 1870 in the ambulance corps, took part in the battles of Gravelotte and Saint-Privot and was in Metz during its siege and capitulation. In 1874, he became *agrégé* at the military medical school of Val-de-Grâce. From 1878 to 1883, he served with the army in Algiers, and, in 1880 while stationed at Constantine, he discovered the malarial parasite—one of the great discoveries of modern medicine. His announcement of the discovery in a communication sent to the Academy of Sciences in 1880 was received with great skepticism. In 1882, he went to Rome, where he demonstrated the parasite in the blood of malarial patients.

From 1884 until 1894, Laveran was professor of military hygiene at Val-de-Grâce and, in 1896, resigned from the army and went to the Pasteur Institute, where he continued his scientific work, including his research on malaria and also the study of other diseases of protozoan origin, notably trypanosomiasis, leishmaniasis, toxoplasmosis and piroplasmosis. He received the Nobel prize for medicine in 1907.

Laveran was the author of more than 600 publications. In addition to more than 100 articles on malaria, he wrote *Traité des fièvres palustres*, 1884, and *Du Paludisme et son Hematozoaire*, 1891. He was also the author of *Traité des Maladies et Epidémies des Armées*, 1875; *Nouveau elements de Pathologie et de Clinique médicales*, 1879 (with T. Tessier); and *Traité d'Hygiène militaire*, 1896. In addition, he wrote more than 40 articles on leishmaniasis, more than 150 on trypanosomiasis, and more than 100 on pathological subjects.

1845-1923—Wilhelm Conrad Röntgen was born in Lennep, Rhineland, and received his early education in Holland, where his family moved when he was three years of age. He attended school at Apeldoorn and studied at the Technical School of Utrecht, from which he was expelled for a youthful prank. In 1865, he matriculated at the University of Utrecht and later at the Zürich Polytechnical School, where he received his Ph.D. degree in 1869. He became *Privatdozent* for physics at Strassburg in 1874, the following year was professor of physics at the Agricultural Academy of Hohenheim, then returned to Strassburg as associate professor in 1876. Three years later, he was appointed professor at Giessen and in 1885, went to Würzburg as professor of physics and director of the institute of physics. Here he discovered in 1895 the Röntgen rays, or, as he called them, the x-rays—one of the greatest discoveries in the history of physics and a discovery of incalculable value to medicine. In 1900, he accepted the chair of physics at the University of Munich, where he taught until his retirement in 1920. He received the Nobel prize for physics in 1901.

1847-1916—Ettore Marchiafava was born in Rome, where he studied medicine, receiving his doctor's degree in 1872. He worked for several years as the assistant of Tommasi-Crudelli in pathology, becoming professor of pathology in 1883. In 1916, he was appointed professor of clinical medicine and held this chair until his retirement in 1921. He was an active student of malaria and, with Celli, differentiated in 1889 the three types of malarial parasites—tertian, quartan, and aestivo-autumnal.

1847-1922—Sir Norman Moore, born in Higher Broughton, Lancashire, was educated at Cambridge, where he received his M.D. degree in 1876. He was physician to St. Bartholomew's Hospital from 1902 to 1911 and president of the Royal College of Physicians from 1918 to 1922. Moore was a great student of medical history, and his scholarly articles and books did much to advance that field. He was the author of *The History of Medicine in Ireland*, 1910; *The History of the Study of Clinical Medicine in the British Isles*, 1913; and *History of St. Bartholomew's Hospital*, 1919; and wrote 459 biographies, mostly for the *Dictionary of National Biography*.

1847-1923—Johannes Orth was a native of Wallmerod, Nassau, and studied medicine at Heidelberg, Würzburg and Bonn, receiving his M.D. degree at Bonn in 1870. In 1873, he was an assistant of Virchow in Berlin, in 1878 was called to Göttingen as professor of pathology, and returned in 1902 to Berlin as Virchow's successor. Orth was an excellent teacher and demonstrator and was the author of two widely used texts on pathology—the *Compendium der pathologisch-anatomischen Diagnostik,* 1876, which ran through eight editions; and his *Lehrbuch der speziellen pathologischen Anatomie,* 1886-1906.

1849-1914—Thomas Morgan Rotch was born in Philadelphia, graduated at Harvard Medical School in 1874, and, after two years' study in Germany, returned to Boston, where he devoted himself to the practice of pediatrics. In 1888, Harvard established a department of pediatrics, and Rotch was chosen head of the department with rank of assistant professor. In 1893, he became professor, holding this position until his death.

Rotch was a pioneer in infant feeding and in introducing x-ray diagnosis in pediatrics and founded the Infants' Hospital in Boston and the first milk laboratory, the Walker-Gordon Laboratory. His textbook, *Pediatrics,* published first in 1896, passed through three editions. He is remembered for "Rotch's sign" in pericarditis with effusion.

1849-1920—William Osler, one of the most influential physicians of his generation, was born in Bond Head, Canada, the son of a missionary. He entered Trinity College, Toronto, with the intention of becoming a clergyman, but, at the beginning of the second year, switched to medicine, and, the following year, entered the medical school of McGill University in Montreal. He received his medical degree in 1872 and, after two years' postgraduate study in London, Berlin, Leipzig and Vienna, returned to Montreal, where he was first appointed lecturer and then, at the age of 26, became professor of the "institutes of medicine" (physiology) at McGill University and pathologist to the Montreal General Hospital. In 1884, he was called to the University of Pennsylvania as professor of clinical medicine. He remained in Philadelphia five years and, in 1889, was called to Baltimore as professor of medicine in the newly founded Johns Hopkins Medical School.

Osler was in Baltimore 16 years, soon becoming a commanding figure in American medicine. A man of great personal charm, a born teacher, a forceful speaker, a fascinating writer, and a scholar of wide interests, endowed with great intellectual powers as well as abounding kindliness, sympathy and tact, he was the idol of his students and the friend of the high and the low, the rich and the poor. At Johns Hopkins, he introduced a combination of the English and German methods of medical teaching, which made his clinic the outstanding one of his period on the American continent and a model widely imitated. He was the living example of his own statement that the fate of an institution "lies in the men who work in its halls, and in the ideals which they cherish and teach." Two years after his arrival in Baltimore, Osler began writing his textbook, the *Principles and Practice of Medicine,* which appeared in 1892. It was the most popular and widely read text of its time, went through eight editions during the author's life-time, and was translated into French, German, Spanish and Chinese.

In 1905, Osler was called to Oxford as Regius Professor of Medicine and, in his new home, exercised the same extraordinary powers of stimulating and revitalizing everything and every person with whom he came in contact. He was created a baronet in 1911 and received honorary degrees during his career in America and England from McGill, Toronto, Harvard, Johns Hopkins, Edinburgh, Oxford, Leeds, Christiania, Dublin, Durham and Cambridge. The death of his son in the World War was a great blow to the devoted father, who bore the sorrow true to his ideal, "to cultivate such a measure of equanimity as would enable me to bear success with humility, the affection of my friends without pride, and to be ready when the day of sorrow and grief came to meet it with the courage befitting a man."

Osler was eminent as a teacher, investigator, author, scholar, bibliophile, and public spirited citizen. He was one of the first to investigate blood platelets (1873), discovered the filaria causing canine bronchitis (*Filaria Osleri*, 1877), described polycytemia rubra (1903) but later learned of and insisted upon the priority of Vaquez, noted hereditary telangiectasis with recurrent hemorrhages (1908), and called attention to "Osler's nodes" in endocarditis. He was editor of *Modern Medicine,* 1910, and editor and founder of the *Quarterly Journal of Medicine,* 1908.

His numerous addresses on a wide range of subjects are an enduring monument of his comprehensive knowledge, and his historical papers on Servetus, Linacre, Beaumont, Elisha Bartlett, the Alabama Student, Louis, and other notables in the history of medicine called forth the admiring remark of Sudhoff, "An essay of Osler's is worth many ponderous tomes of dry erudition." The collection of his addresses published under the title of *Aequanimitas,* 1904, has been a source of inspiration to innumerable physicians and medical students, and his *Evolution of Modern Medicine,* 1921, is unrivaled as "an aeroplane flight over the progress of medicine through the ages" —to employ Osler's own description of his work. He was the master of a clear vigorous style, and his numerous quotations, as well as his chaste diction, show the influence of the Bible and the Book of Common Prayer. He was an inveterate collector of books and bequeathed the bulk of his magnificent library to his alma mater, McGill University. The description of his books, with innumerable details regarding the individual volumes and their authors, was incomplete at the time of his death but was finished by his nephew, Dr. W. W. Francis. It was published under the title of *Bibliotheca Osleriana* in 1929, contains more than 7,500 entries and is "probably the most complete well-annotated bibliography in the history of medicine" (Garrison).

With all these achievements to his credit, the influence of Osler as a local and national propagandist for better public health has often been overlooked. He directed his shafts particularly at pneumonia, typhoid fever and tuberculosis, and his vigorous championship of measures to improve public health had a lasting influence.

As Shattuck remarked, Osler "has

made no profound or fundamental discovery; but no one of our day has, in his life, teaching, and example, so radiated, far and near, an inspiration to his fellow physicians."

1850-1934—William Henry Welch was born in Norfolk, Connecticut, the son of a physician, and received his A.B. degree from Yale in 1870. His early interests were in the humanities, and his ambition was to be professor of Greek. Unable to obtain a suitable post, he turned to medicine, entering the College of Physicians and Surgeons in New York and receiving his doctor's degree in 1875. After a year's internship in Bellevue Hospital, he went to Germany, where he studied with Hoppe-Seyler, Waldeyer and von Recklinghausen in Strassburg, with Wagner and Ludwig in Leipzig, and with Cohnheim in Breslau. In Breslau, he carried out an important piece of research, producing edema of the lungs by pressure on the left ventricle, an investigation which was published in Virchow's *Archiv*, 1878. While in Breslau, Koch came to Cohnheim's laboratory to present his finished work on the anthrax bacillus, and Welch describes how "Cohnheim came through flushed and realizing the significance of this great work."

Welch returned to America with a thorough training in microscopic anatomy and pathology, also with a new and deep appreciation of scientific medicine. He began practice in New York and organized a small pathological laboratory at the Bellevue Hospital Medical College, where he conducted courses in pathology. In 1884, he was appointed professor of pathology in the new Johns Hopkins University and arrived in Baltimore the following year. Even before the new pathological laboratory was completed, he gave a course of lectures on "Microorganisms in Disease." With the completion of the laboratory, he began regular courses in pathology and bacteriology, which drew many young physicians, among them Walter Reed, James Carroll, Simon Flexner, J. H. Wright, Reid Hunt, Philip H. Hiss, Jr., and E. R. LeCount, all of whom later achieved fame as pathologists and bacteriologists. In Baltimore, Welch found another kindred spirit, William T. Councilman, who was interested in pathology and became Welch's lifelong friend and his associate until he departed for Boston to become professor of pathology at Harvard.

The Johns Hopkins Hospital was opened in 1889, but four years were to elapse before the medical school was opened, eight years after Welch's arrival in Baltimore. Meanwhile, Welch had been quite active in teaching and research, had founded an outstanding school of pathologists, established pathology in America as an important and independent science, and had discovered in 1892 the well-known *Bacillus aerogenes capsulatus,* or Welch bacillus, and the *Staphylococcus epidermidis albus.*

The role of Welch in establishing the Johns Hopkins medical school and charting its course through its early history soon marked him as a most unusual person. His later influence and activities in medical education, in medical research, and in public health demonstrated that he was a medical statesman of the first rank. He was the first dean of the medical school and held the chair of pathology until 1916, when he became director of the newly founded School of Hygiene and Public Health. In 1926, he was made professor of the history of medicine, holding this chair until 1932.

Welch was a man with a prodigious memory and a wide knowledge of medical, scientific and historical literature, an excellent teacher, and a fascinating lecturer. He had an unusual facility in public speaking, and many of his thoughtful and polished public addresses, which seemed the result of hours of toil and repeated corrections of a manuscript, were entirely extemporaneous. He invariably made a profound impression on those who either met him or heard him speak in public.

1850-1905—Johann von Mikulicz-Radecki was born in Czernowitz, received his medical degree in Vienna in 1875, and was for several years assistant to Billroth. He was professor of surgery at Cracow (1882-1887), Königsberg (1887-1890), and Breslau from 1890 until his death. Mikulicz was one of the outstanding surgeons of his period, scientific as well as practical. He did much to improve antiseptic methods in surgery and introduced cotton gloves, which were later replaced by rubber. He improved the methods of narcosis and local anesthesia, made both esophagoscopy and gastroscopy practical methods, and introduced new and improved operations for goitre, pyloroplasty, and resection of the esophagus, stomach and intestines. In 1892, he described symmetrical enlargement of the lachrymal and salivary glands—Mikulicz disease.

1850-1929—Leon Bouveret was born in St. Julien-sur-Reyssouze and studied medicine at Lyon and Paris, where he received his doctor's degree in 1878. The same year, he returned to Lyon, where he became professor *agrégé* and spent his professional life. He wrote several books, the best known of which was his *Traité des maladies de l'estomac,* published in 1893. He was one of the earliest physicians to call attention to paroxysmal tachycardia, which, since his paper of 1889, is often called by French physicians *"la maladie de Bouveret."*

1851-1912—Julius Leopold Pagel, noted medical historian, was born in Pollnow, Pomerania, and studied medicine at Berlin, receiving his degree in 1875. His doctor's dissertation on the history of Göttingen medical school in the eighteenth century showed his early interest in the history of medicine. He settled in Berlin as a practicing physician but soon devoted himself mainly to historical studies and, in 1898, received the title of professor in charge of the department of medical history at the University of Berlin. He was an editor of the encyclopedic *Biographisches Lexikon der hervorragenden Ärzte,* issued editions of Henri de Mondeville (1889, 1892) and of Joannes Mesuë (1893), and, in 1898, published a scholarly *Einführung in die Geschichte der Medicin.* With Max Neuburger, he was editor of the *Handbuch der Geschichte der Medizin,* in three volumes, which was published in 1902-1905 and remains a monument to German scholarship in this field.

1851-1942—Graham Steell was born in Edinburgh, where he graduated in medicine with the degree of M.B.

in 1871. He later moved to Manchester, becoming professor of clinical medicine at Victoria University. He was an acute clinician, an excellent teacher, and a man of many interests. He is remembered especially for his description of the pulmonary diastolic murmur in mitral stenosis—the Graham Steell murmur—which he described in an article published in the *Medical Chronicle*, 1888.

1851-1902—Walter Reed was born in Gloucester County, Virginia, and received his medical degree at the University of Virginia at the early age of 18 in 1869. He then entered the Bellevue Medical College in New York, where he obtained his second M.D. the following year. He was commissioned in the Medical Corps of the United States Army in 1875 and, after serving 13 years in various army posts, was ordered to Baltimore in 1890 and worked under Dr. William H. Welch in the pathological laboratory of the Johns Hopkins Hospital. In 1893, he was appointed curator of the Army Medical Museum and professor of bacteriology in the Army Medical School in Washington.

During the Spanish-American War in 1898, Reed was made chief of the commission to study the origin and spread of typhoid fever in the army camps. This exhaustive report demonstrated that flies were the most important carriers of the infection, aided by dust and the uncleanliness of the attendants. In 1900, he was appointed chief of the Yellow Fever Commission, which investigated an epidemic among the American troops in Cuba. This commission, consisting of Dr. Reed, Dr. James Carroll, Dr. Jesse W. Lazear, and Dr. Aristide Agramonte, proved that yellow fever was transmitted by the bite of the stegomyia mosquito. Reed died from acute appendicitis and was buried in Arlington with the simple inscription over his tomb: "He gave to man control over that dreadful scourge—Yellow Fever."

1852-1922—William Stewart Halsted, born in New York, graduated from Yale College, where he distinguished himself as an athlete and captain of the football team rather than as a student, and received his medical degree from the College of Physicians and Surgeons of New York in 1877. After a year's internship in the New York Hospital, he went abroad for two years, working mostly in Billroth's clinic in Vienna but also with von Bergmann in Würzburg and in Leipzig and Halle. On his return to New York in 1880, he began the practice of surgery and, for five years, was an extremely busy young surgeon, serving on the staffs of no less than six widely separated hospitals. During this period, he met Dr. William H. Welch, who was teaching pathology at Bellevue Hospital, and the two became close friends.

In 1881, Halsted saved his sister's life by a reinfusion of aerated blood and, the same year, introduced the well known "cigarette" drain for wounds. Four years later, he discovered the principle of conduction or block anesthesia by the injection of cocaine into a nerve trunk. His priority in this discovery, later claimed by others, was finally established in 1922, 37 years later, when the American National Dental Association, after an exhaustive investigation, conferred a gold medal on Halsted for this achievement. In his work on this problem, he carried out experiments upon himself, became addicted to cocaine, wrecked his health, and retired from practice. He soon overcame the habit, however, and regained his health.

Halsted went to Baltimore in 1887 at the invitation of Welch and worked in the pathological laboratory, studying first intestinal sutures and then the thyroid gland. In 1889, he was appointed associate professor of surgery and, the following year, professor of surgery and surgeon-in-chief to the Johns Hopkins Hospital. He held this position for 32 years.

Halsted was one of the greatest scientific surgeons in his time. A deep thoughtful student with a profound knowledge of anatomy, physiology and pathology, he worked out many of his fundamental surgical advances in the experimental laboratory before employing them in the operating room. Seeing the splendid results following the use of boiled instruments and surgical dressings in operations, he began to think of the "boiled hand" and, in 1890, introduced rubber gloves in the operating room. In 1889, he devised his well-known operations for hernia and carcinoma of the breast. In 1892, he ligated the subclavian in its first division, performed in 1898 the first successful operation for a primary carcinoma of the ampulla of Vater, and carried out over a series of years clinical and experimental observations on the thyroid and parathyroid glands. As a surgeon, Halsted was a perfec-

tionist, never sacrificing meticulous care for speed at operation, abhorring the spectacular and dramatic, and stressing the gentle handling of living tissue. "In every advance that has marked the progress of surgery in the last 30 years," Matas said in a memorial address, "we find the impress of his hand and the reflex of his brain."

It was Halsted's belief that competent surgeons could be trained only by years of experience under the guidance of more experienced surgeons. One of his great practical achievements was the introduction of surgical residencies, which have now become the established norm in American surgical clinics.

1853-1925—James Mackenzie.

1854-1925—Giovanni Battista Grassi, born in Rovellasca, Como, graduated at Pavia in 1878 and was professor of zoology at Catania from 1883 until 1895, when he was called to Rome as professor of comparative anatomy, holding this position until his death. He was prominent in the study of malaria and claimed priority in the discovery of the role played by the anopheles mosquito in the transmission of malaria, a claim that involved him in an acrimonious dispute with Ross, whose claims were supported by Laveran and Koch. Grassi made many observations on the role of insects, particularly flies, in the spread of disease and studied ancylostomiasis, showing that the disease could be diagnosed by the presence of ova in the stools.

1854-1907—James Carroll was born in Woolwich, England, emigrated to Canada at the age of 15, and, for several years, lived the life of a backwoodsman. In 1874, he enlisted in the United States Army as a private, then studied medicine and graduated at the University of Maryland school of medicine in 1891, after which he did postgraduate work in pathology and bacteriology at the Johns Hopkins Hospital. He was a member of the Yellow Fever Commission headed by Walter Reed and submitted to the bite of a stegomyia mosquito which had fed on four cases of yellow fever. Carroll developed the disease but recovered. This was the first carefully controlled successful experiment proving the transmission of yellow fever by the mosquito.

1854-1917—Ernst von Behring was born in Hansdorf, Prussia, and studied in Berlin, graduating in 1878. He entered the army, served as an army physician for seven years, and, in 1888, was ordered to Berlin, where he taught for a year. Resigning from the army, he went to Koch's Institute for Infectious Diseases in 1890 and studied first the bacteriacidal properties of blood serum. In 1892, he discovered with Kitasato diphtheria antitoxin and, the same year, prepared tetanus antitoxin. He was called in 1894 to Halle as professor and in 1895 to Marburg, where he established an institute for the production of diphtheria antitoxin. He continued to study diphtheria and, before his death, recommended immunization of children with a mixture of toxin and antitoxin.

1854-1915—Paul Ehrlich.

1854-1920—William Crawford Gorgas was born in Touminville, Alabama, the son of General Josiah

Gorgas, a graduate of West Point, who cast his lot with the South in the Civil War and became Chief of Ordnance in the Confederate Army. William Gorgas wished to become an army officer but, failing after repeated attempts to secure an appointment to West Point, studied medicine at Bellevue Medical College in New York, and, after graduation, entered the army medical service in 1880. In 1898, he was sent to stamp out an epidemic of yellow fever in Havana. At first skeptical of the mosquito theory of Carlos Findlay, he was convinced by the work of Reed's Yellow Fever Commission and carried out such a thorough campaign of mosquito extermination that yellow fever was soon eradicated in Havana and, in three months, the city became free of the disease for the first time in 150 years.

After the United States began the construction of the Panama Canal, Gorgas was sent in 1904 to take charge of sanitation in the Canal Zone. In spite of the powerful opposition of the army and, for a time, of the secretary of war, he persisted in his campaign of mosquito extermination and stamped out yellow fever, the nemesis of all previous attempts to build a canal, and the canal was successfully completed. The comprehensive sanitary methods he introduced soon made Panama, formerly a notoriously unhealthy spot, one of the healthiest communities in the world.

Gorgas became Surgeon-General of the Army in 1914. His counsel in matters of sanitation was sought far and wide, and he became known as "Physician to the World."

1855-1931—Sir David Bruce was born in Melbourne, Australia, graduated at Edinburgh in 1881, and entered the army medical service in 1883. While stationed in Malta, he studied Malta fever and discovered in 1887 the causal organism at first called the *Micrococcus melitensis,* later renamed *Brucella melitensis.* In 1898, he investigated the "tsetse fly disease," or nagana, a disease of cattle, demonstrating a trypanosome (*Trypanosoma brucei*) in the blood of infected animals and also proving that the disease was transmitted by the bite of a tsetse fly (*Glossina morsitans*). He found that wild game were reservoirs of infection but did not suffer any disease from the presence of parasites in their blood.

From 1903 to 1906, Bruce studied sleeping sickness in Africa and demonstrated that it was caused by the *Trypanosoma gambiense* and that it was transmitted from man to man by another tsetse fly (*Glossina palpalis*). He was knighted in 1908. In 1912, he became a major general and, from 1914 until his retirement in 1919, was commandant of the Royal Army Medical College.

1857-1938—John Jacob Abel was born near Cleveland, Ohio, and received the degree of Ph.D. at the University of Michigan in 1883. He then spent seven years abroad studying at the universities of Leipzig, Strassburg, Heidelberg, Vienna, Bern, Würzburg and Berlin. He received his M.D. degree from the University of Strassburg in 1888 and was called in 1891 to the chair of materia medica and therapeutics at the University of Michigan. In 1893, he was appointed the first pro-fessor of pharmacology in the new medical school of Johns Hopkins University and spent the rest of his life in Baltimore.

Abel was soon recognized as an outstanding pharmacologist. He was the first to isolate epinephrin (1898), the first chemical isolation of a hormone, and bufagin (1911), made intensive investigations on the pharmacological properties of the phthaleins, studied the active principles of the pituitary gland, invented with Rowntree an artificial kidney, with which they extracted from the blood many substances, including amino acids (1912-1914), devised the method of plasmaphaeresis (1914), and, in 1926 at the age of 69, crystallized insulin. He retired from his chair in 1932 at the age of 75 years but continued his research work, and his last paper, one on tetanus toxin, was published the year of his death.

Abel was quite active in encouraging the establishment of American scientific journals and acted as godfather to a number of journals, including the *Journal of Biological Chemistry,* the *Journal of Experimental Medicine,* the *Journal of Pharmacology and Experimental Therapeutics,* the *Journal of Bacteriology,* the *Journal of Immunity,* and the *Journal of Cancer Research.*

1857-1932—Sir Ronald Ross, one of the greatest of modern sanitarians and of investigators in tropical medicine, was born in Almora, India, the son of Major Ross, a distinguished officer of the British Army, who became later General Sir Campbell Ross. Ronald Ross, the eldest of 10 children, was sent to England at the age of eight for his education and, at 17, began the study of medicine at St. Bartholomew's Hospital. In 1881, he passed his examinations "without distinction," was commissioned surgeon in the Indian Medical Service, and sailed for India.

In India, he became interested in the study of malaria but, because of faulty technique, was never able to see in the blood the parasites which had been described by Laveran in 1880. While on leave in London in 1894, he was shown by Sir Patrick Manson the parasites in the blood of a patient in Charing Cross Hospital. Manson expressed to him his own belief that malaria was transmitted by mosquitoes, a theory advanced by King in America in 1883 and supported by Laveran himself. On his return to India, Ross began work again with renewed enthusiasm. In 1895, he found the so-called flagella (sexual forms) of the parasite in the stomach of an anopheles mosquito which had fed on a patient with malaria and, in 1897, the pigmented cells of the parasites also in a mosquito's stomach; and, in 1898, he demonstrated sporozoites in the salivary glands of mosquitoes. These discoveries indicated the transmission of malaria by the mosquito.

Retiring from the Indian Medical Service in 1899, Ross was appointed lecturer on tropical diseases at the Liverpool School of Tropical Medicine and went to London in 1912 as a consultant on tropical diseases. In 1902, he received the Nobel prize in medicine; the order of knighthood was conferred on him in 1911; he was made in 1923 director of the Royal Institute and Hospital for Tropical Diseases; and, in 1926, he became director of the new Ross Institute, named in his honor.

Sir Ronald Ross was a remarkably versatile man. Besides his scientific researches in medicine, he was a first-rate mathematician who contributed important articles to mathematical journals, a talented musician who composed chamber music, a novelist who wrote stories which belong to real literature, and a poet whose poems were highly praised by John Masefield. He also invented a system of shorthand and devised a method of phonetic spelling, in which some of his poems are written.

1857-1914—Angelo Celli was born in Cugli, Pesaro, and studied at Rome, where he received his doctor's degree. In 1886, he became professor of hygiene in Palermo and established there a Pasteur institute. In 1887, he was made associate professor of hygiene at Rome and, in 1890, full professor. He saw in 1884 the meningococcus, later studied by Weichselbaum, and also apparently saw the dysentery bacillus before Shiga. In 1889, Celli and Marchiafava differentiated the tertian, quartan, and aestive-autumnal types of malarial parasites. Celli was quite active in the work of malarial control and of freeing the Roman Campagna from malaria. He wrote many papers on hygienic subjects and was the author of *Manuale dell'uffiziale sanitario,* 1899; *Manuale d'igienista,* 1906-1907; and a noteworthy historical monograph, *Die Malaria in ihrer Bedeutung für die Geschichte Roms und der römischen Campagna,* 1929.

1858-1931—Oskar Minkowski was born in Alexoten, Russia, and received his degree in medicine at Königsberg in 1881. There he was a pupil and assistant of Naunyn and followed his chief to Strassburg, where he was appointed associate professor in 1891. In 1905, he was made professor of medicine in Greifswald and, in 1909, became professor at Breslau, remaining there until his retirement in 1926.

Minkowski was a favorite pupil of Naunyn, who praised his great intelligence, his clear understanding, and his unusual ability to grasp the significance of problems he encountered in his research work. At the age of 26, he demonstrated β-oxybutyric acid in the urine of severe diabetics, later proved the lowered carbon dioxide tension of the blood in diabetic coma, and introduced alkali therapy for this condition. In 1889, he produced diabetes in a dog by complete extirpation of the pancreas. This work was published with von Mehring, but Naunyn assigns the major credit to Minkowski. In 1900, Minkowski described hemolytic icterus. He also made important contributions in the fields of gastric disease, employing gastric lavage for pyloric stenosis, and of neurology, describing Korsakoff's syndrome before Korsakoff. Three years before Marie's publication on acromegaly, he suggested the pituitary origin of this disease.

1858-1943—Howard Atwood Kelly was born in Camden, New Jersey, and received his medical education at the University of Pennsylvania, where he graduated in 1882. In 1888, he became professor of obstetrics in the University of Pennsylvania, resigning this position in 1889 to take the chair of obstetrics and gynecol-

ogy at Johns Hopkins. He soon became one of the leading gynecologists of his time. He was a pioneer in the development of local anesthesia and devised many new operative procedures and instruments. The Kelly pad, the Kelly clamp, and the Kelly rectoscope were his inventions. In addition to numerous medical articles, more than 460 at the time of his retirement in 1919, Kelly's Operative Gynecology, 1898, and Medical Gynecology, 1908, both illustrated by the incomparable medical artist, Max Brödel, were outstanding books in their field, as well as his Vermiform Appendix, 1905, and Gynecology and Abdominal Surgery, 1907-1908. He was also an avid collector of old medical books and a life-long student of medical history. He wrote many articles on historical topics and was the author of Walter Reed and Yellow Fever, 1906, and editor of A Cyclopedia of American Medical Biography, 1912, a most valuable and accurate source book.

1860-1904—Niels Finsen was born in Thorshavn on the Faeroe Islands and studied medicine at Copenhagen, where he received his medical degree in 1890. He was assistant at the anatomical institute from 1890 until 1893 and, in 1893, published his first paper on the value of red light in the treatment of smallpox. In 1896, he founded the Light Institute of Copenhagen (Finsen's medicinske Lysinstitut) for the study of the biological and therapeutic effects of light. He had great success with the treatment of smallpox and tuberculosis and received the Nobel prize for medicine in 1903. His results were published in

La photothérapie, Paris, 1899, and *Ueber die Bedeutung der chemischen Strahlen des Lichtes für Medicin und Biologie,* Leipzig, 1899.

1860-1936—Henri Vaquez was born in Paris and received his medical degree at Paris in 1890. He became professor *agrégé* in 1898 and professor in 1918. He devoted himself especially to the study of diseases of the blood and of the heart and was soon recognized as one of the leading French internists. He first described in 1892 *polycythemia vera,* since called Vaquez's disease, and published in 1920 his *Maladies du coeur,* one of the best books on heart disease. He was a founder and editor of the well-known *Archives des maladies du coeur, des vaisseaux et du sang.*

1860-1945—William Henry Howell was born in Baltimore and received his Ph.D. degree from Johns Hopkins University in 1884, majoring in biology. He became successively assistant, associate, and associate professor of biology in Johns Hopkins and was professor at Michigan from 1889 until 1892, when he went to Harvard as associate professor of physiology. The following year, he was appointed professor of physiology at Johns Hopkins, holding this position until 1918. From 1918 until 1931, he was professor in the School of Hygiene. After retirement, he continued investigative work until the day of his death.

Howell carried out important investigations on the circulation and coagulation of the blood, discovered and isolated heparin. His *Text-book of Physiology,* first published in 1906, went through 14 editions during his life-time.

1862-1917—Franklin Paine Mall was born in Belle Plain, Iowa, and graduated from the University of Michigan with the degree of M.D. in 1883. He then went abroad with the ambition of becoming an ophthalmologist but presently abandoned this plan, working instead with His in Leipzig in embryology and later with Ludwig in physiology. He was appointed fellow in pathology at the Johns Hopkins Hospital in 1886, adjunct professor of anatomy at Clark University in 1889, and professor of anatomy at Chicago in 1892 and, in 1893, went to Johns Hopkins as the first professor of anatomy in the new medical school. Mall's anatomical work was mainly in the field of embryology, and he made important contributions to the subject of monsters and the pathology of early human embryos and on the microscopic anatomy of the liver. He was the co-editor with Keibel of a *Manual of Human Embryology,* 1910-1912.

1862-1929—Amico Bignami was born in Bologna and received his medical degree in 1882 at Rome, where he was appointed professor of pathology in 1906. His earlier work was on the pathology of the brain, acromegaly and leukemia, but later he worked mainly on malaria. He became a believer in the mosquito theory of transmission and, in 1898, produced malaria in a man by subjecting him to the bite of an infected mosquito. The same year, he worked out, in collaboration with Grassi and Bastianelli, the plasmodium cycle in the anopheles mosquito and in man.

1865-1939—George Redmayne Murray was born in Newcastle-upon-

Tyne and educated at Eton, Cambridge, and University College, London. After postgraduate study in Berlin and Paris, he was appointed professor of pathology at Durham University and later professor of medicine at Victoria University, Manchester. He was the first physician to treat with thyroid extract a patient suffering from myxedema. His patient was successfully maintained on thyroid extract for 28 years until her death at the age of 74.

1865-1926—Sir William Boog Leishman was born in Glasgow, the son of William Leishman, professor of obstetrics in the University. After graduation at Glasgow in 1886, he entered the army medical service. He served in India from 1890 until 1897 and later returned to England, where he was appointed professor of pathology in the Army Medical School. In 1903, he discovered the causal organism of kala-azar in the spleen of a soldier, who had contracted the disease in India and died later in England. Almost simultaneously, Charles Donovan found the same organism after a splenic puncture, and the parasite has been named the Leishman-Donovan bodies, or the *Leishmania donovani*.

Leishman also devised a stain for parasites, made important observations on phagocytosis, and was quite active in the introduction of anti-typhoid vaccination in the British Army. He was knighted in 1908 and, the following year, was elected Fellow of the Royal Society. In 1918, he received the rank of major-general.

1872-1917—Oswaldo Cruz was born in 1872 in Sao Luiz de Parahytinga, Brazil, and received his medical degree at Rio de Janeiro in 1892. After working three years in Paris at the Pasteur Institute, he returned to Rio de Janeiro and began to practice medicine, carrying on bacteriological studies in his private laboratory. In 1901, an *Instituto Serotherapico Federal* was established with Cruz as director. The name of this Institute was changed in 1908 to *Instituto Oswald Cruz*. Cruz carried out many original investigations, was an able and efficient administrator and sanitarian. He died at the age of 45, honored by his countrymen as one of the greatest benefactors Brazil had ever produced.

The Twentieth Century

I T IS HAZARDOUS to judge any period in medical history except in retrospect. Medical history is filled with the names of physicians who were among the greatest in their time. Medical discoveries have at times shown a similar as well as a reverse pattern. Many observations which excited admiration and applause among contemporaries have been relegated to the limbo of forgotten things by succeeding centuries. In attempting to assess the medical progress of the twentieth century, these mistaken appraisals should be kept in mind. The first half of the twentieth century witnessed some startling medical discoveries. However, many of the great medical discoveries of the twentieth century would have been impossible without those of the nineteenth.

The relative brevity of this chapter as compared with some earlier ones is due to the difficulty of presenting contemporary events in medical history in their proper perspective. An equally important deterrent to an extended chapter on medicine of the twentieth century is the profusion of names and the plethora of discoveries. As a result of this dual dilemma, it seems advisable to record only the most outstanding medical discoveries and the most momentous medical events in the first half of this century, which may, judging by its spectacular advances so far, close as the greatest century in the history of human progress.

The opening years of the century saw Germany still in the forefront of medical progress. Her hospitals and universities continued to be centers of intense scientific activity. Important discoveries in chemistry, bacteriology, pathology, physiology, physics and pharmacology made this period the Golden Age of German medicine.

In chemistry, Emil Fischer (1852-1919) carried on the great traditions of Liebig, Wöhler and Kekulé. Fischer, who was successively professor of chemistry at Munich, Erlangen, Würzburg and Berlin, devoted most of his life to the synthesis of proteins from amino acids. He discovered, isolated and worked out the formulae of a host of chemical compounds, including phenylhydrazine, the aliphatic hydrazins, mannose and isomaltose. He synthetized the purin compounds, caffeine, xanthine and theobromine and clarified the relationship of these purin compounds to gout. He synthetized and

921

worked out the formulae for most of the sugar groups and, in his
studies on proteins, linked together chains of animo acids to produce polypeptids, which he showed to be essential parts of different
protein molecules. He demonstrated that enzymes are specific in
their action, affecting only certain chemicals to which they are related—as he phrased it, like "a key to a lock." In his search for a
reliable hypnotic, he synthetized veronal and initiated the work on
the pharmacologic and therapeutic effects of the barbiturates. In
his later years, he was occupied in the creation of synthetic sub-
stitutes for nitrogenous products, animal fats, and various other food
stuffs. "No chemist of modern times," wrote Garrison, "better deserved the honor of the Nobel prize, which he received in 1902."

Medical clinics in Germany were models for the world. In Berlin,
Wilhelm His, Jr., was director of the First Medical Clinic. "He
was," in the words of Külbs, "a fluid, spirited and witty social
character who could converse with charm and grace. His listeners
were always intrigued and realized the depth of his training
and knowledge." The son of Wilhelm His, the great anatomist
of Leipzig, he was brought up in a cultured environment, was an
excellent musician and a talented painter. As a medical student
in Strassburg, he had carried out important investigations on the
metabolism of pyridine (1886), and he had already discovered the
auriculo-ventricular bundle—the bundle of His, one of the great
discoveries of cardiology (1893). Later, he carried out notable investi-

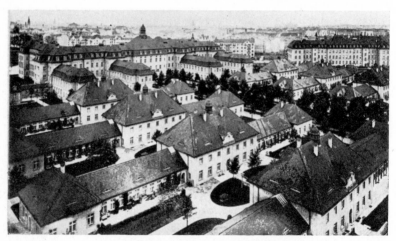

RUDOLF VIRCHOW HOSPITAL
General view looking toward the entrance.

gations on gout and arthritis. "He was a master of his profession, a great physician, investigator, and a highly cultured gentleman" (Petow).

The Second Medical Clinic was directed by Friedrich Kraus, who had been professor in Graz, a dramatic and most interesting teacher, who usually filled the auditorium to overflowing. Kraus was interested in all fields of medicine, had written extensively on diseases of metabolism, blood, heart, lungs, and on infections, was deeply interested in studies of the constitution of patients and its relation to disease, and was the editor with Brugsch of an extensive *Spezielle Pathologie und Therapie* in 19 volumes.

In Leipzig, Adolf Strümpell, who had resigned his chair in Vienna to come to the Saxon metropolis—"to leave all the splendor of Vienna and to return to the German home"—had made important contributions to medicine with the first descriptions of spondylitis deformans and of polioencephalomyelitis. His textbook of medicine went through 30 editions and held the same position in German medical literature that Osler's textbook did among English readers.

In Halle, Franz Volhard, who had described the first complete pericardiectomy for constrictive pericarditis and had written with Fahr a well-known treatise on Bright's disease, was a commanding figure.

In Munich, Ernst von Romberg, who had been a colleague of His, Jr., at Leipzig and later professor at Marburg and Tübingen, was director of the First Medical Clinic. The author of a noted book on diseases of the heart, he was an excellent clinician and teacher, whose public clinics were conducted with such perfection in demonstration that they seemed almost rehearsed before presentation.

The Second Medical Clinic was directed by Friedrich von Müller, whom Garrison described in 1912 as "perhaps the most scientific teacher of internal medicine today." Müller was a great favorite of American students, and many of the outstanding clinicians in the United States today, worked at one time in his clinic. Many well-known professors of internal medicine in Germany had been his former assistants. After visiting Müller's medical clinic in Munich in 1912, Abraham Flexner described in vivid terms his stimulating experience:

The professor reads the history, displays on the blackboard the temperature chart, then in quick, clear fashion explores the patient, pointing out what he finds, discoursing on its significance, suggesting alternate explanations. . . . The etiology, the pathology, the therapeutics of the condition are set forth with wonderful vigor and lucidity. . . . A master mind at work is exhibited daily to 200 students or more.

In the field of medical history, a new era had been inaugurated by the establishment of the *Institut für Geschichte der Medizin* in Leipzig in 1905, with Professor Karl Sudhoff as its director. This foundation was endowed by a bequest of 500,000 marks left by the widow of Professor Theodor Puschmann (1844-1899), who had lec-

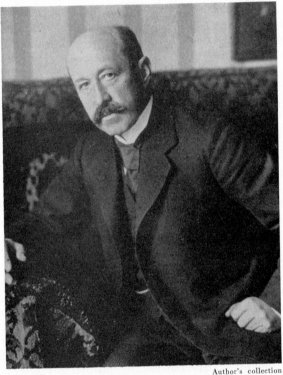

Author's collection

FRIEDRICH MÜLLER
Photograph taken in 1912.

tured on medical history in Leipzig from 1878 until 1888, when he was called to Vienna as professor of this subject.

Karl Sudhoff (1853-1938), a native of Frankfurt-am-Main and a graduate of Erlangen in 1875, had practised medicine 30 years before going to Leipzig and, although entirely self-taught in medical history, was an accomplished classical scholar as well as a Germanic philologist. In 1876, he began a study of Paracelsus's manuscripts, a study crowned in 1933 with his edition of Paracelsus in 15 volumes.

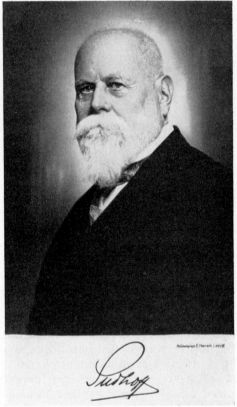

Photo E. Hoenisch, Leipzig

KARL SUDHOFF

An indefatigable worker, he spent much time in Italy investigating libraries and museums and published more than 500 monographs, many of them appearing in the *Archiv für Geschichte der Medizin,* which he founded in 1908. His writings include the history of dentistry, the School of Salerno, German medical incunabula, anatomical illustrations in the Middle Ages, and a history of medicine. Sudhoff was the greatest medical historian of modern times.

The surgical clinics of Germany were in every respect the equals of the medical. In Berlin, the professor of surgery, August Bier, having made the first successful clinical use of spinal anesthesia (1898), had introduced venous local anesthesia and had demonstrated the value of local hyperemia in the treatment of infections. Albert Hoffa, the celebrated orthopedic surgeon, had only recently left Würzburg for Berlin. Julius Hirschberg, former assistant to von Graefe, was now professor of ophthalmology and eminent both as an ophthalmologist and medical historian. In Leipzig, Friedrich Trendenburg, a man of great ability who left a deep impress on surgery, and Erwin Payr, well known for his work on intestinal sutures and thyroid transplantation, were professors of surgery. Erich Lexer, director of the surgical clinic at Jena, was an authority on osteomyelitis and had written a textbook on surgery, translated into English by Dean Lewis and widely used by American students.

The University of Freiburg, at the beginning of the century, had a world famous pathologist in Ernst Ziegler. His fame was even excelled by that of his successor, Ludwig Aschoff. In obstetrics, there was Ernst Bumm in Berlin, Albert Döderlein in Munich, and, in Stuttgart, Gustav Walcher, whose description of "Walcher's position" is well known.

In German-speaking Vienna, a large group of outstanding men made the old capital one of the most active centers of medical teaching and research in the world. Carl von Noorden, a native of Bonn, made a great reputation through his systematic study of the dietetic treatment of metabolic diseases and had been called from his position as physician to the municipal hospital of Frankfurt-am-Main to the directorship of the First Medical Clinic in Vienna. Von Noorden's works had been translated into English and were almost as well known in America as in Germany. Karel Wenckebach, a Hollander from The Hague, who had been previously professor at Groningen and Strassburg, was another Vienna luminary. He achieved a world-wide reputation as a cardiologist and described the Wenckebach bundle and the well-known Wenckebach phenomenon in cardiac arrhythmia. Other prominent internists and teachers of internal medicine were Edmund von Neusser, Franz Chvostek, and Nikolaus von Jagić, whose skill in physical diagnosis was reminiscent of Skoda. In the pediatric clinic, Clemens von Pirquet and Bela Schick were laying the corner-stones of allergy, the former discovering the cutaneous, or von Pirquet, test for tuberculosis, the latter discovering the Schick test, a test for susceptibility to diphtheria infection. Both have had world-wide application and have been of such tremendous value in the control of tuberculosis and diphtheria.

Surgery was represented by two men of international reputation. Anton Freiherr von Eiselsberg, an old pupil of Billroth, a brilliant surgeon, an excellent teacher, and a noteworthy investigator, was professor of surgery. He made important contributions to bacteriology, particularly on streptococcic infections and tetanus, was a pioneer in neurological surgery, especially of the pituitary gland, and studied tetany, a common complication in thyroidectomy, producing it experimentally by removal of the parathyroids. Many sided in his surgical interests, he was also one of the founders of modern

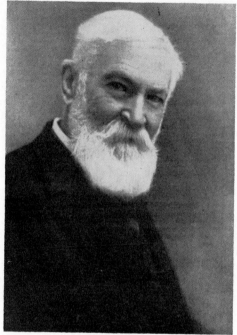

Lorenz, *My Life and Work*, New York, 1936

ADOLF LORENZ

surgery of the stomach and intestines. Adolf Lorenz, professor of orthopedic surgery, made important contributions to the treatment of flat foot and especially of congenital dislocation of the hips. He was widely known in America and featured by the press as "the discoverer of bloodless surgery." In addition, there was Julius von Hochenegg, a scholarly and scientific surgeon, who was the editor of a book on operative surgery and chief of the Second Surgical Clinic. Ernst Fuch in ophthalmology and Gustav Riehl in dermatology were outstanding.

In pathology, Anton Weichselbaum, the discoverer of the menin-

gococcus and co-discoverer of the pneumococcus, was still active as
a teacher and investigator. Carl Toldt, whose atlas of anatomy was
widely used by American students, was professor of anatomy. He
had assembled a large museum, and his institute was an active
center of histological and anthropological research. In medical history, Max Neuburger had founded an institute, from which came
some of the noteworthy publications of the time. From 1906-1910,
he published his well-known *Geschichte der Medizin,* which has
been translated into English and has taken its place on the shelves
of medical libraries throughout the world as one of the most
scholarly histories ever written. Pharmacologists flocked to the institute of Hans Horst Meyer, upon whom, by common consent, the
mantle of the aging Schmiedeberg had fallen. Meyer's investigations
covered almost the entire field of pharmacology—poisoning with
heavy metals, pharmacology of cathartics, diuresis, narcosis, tetanus
and diphtheria toxins, the effect of various drugs on heat regulation
and upon the sympathetic nervous system.

American medical students came to Vienna in such numbers that
they founded the American Medical Association of Vienna. Regular
meetings addressed by members of the Vienna faculty were held.

At this period in Vienna, there were two psychiatrists who have
left a deep impress on posterity—Julius Wagner von Jauregg and
Sigmund Freud. Julius Wagner von Jauregg, a native of Wels in
Upper Austria, was born in 1857 and received his doctor's degree
at Vienna in 1880. In 1833, he joined the staff of the psychiatric
clinic there, where he presently noted, with curious interest, the disappearance of mental symptoms in some patients who had contracted typhoid fever. In 1887, he wrote an article suggesting the
treatment of patients suffering from psychoses by infecting them
with a febrile disease, such as malaria or erysipelas. He himself attempted to treat some of these patients by injecting a culture of
streptococci but failed to produce erysipelas. After Robert Koch
discovered tuberculin, he employed this to produce fever but abandoned it as too dangerous a preparation.

In 1893, Wagner von Jauregg went to Vienna as professor of
psychiatry. Here he resumed his work with tuberculin and found
that some psychotic patients, notably paretics, were improved. He
continued to toy with the idea of using malaria but was unable to
obtain any malarial blood. In 1917, when a shell-shocked soldier
suffering from malaria was admitted to his clinic, he regarded it, as
he said, as "a sign of destiny." On June 14, 1917, he inoculated
three patients suffering from paresis with malaria. All three showed

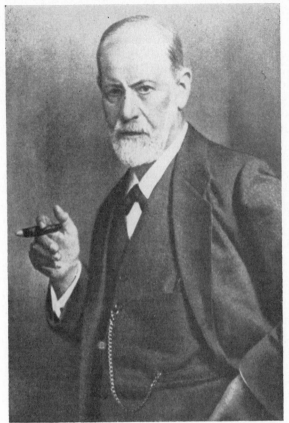

Les Médecins Célèbres, Paris, 1947

SIGMUND FREUD

marked improvement in a short time. He published his results on these and other patients in 1918, and soon this method of treatment spread around the world.

Sigmund Freud was born in Freiberg, in Moravia, in 1856 and came to Vienna when a child of four. He began the study of medicine at Vienna and at first was chiefly interested in botany and chemistry. From 1876 to 1881, he worked in the physiological laboratory with Brücke and received his doctor's degree in 1881. He then worked in the Institute of Cerebral Anatomy under Meynert. During this period, he published several excellent articles dealing mainly with neurological pathology and became a *Privatdozent* for neuropathology in 1885. In 1884, he studied with Carl Koller the pharmacologic effects of cocaine, hoping to cure patients addicted to morphine by substituting cocaine. However, Freud soon turned his attention to other problems, while Koller continued his investigations, introducing the same year cocainization of the eye for the production of local anesthesia.

In 1884, Josef Breuer, a Viennese physician, related to Freud an interesting experience in which a patient was relieved of her hysterical symptoms by having her recollect, while in a state of hypnosis, the circumstances of their origin and the attending emotions. Nine years later, Freud collaborated with Breuer in a book, *Studien über Hypnose,* which records the discovery of the "unconscious mind." Soon afterwards, Freud replaced hypnotism as a method of reviving buried memories by the method of "free-association," the keystone of the method of psychoanalysis—a method described as mental catharsis.

Freud's further investigations on the nature of the psychoneuroses led him to his three fundamental conclusions—the existence of the subconscious and its influence on the conscious; the splitting of the mind into layers due to an intrapsychical conflict, especially repression; and the existence and importance of infantile sexuality. The young child's sexual attitude towards its parents, with the accompanying jealousy and hostility, was described as the "Oedipus complex." Freud also developed a theory of the significance of dreams, holding them to be often the key to subconscious mental processes. John Rickman states, "Freud's theory of dreams provides the main conceptual structure on which psychodynamical research is built, and therefore on which therapy is based."

Freud had and still has enthusiastic and almost fanatical followers, as well as bitter and relentless enemies. Yet, no one can deny the powerful impact his teachings have had upon psychiatry and psychology, an impact not limited to the confines of medicine, but extending far beyond into other fields of intellectual activity.

In bacteriology, the *Kaiserliches Gesundheitsamt* (Imperial Health Office) in Berlin, where Koch, Löffler, Gaffky, Pfeiffer, Behring and Kitasato had made epochal discoveries, continued as a world center of bacteriologic research. A crowning achievement of this institute was the announcement in 1905 by one of its members, Schaudinn, that the causative agent of syphilis had been discovered.

Fritz Schaudinn (1871-1906), the son of an inn-keeper in East Prussia, took his doctor's degree in zoology at Berlin in 1894 and devoted himself to the study of protozoa. He isolated and studied many new species of amoeba, differentiated the harmless *Entamoeba coli* from the pathogenic *Entamoeba histolytica* of amoebic dysentery, and carried out classic investigations on coccidia, eimeria, hemosporidia and trypanosomes. In 1898, he became *Privatdozent* for biology at the University of Berlin and, in 1904, having achieved a reputation as an outstanding protozoologist, was appointed direc-

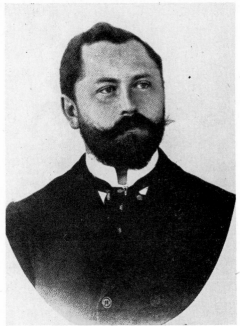

Surgeon General's Library, Washington, D.C.

FRITZ SCHAUDINN

tor of the laboratory of protozoology at the *Kaiserliches Gesundheitsamt*. A year later, working with Erich Hoffman, he demonstrated by a special staining technique a spirochaeta in syphilitic lesions, the *Spirochaeta pallida,* a pale-staining spirochaeta, which he believed was the etiological agent of syphilis. This causal relationship was soon demonstrated by observers throughout the world.

The causal agent of syphilis had been sought for more than two decades by numerous bacteriologists. In 1905, Lassar remarked, "One hundred and twenty-five causes of syphilis have been established during the last 25 years." Schaudinn's discovery of the *Spirochaeta pallida* was an achievement which ranked with Koch's discovery of

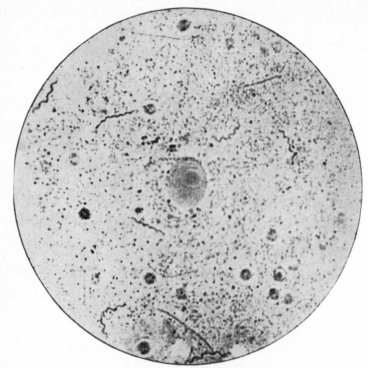

Arbeit a.d. Kaiserl. Gesundheitsamte, 1905

SPIROCHAETE PALLIDA

This discovery of the *Spirochaete pallida* (*Treponema pallida*) was one of the greatest triumphs of microbiology. This photograph from Schaudinn's original paper shows a red blood cell in the center of the microscopic field and seven spirochaete.

the tubercle bacillus. It marked the beginning of a new era in the study of syphilis.

The following year, the study of syphilis received a second great impetus through the discovery of the Wassermann reaction, which was announced by Wassermann, Neisser and Bruck in 1906. August von Wassermann (1866-1925) was a native of Bamberg, received his doctor's degree at Strassburg in 1888, and worked at the Robert Koch Institute for Infectious Diseases in Berlin from 1890 until 1906. He carried out important investigations on toxins and antitoxins and diphtheria antitoxin and, before working on syphilis, had devised a complement fixation test for the diagnosis of tuberculosis based

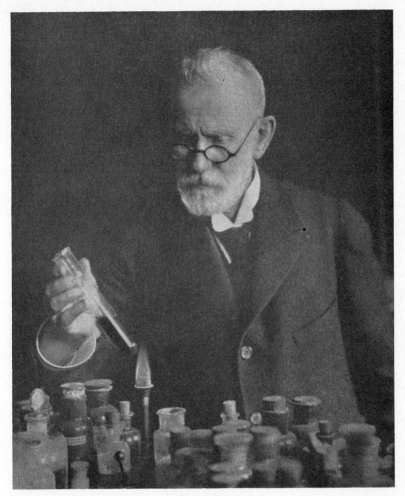

PAUL EHRLICH

on the complement fixation reaction discovered by Bordet and Gengou in 1901. The importance of the Wassermann reaction in the
modern practice of medicine can scarcely be exaggerated.

These startling discoveries stimulated, as never before, an intensive study of syphilis. Among those, whose interest was aroused anew,
was Paul Ehrlich, one of the outstanding personages in medical science during the closing years of the nineteenth and the early years
of the twentieth century.

Paul Ehrlich was born in Strehlen, a small town in Silesia, and finished the *Gymnasium* in Breslau, where he was an excellent mathematical and Latin scholar. He began the study of medicine at Breslau and then studied at Strassburg, Freiburg and Leipzig, where he received the doctor's degree in 1878. While a student at Strassburg, he became interested in lead poisoning and devised a fuchsin stain to demonstrate lead in the tissues. This experiment convinced young Ehrlich that certain tissues had a selective affinity for certain chemicals—a *leitmotif* that dominated all of his subsequent medical thinking.

In 1878, Ehrlich went to Berlin as assistant to Frerichs and, while there, continued his studies on the relationship between the structure of chemicals, their distribution in the body, and their effects. During this period, he devised his well-known stain for the blood and demonstrated by the specific staining of the granules in the polymorphonuclear leukocytes the three types we recognize today. This work of Ehrlich was the foundation stone of modern hematology. During this earlier period, he also devised his diazo reaction, began the study of vital staining, and greatly improved staining methods for the tubercle bacillus by demonstrating that it was acid fast.

The second period of Ehrlich's scientific life opened in 1890, when he began to work in Koch's Institute for Infectious Diseases, having meanwhile received the title of associate *(ausserordentlicher)* professor. Here he studied the chemistry of diphtheria antitoxin, devising improved techniques for its production and concentration as well as introducing methods of standardization, which contributed greatly to the accuracy of dosage. His *Das Sauerstoffbedürfnis des Organismus* (The oxygen requirement of the organism), published in 1885, contains his view that there is a selective affinity between chemical substances and certain body tissues and outlines his famous "side-chain theory." This theory was suggested by Kekulé's hypothesis of the benzene ring, in which the six carbon atoms of this compound (C_6H_6)

form a stable hexagonal nucleus among themselves while linked also with unstable "side chains" of easily replaceable hydrogen.

Ehrlich assumed that the living protoplasmic molecule consists of a stable nucleus with unstable side chains or receptors, which enable it to combine with food stuffs and to neutralize toxins by throwing off detached side chains into the blood. "In spite of the enormous amount of criticism which has been heaped upon this theory and its author, it may safely be affirmed that, as based upon a fundamental postulate in organic chemistry, it has proved to be a valuable 'heuristic principle' in developing the science of immunity and serumreactions" (Garrison). Wassermann declared that, without the side-chain theory, he would never have discovered the Wassermann reaction.

In 1899, Ehrlich went to Frankfurt-am-Main as director of the *Kgl. Institut für Experimentelle Therapie* (Royal Institute of Experimental Therapy), where he continued his work on immunity and toxins and carried out important investigations on cancer, demonstrating that carcinomata, on repeated passage through animals, increase in virulence and that it is possible to transform a carcinoma into a sarcoma. In 1906, a special institute was erected for him, the Georg Speyer Haus, where he realized his long ambition of devoting himself entirely to the systematic study of chemotherapy. Here he worked at first with trypanosomiasis and demonstrated the curative effects of the dye trypanrot in the treatment of experimental trypanosomiasis in animals. The most outstanding work was his study of the therapeutic effects of arsenical compounds in experimental syphilis, a work crowned by his discovery of Salvarsan, or 606, in 1910. The work on Salvarsan was guided by Ehrlich's maxim, *corpora non agunt nisi fixata*—that a chemical substance is effective only on tissues by which it is fixed. Ehrlich had found, however, in his earlier work with trypanosomes that, when the doses of certain dyes which were insufficient to produce complete sterilization were administered, the parasites were able to immunize themselves against later doses. The same phenomenon occurred with Salvarsan, and Ehrlich's dream of a *therapia magna sterilisans* was never completely realized. But it was a great advance. Salvarsan is a remarkable drug and for a generation was the most potent and widely used drug in the treatment of syphilis.

Ehrlich died in 1915. He received the Nobel prize in 1908 and was created in 1911 *Wirklicher Geheimrat* and *Excellenz*. He did the most fruitful work in infectious diseases since Pasteur and Koch and created a new science—chemotherapy.

In addition to Schaudinn's discovery of the *Spirochaeta pallida,* other important disease-producing microorganisms were discovered in the early years of the twentieth century. In 1906, Howard T. Ricketts, of Chicago, studying Rocky Mountain spotted fever, transmitted the disease to guinea pigs by the bite of a tick and, in 1909, described, in the blood of infected guinea pigs and monkeys and in the eggs of infected ticks, an organism which he thought had a specific relationship to the disease, "a bipolar-staining bacillus of minute size." Charles Nicolle, director of the Pasteur Institute of Tunis, found that typhus fever could be transmitted to a chimpanzee by the injection of a small quantity of blood from a patient in the acute stage of the disease and announced in 1909 that typhus fever could be transmitted from an infected monkey to a healthy animal by the bite of the body louse. In 1910, Ricketts went to Mexico with Russell Wilder to investigate an epidemic of *tabardillo,* or typhus fever, where he found the disease was transmitted by the body louse and also reported that he had seen small bacilli resembling those found in Rocky Mountain spotted fever in the stools of infected lice and in the blood of infected monkeys.

In 1913, von Prowazek, studying typhus fever in Serbia, found the same organisms in lice who had fed on typhus patients. Both of these observers were martyrs to medical science—Ricketts dying of typhus fever in Mexico in 1910 and von Prowazek succumbing to the same disease in 1915. The following year, da Rocha-Lima, who was von Prowazek's colleague in this work and had also contracted the disease but recovered, published the first adequate description of the new organisms, to which he gave the name *Rickettsia prowazeki,* and pointed out the differences between rickettsia and bacteria.

Since da Rocha-Lima's work, rickettsia have been recognized as a distinct type of micro-organism. At least five diseases are caused by rickettsia—typhus fever caused by the *Rickettsia prowazeki,* Rocky Mountain spotted fever by the *Rickettsia rickettsi,* trench fever or Volhynian fever by the *Rickettsia quintana,* murine typhus or the Mexican tabardillo by the *Rickettsia muricola,* Tsutsugamushi, Japanese river fever or scrub typhus, by the *Rickettsia orientalis,* and "Q" fever by the *Rickettsia burneti.* Rickettsial diseases now take their place in standard textbooks as a group distinct from bacterial diseases.

Another group of diseases soon took their place as distinct from bacterial diseases—diseases due to viruses. The first discovery that an ultramicroscopic virus could produce disease was made by Löffler in 1898 in the course of some experiments on foot-and-mouth disease. He found that the contents of vesicles formed in this disease, after being passed through a filter of infusorial earth, produced the disease in animals, although the fluid showed no particles or organisms on microscopic examination and no bacteria could be cultivated. This method of study was continued during the following years, and some forty types of viruses producing disease in men and animals were described. Among the diseases now recognized as due to filtrable viruses are cowpox, smallpox, psittacosis, rabies, yellow

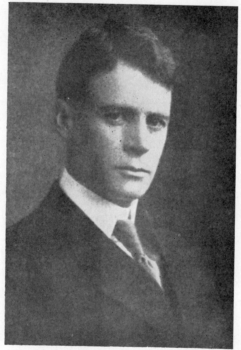

J.A.M.A., 1910

HOWARD T. RICKETTS

fever, influenza, encephalitis, measles, poliomyelitis, mumps, chickenpox, herpes and the common cold. The viruses vary greatly in size from 275 mμ, the diameter of the psittacosis virus, to 10 mμ, the diameter of the virus of foot-and-mouth disease. The virus of vaccinia measures 225 mμ, of rabies 125 mμ, of poliomyelitis 12 mμ, and of influenza 11 mμ. An idea of the minuteness of these organisms can be gained from the size of the red blood cell, which is 7500 mμ, or 750 times the diameter of the foot-and-mouth disease virus. Viruses have been postulated as the causative agents in certain tumors,

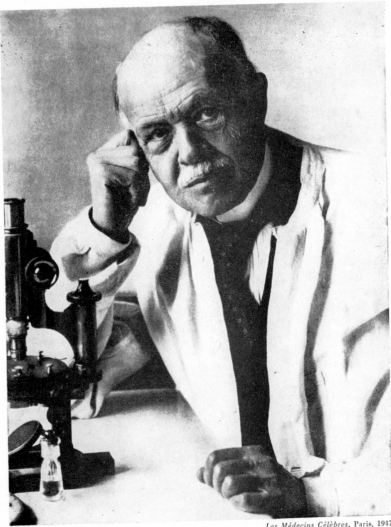

Les Médecins Célèbres, Paris, 1947

CHARLES NICOLLE

and Stanley has described a remarkable virus, the etiological agent
in tobacco mosaic, a plant disease, which he has crystallized and
which has the properties of an inanimate chemical substance although it multiplies like living molecules.

The development of our knowledge of vitamins is also an achievement of the twentieth century. The beginning of this knowledge dates back to 1753, when Lind's *A Treatise of the Scurvy* appeared, and to 1794, when the British fleet reached Madras after a voyage of 23 weeks without a single case of scurvy on board, thanks to the daily ration of lemon juice. The practical results of this procedure 41 years after Lind had advocated it were immediately recognized, and, with the regulation of adding lemon juice to the daily ration the following year, scurvy disappeared from the British Navy. The theoretical value of this demonstration, the first discovery of a deficiency disease, was not, however, fully appreciated.

Nearly a century later, Christian Eijkman, who had gone to Java as a member of a commission to study beriberi, published in 1890 a paper on "Polyneuritis in Chickens." He pointed out the similarity between beriberi and a polyneuritis in chickens, which could be produced by feeding chickens on polished rice and could be cured by either feeding them unpolished rice or treating them with aqueous or alcoholic extracts of the polishings. Dr. G. Grijns, who succeeded Eijkman as director of the laboratory at Batavia, continued these observations and came to the conclusion that beriberi was due to the lack of some indispensable ingredient in the food. Eijkman's observations on chickens were confirmed on human beings by William Fletcher in 1907. Fletcher fed patients at the Kuala Lumpur lunatic asylum in Malaya on two diets—one of "uncured" husked rice and the other of "cured" unhusked rice. The patients who ate husked rice showed much beriberi, whereas those eating unhusked rice developed no beriberi.

The whole subject of "indispensable ingredients in the food" began to attract increasing attention following the work of F. Gowland Hopkins, who had gone to Cambridge University on the invitation of Sir Michael Foster to lecture on physiological chemistry. In a series of classical experiments in 1906, Hopkins demonstrated that rats failed to grow on a diet of artificial milk, but gained weight and grew rapidly when a small quantity, even one-half teaspoonful, of cow's milk was added to their daily ration. He stated, "No animal can live on a mixture of pure protein, fat and carbohydates," even when mineral salts were added. His conclusion was that there must be present in food some additional substance, to which he gave the non-committal name of "accessory substance." He suggested that scurvy might have been caused by the absence in the sailors' diet of an accessory substance, which was present in lemon juice.

Hopkins's theory of "accessory substances" had actually been advanced 25 years earlier by Lunin of Basel, who found that mice did not thrive on artificially prepared synthetic milk. His conclusion was that natural milk must contain some unknown ingredients necessary for growth. "His remarks met the usual fate accorded to the 'wild notions' of scientific innovations—nobody paid any attention" (Scott).

Meanwhile, it had been found by Casimir Funk, a Polish chemist, that yeast was as effective in curing or preventing beriberi as the

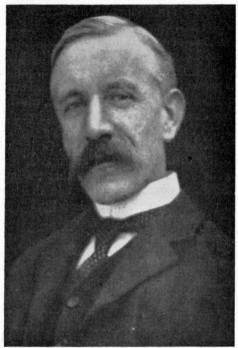

MacCallum and Taylor, *Nobel Prize-Winners*, Zurich, 1938

SIR FREDERICK GOWLAND HOPKINS

extracts of rice husks. He thought that the substance essential for life and growth was an amine and proposed the name "Vitamine," for it in a paper published in 1912 under the title, "The Etiology of Deficiency Diseases." Later, it was discovered that they were not amines, so it was suggested that the name be changed to "Vitamin" in order not to perpetuate this error, a suggestion which has been generally adopted.

An American chemist, Elmer McCollum, working at the Wisconsin Agricultural Experiment Station, found that rats on an artificial diet did not flourish but developed keratomalacia. When butter fat was added to the diet, the rats throve and were cured of their keratomalacia. He suggested the term, "fat soluble A," for this vitamin. Later, he found a similar accessory factor which prevented the development of polyneuritis and, as it was soluble in water, proposed the name, "water soluble B."

In 1907, Holst and Froelich showed that guinea pigs developed scurvy on a deficient diet—the first experimental production of scurvy—but that scurvy could be prevented by the addition of lemon juice. This observation made possible the further study of scurvy in the laboratory.

The development of the subject of vitamins is recorded in a vast literature in which we find a large number of names of investigators who have made notable contributions to this subject. Vitamin A has been extensively investigated and its synthesis accomplished by Fuson and Christ. A diet deficient in vitamin A produces exophthalmia and nyctalopia, or night blindness. Vitamin B, the vitamin concerned in beriberi, has been found to be a complex factor, the best known constituents of which are B_1, or thiamine, the antiberiberi vitamin isolated by Jansen and Donath; and B_2, or riboflavin, a growth factor, isolated by Kuhn. Goldberger proved that pellagra was due to a lack of vitamin B, the exact fraction of which was later shown to be nicotinic acid. Vitamin C, which prevents scurvy, was shown by Szent-Györgyi to be hexuronic acid, also called ascorbic acid, or cevitamic acid. Vitamin D, which is activated ergosterol, was found to prevent rickets. Nicotinic acid is a cure for pellagra. Vitamin E, discovered by Evans, the absence of which leads to sterility, has been shown to be a tocopherol. Thus, in the early years of the twentieth century, much of the mystery surrounding night blindness, beriberi, scurvy, rickets and pellagra has been cleared up.

Another achievement of the early years of the century was the demonstration of the role played by allergy in disease. The peculiar sensitivity of certain individuals to various substances had been noted for centuries. Rhazes described "rose catarrh" in patients who had attacks of sneezing and itching of the nose whenever they came in contact with roses and this phenomena was rediscovered by Botallo in 1565. Later, in the nineteenth century, John Bostock wrote his classic account of "summer catarrh" (1819). In 1831, Elliotson proposed the theory that hay fever was caused by the blossoms of graminaceous plants, and, in 1870, Morrill Wyman demonstrated on himself that an attack of hay fever could be induced by sniffing ragweed pollen. Van Helmont, back in the seventeenth century, had described attacks of asthma caused by house dust and

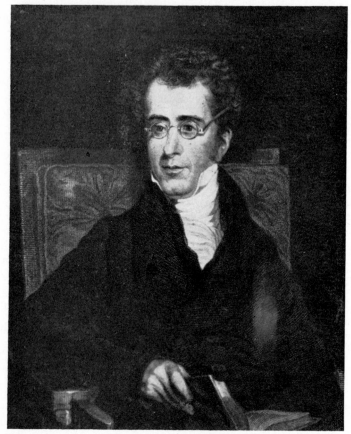

Surgeon General's Library, Washington, D.C.

JOHN BOSTOCK

John Bostock (1733-1846) was a distinguished physician who gave up the practice of medicine and devoted himself entirely to the study of science. He wrote the first systematic treatise in English on physiology, translated Pliny's *Natural History,* and described his own case of hay fever.

by eating fish fried in oil, and similar observations were reported with increasing frequency during the eighteenth and nineteenth centuries.

In 1902, Charles Richet, working with the toxin produced by the Portuguese man-of-war, a species of jelly fish which produces urticaria on contact, found that a single injection of the toxin in ani-

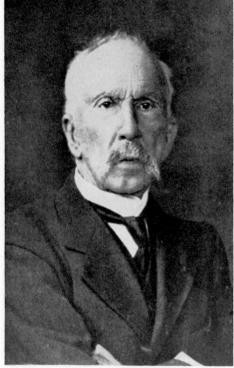

Les Médecins Célèbres, Paris, 1947

CHARLES RICHET

mals produced no effect but a second injection, after the lapse of a few days, was fatal. He called this phenomenon anaphylaxis, "a lifting up or removal of protection," as compared with prophylaxis, "favoring protection." Richet's work was the spark that ignited a train of subsequent researches.

Von Pirquet noted that patients receiving a second injection of horse serum several days after an initial injection often developed attacks of urticaria and asthma. He studied this phenomenon intensively and proposed that the term, anaphylaxis, be dropped as inaccurate since it was not a diminution in protection. He suggested the term, allergy, or a changed state, a suggestion that has been almost universally followed. In the course of his work, he developed his well-known skin test for tuberculosis, which he regarded as caused by allergy to the tubercle bacillus.

Knowledge of allergy now advanced at a rapid pace through the

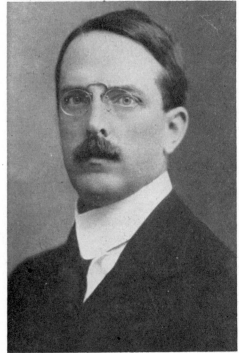

CLEMENS VON PIRQUET
Photograph taken in 1912.

work of Arthus, Theobald Smith, Coca, Otto, Vaughan, Weichardt,
Schick, Wolff-Eisner, Rosenau and Anderson, Auer, Duke and
Lewis—to mention but a few names. In 1910, Meltzer pointed out
that asthma was an allergic process, and the role of allergy as a
cause of asthma, hay fever, certain skin diseases and as a factor in
certain infectious diseases was clearly demonstrated.

Medicine in the twentieth century profited from the great advances in the physical sciences. The discovery of radium was one.
The investigations which led to the discovery of radium began
with the chance observation of Henri Becquerel, the French physicist, that a piece of uranium ore, lying on a photographic plate in
the dark-room, affected the plate on the spot where the ore lay.
Investigating the problem further, he found that pitchblende, the

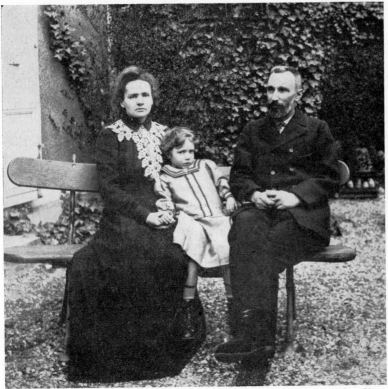

PIERRE AND MARIE CURIE WITH THEIR ELDEST DAUGHTER, IRÈNE

Irène in 1935 received the Nobel prize for chemistry with her husband, Frédéric Joliot. Photograph taken in 1904.

ore which was the chief source of uranium, was much more powerful than could be explained by its content of uranium. Becquerel concluded there must be a new element with powers of affecting photographic plates and asked Pierre and Marie Curie to work on the problem. On July 18, 1898, a paper, *Sur une substance nouvelle radio-active, contenue dans la pechblende,* by P. Curie and Mme. S. Curie was presented to the *Académie des Sciences* by Becquerel. It announced the discovery of radium.

This spectacular discovery of an element possessing radioactivity aroused both interest and enthusiasm. The employment of radium in medicine is said to have been the result of an accidental burn which Becquerel received while carrying a fragment of uranium in his waistcoat pocket. The similarity between this burn and those produced by x-rays suggested the use of radium for the same conditions in which x-rays were found to have therapeutic effects. It was soon observed that the same disease which had been successfully treated with x-rays responded also to radium. In addition, radium could be administered intravenously in the form of its salts and, in some diseases, offered a more convenient form of treatment.

The string galvanometer was another development in physics which was of extreme value to medicine. It had been known since the observations of Matteucci in 1843 and of Kölliker and Müller in 1856 that the frog's heart, on contraction, produced an electric current. In 1887, Waller showed that a similar current could be demonstrated in the human heart by connecting electrodes placed on the surface of the body with a capillary electrometer. Willem Einthoven, professor of physiology at the University of Leyden, devised in 1903 a very delicate string galvanometer and constructed the first electrocardiograph. Einthoven's instrument, very sensitive yet practical, gave clear records of the electrical changes in the beating heart and inaugurated a new era in the study of cardiovascular disease. This discovery came at a period which saw a renewed interest in cardiology, largely as the result of the studies made by Sir James Mackenzie.

Few physicians of the twentieth century had a more picturesque career or made more solid contributions to the field of cardiology than James Mackenzie. He was born on a farm in the parish of

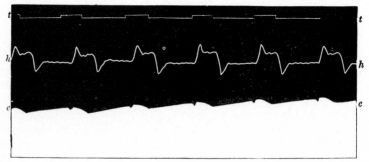

Fig. 1. Man. Heart led off to electrometer from front and back of chest (front to Hg; back to H₂SO₄).

e.e. electrometer.   h.h. cardiograph.   t.t. time in seconds.

ELECTROCARDIOGRAPHIC TRACING OBTAINED BY WALLER IN 1887

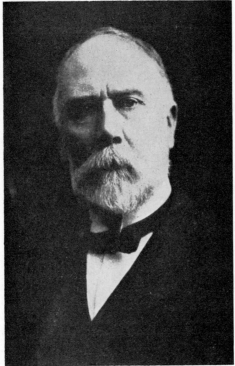

Wilson, *The Beloved Physician*, London, 1926

JAMES MACKENZIE

Scone in Perthshire, Scotland, in 1853. His early schooling was received at the Academy of Perth, where he says, "I was considered a dunce," and which he left at the age of 15, profoundly disturbed because memory tests were considered the final test of intellectual capacity. After working for several years as an apprentice to a chemist (druggist) of Perth, he entered the medical school at Edinburgh, where he graduated in 1878. During his first years in medicine, he found again that memory seemed to be a criterion by which intellectual capacity was judged. As he proceeded in his course, he found that the power of reasoning was equally important and gradually realized that he himself was endowed with such powers. After graduation, he settled in Burnley, a manufacturing town in Lancashire, as assistant to Drs. Briggs and Brown, who had a large general practice.

In Burnley, Mackenzie saw many patients with irregularities of the pulse. Some of these patients died of heart failure while others seemed not in the least inconvenienced. Realizing his own ignorance of the subject, he studied a huge encyclopedia of medicine and, failing to find an explanation there, finally went to Edinburgh, where he consulted his old professors. Receiving no answer to his queries from either books or professors, he was forced to adopt the method of "wait and see." In 1883, he embarked upon a program of careful study of his own cardiac patients, but his conclusions were not published until 1902—nearly 20 years later.

Mackenzie purchased a Dudgeon sphygmograph and took many tracings of the radial pulse. He amassed an enormous number of tracings, which confirmed his idea that there were several different kinds of irregularity of the heart, but which failed to answer his question as to which were the dangerous kinds of waves and which were the harmless. The idea then occurred to him that, if he could simultaneously record the waves of the radial pulse and the waves in the jugular vein, he would have a complete picture of the heart's activity—the jugular waves recording the activity of the auricles and the radial pulse, the activity of the ventricles. He worked for a time with a crude instrument of his own and presently, with the aid of a watchmaker, devised the well-known "Mackenzie Ink Polygraph."

In 1902 Mackenzie's *The Study of the Pulse* was published, the first scientific treatise on irregularities of the pulse. It classified irregularities as the "youthful type" (sinus irregularity), the "adult type" (extra-systole), and the "dangerous type," called at first by Mackenzie "auricular paralysis" and later "auricular fibrillation." This work was an immediate success and established his reputation. After 28 years of practice in Burnley, he moved to London in 1908 and, the same year, published his *Diseases of the Heart,* a classic in cardiology, which was soon translated into French, German, Italian and Russian. He was elected a Fellow of the Royal Society, and knighthood was conferred on him. After a successful career as a heart specialist in London for 10 years, he left London for St. Andrews, to "return to general practice." He died in London in 1925.

Mackenzie found cardiology a welter of conflicting theories and left it an organized subject endowed with facts, many due directly to his own labors. His polygraph is no longer widely employed but has been superseded by the electrocardiograph. However, with his polygraph, he established the fundamental differences in the various types of cardiac irregularities and erected a milestone in the history of cardiac disease.

Mackenzie's polygraph and Einthoven's electrocardiograph opened a new era in cardiology, the first momentous advance since Laennec discovered auscultation. The polygraph in Mackenzie's hand had already demonstrated the "youthful," the "adult," and the "dangerous" types of cardiac irregularity. The electrocardiograph in the hands of Thomas Lewis, Mackenzie's pupil, showed that the "dangerous type" of irregularity was due to fibrillation of the auricles.

Another interesting heart condition was satisfactorily explained about the same time—Stokes-Adams disease, as it was usually called, although Morgagni earlier, in 1761, had described a similar case, which he designated "epilepsy with a slow pulse." Morgagni found nothing at autopsy to explain the symptoms of his patient; Adams found "no morbid appearance of any consequence." Other physicians, for more than a century, had the same experience.

In 1893, Wilhelm His, Jr., an assistant in the medical clinic at Leipzig, published in the *Arbeiten aus der Medizinischer Klinik zu Leipzig* an article in which he described "a muscle bundle which unites the auricular and ventricular septal walls"—the now well-known bundle of His. As His himself wrote later, "Very few people have read this article." The same year, he produced dissociation of the auricular and ventricular beats by severing this bundle and reported these results in the *Wiener Medizinische Blätter,* 1894.

Mackenzie made no mention of the bundle of His in the *Study of the Pulse,* although he published some curves showing clearly two and three beats of the auricle to one of the ventricle. With the introduction of the electrocardiograph, the mechanism of the slow pulse became obvious, and, as Vaquez noted, "By 1910, the positive observations were so numerous and so concordant, that by almost unanimous consent the Adams-Stokes syndrome became synonymous with changes in the auriculoventricular bundle."

Dr. James B. Herrick of Chicago made cardiac history in 1912 with his notable paper on "The Clinical Feature of Sudden Obstruction of the Coronary Arteries." He pointed out that coronary occlusion was a frequent cause of death and gave "the earliest complete clinical description of sudden coronary occlusion" (White). His pupil, Fred Smith, in a study of experimental coronary occlusion, described certain changes in the electrocardiogram which were subsequently seen in one of Herrick's patients in whom the diagnosis of coronary occlusion had been confirmed by necropsy.

Herrick is an outstanding figure in American medicine. In 1910, he described the first case of sickle-cell anemia and called attention

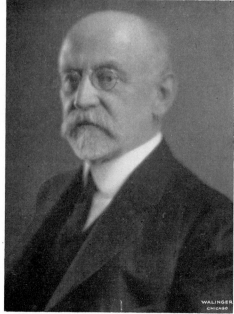

Photo by Walinger

JAMES B. HERRICK

to this new and interesting type of anemia. His work on coronary disease remains one of the great contributions to cardiology. In the midst of an active life as a consultant and teacher, he found time to write an excellent *Short History of Cardiology,* 1942, in which, with characteristic modesty, he dismisses all reference to his own work with the remark, "These developments are so recent that they cannot be considered as having become a part of history." A man of broad culture and reading, Herrick has written some charming essays, such as *Why I Read Chaucer at Seventy,* 1931; and his recent *Memories of Eighty Years,* 1949, belongs to the enduring contributions to autobiography.

Chicago, at this period, was a very active medical center. In addition to Herrick, there was an outstanding group of internists and surgeons who made medical history. Frank Billings (1854-1932), a dynamic teacher, outstanding clinician, and medical statesman, was a powerful influence in medical education and stimulated, more than any other man, the study of focal infection. After the departure of Osler for Oxford, he was by common consent the dean of American physicians. Among his pupils and associates, Joseph Capps, Ernest Irons, Edward C. Rosenow, and Joseph Miller have added to the lustre of Chicago medicine. Capps has contributed important studies on the localization of pain and on red cell volume, while Rosenow's work on the selective localization of bacteria is well known. Two other associates, George Dick and Gladys Dick, demonstrated that scarlet fever is caused by hemolytic streptococci and devised the well-known Dick test for the determination of individual susceptibility to this disease. Among the younger generation, Walter Palmer has made notable contributions, particularly in the field of gastroenterology, Louis N. Katz enjoys a great and deserved reputation in cardiology and R. T. Woodyatt in diabetes.

In pathology, Chicago was represented by such outstanding pathologists as Ludvig Hektoen, E. R. Le Count, D. J. Davis, H. Gideon Wells, and Paul Cannon. In surgery, Nicholas Senn, John B. Murphy, A. J. Ochsner, Arthur D. Bevan, and Dean Lewis enjoyed national and international reputations. Of the younger generation, Dallas Phemister and Herman Kretschmer have carried on in the tradition of their predecessors and have earned enviable reputations as conservative, sane and scientific surgeons. Casey A. Wood had a wide reputation as ophthalmologist and medical historian.

Chicago also achieved a certain leadership through the location there of the offices of the American Medical Association. This Association, which was organized in 1847, largely through the efforts of Nathan Smith Davis, to improve the then disgraceful status of medical education in the United States, devoted itself during the first 50 years of its existence more to discussion rather than accomplishment. In 1901, the Association was reorganized on its present basis and, for the past half century, has carried on, through its Council on Pharmacy and Chemistry, a vigorous campaign against patent medicines, nostrums, medical frauds, and misbranded drugs and has been, through its Council on Medical Education, a powerful influence in improving the standards of medical education and in bringing about the disappearance of numerous diploma mills, propriety medical "colleges," and poor medical schools. *The Journal of the American Medical Association* was founded in 1883. In 1889, George H. Simmons became editor, and, as Garrison wrote in 1924, the Journal "has steadily advanced to a position corresponding with that of the *British Medical Journal* in England or the *Deutsche medizinische Wochenschrift* in Germany." On Simmon's retirement in 1924, his successor, Morris Fishbein, an able and brilliant medical journalist, improved the *Journal* even more and made it one of the

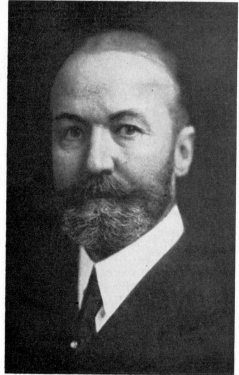

Davis, *J. B. Murphy*, New York, 1938

JOHN B. MURPHY

greatest, in the opinion of many the greatest, medical journal of its time.

Many American cities had noteworthy physicians. In Boston, Henry Christian, Richard Cabot, and Elliott P. Joslin were men of international reputation. Christian was a teacher, scholar, and inspirer of young men. Cabot was a teacher of physical diagnosis and an enthusiastic advocate of case history teaching. Joslin, an old student of Naunyn, has devoted his life to a study of diabetes mellitus, has had the greatest experience in treating diabetes of any physician in modern times, and has written the classic treatise on diabetes in the English language, *The Treatment of Diabetes Mellitus.* Among the younger group, Paul D. White and Samuel Levine became cardiologists of international reputation; James H. Means, a leader in

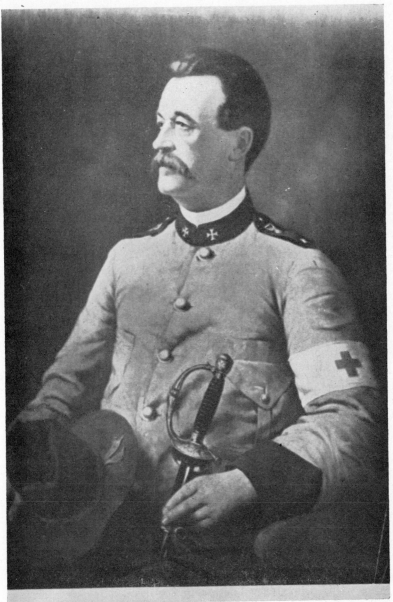

Surg. Gynec. & Obst., 1908

NICHOLAS SENN AT THE AGE OF FIFTY-FOUR

the study of thyroid disease; and Elliott Cutler, a pioneer in cardiac surgery.

Harvard Medical School at this period had two noteworthy anatomists in Frederick T. Lewis and Charles S. Minot, whose microtome is well known to all workers in normal and pathological histology. In pathology, Frank B. Mallory, Homer B. Wright, and S. Burt Wolbach made important contributions with which their names are associated. Reid Hunt in pharmacology was an acknowledged leader in this field, and the work of Otto Folin and of Edwin J. Cohn created a new era in biochemistry.

Among the surgeons, Frank Lahey, successively professor of surgery at Tufts and at Harvard, is one of the outstanding surgeons of his time. A scholar with an unusual grasp of surgical literature, a brilliant yet conservative surgeon, a forceful and dynamic teacher, he founded in Boston the Lahey Clinic, an institution which is, in certain respects, the counterpart in New England of the older and larger Mayo Clinic in the midwest.

In Cleveland there developed at Western Reserve a noteworthy group—C. F. Hoover, a keen clinician, able teacher, and persistent investigator; the well-known surgeons George Crile and Carl A. Hamman; and Howard T. Karsner, for a generation one of the leading American pathologists. Washington University in St. Louis, wrote Abraham Flexner in 1910, "bids fair shortly to possess faculty, laboratories, and hospital conforming in every respect to ideal standards." Mr. Flexner proved a good prophet. Here, George Dock, one of the great figures of contemporary American medicine, who had described in 1896 the first case of coronary occlusion in America proved by autopsy, established a new tradition of teaching and investigation, ably carried on by his successor, David Barr. In surgery, Evarts Graham was a pioneer in lung surgery and created a new epoch in the history of hepatic diseases by his discovery, with Cole, of a practical method for visualizing the gallbladder. Washington University also had on its faculty Joseph Erlanger, professor of physiology, who, in 1944, shared the Nobel prize in medicine with Herbert S. Gasser, professor of pharmacology. Carl F. Cori, professor of pharmacology and biochemistry in 1947, shared that year with Gerty Cori the Nobel prize in medicine.

The University of Kansas in 1905 established a four-year medical school in Lawrence and Kansas City. Among members of the Lawrence faculty who attained national recognition were George E. Coghill, professor of anatomy, Noble P. Sherwood and Marshall A. Barber, professors of bacteriology. The latter devised the ingenious method of isolating individual bacteria with a very fine capillary tube and proved that the dose of a single anthrax bacillus may prove fatal to experimental animals. He later became one of the world's outstanding malariologists. In Kansas City, John Fairbairn Binnie, Thomas Grover Orr, Frank Teachenor, and Earl Padgett became surgeons of international prominence; Logan Clendening was a recognized authority on medical history; and William Waddell Duke made outstanding contributions to hematology and allergy. Duke devised the well-known method for estimating the bleeding time and discovered a new type of allergy—physical allergy. Richard L. Sutton and Charles C. Dennie attained wide reputations as dermatologists, Frank C. Neff as a pediatrician, Russell Haden as an internist, H. Roswell Wahl as a pathologist, E. J. Curran as an ophthalmologist, and Edward H. Hashinger has become well known as a pioneer in geriatrics. In Kansas City, Edward Holman Skinner was an early pioneer and authority on roentgenology. In nearby Topeka, Karl Menninger founded a nationally known psychiatric clinic.

In Philadelphia, Musser, Pepper, Wood, Hare, Abbott, Anders, Wolferth, and many others kept aloft the high tradition of Pennsylvania. Krumbhaar achieved an international reputation both as a pathologist and as a medical historian. In Baltimore, Osler had been succeeded by Barker, who, with Thayer, McCrae, Futcher, and an able staff, carried on in the best tradition of Osler. John Howland, one of the ablest pediatricians of his generation, had been called to Johns Hopkins as professor in succession to von Pirquet, who had returned to Europe. Somewhat later, William H. Wilmer, the well-known ophthalmologist, left a very large practice in Washington, D.C., to accept a chair at Johns Hopkins and head a new Institute of Ophthalmology.

New York showed, during this period, medical activity and progress worthy of this great American metropolis. At the Hospital of the Rockefeller Institute, Rufus Cole, Frederick M. Allen and Homer Swift were outstanding clinicians and research workers. At Columbia University, Alphonse Dochez carried out his well-known investigations on pneumonia, the common cold, and scarlet fever; Russell Cecil worked with distinction in the field of arthritis; and Robert Levy's studies on diseases of the heart elevated him to the rank of one of the foremost cardiologists of America. At Cornell, clinical medicine was ably represented by Lewis A. Conner and B. S. Oppenheimer, pathology by James Ewing, and pediatrics by Emmett Holt. Emanuel Libman, whose studies on cardiac disease, notably on endocarditis, belong to the classics in American medical literature, was a powerful stimulus at Mt. Sinai Hospital. At the same institution, Henry Koplik, discoverer of "Koplik's spots" in measles, gave distinction to the department of pediatrics, and George Baehr achieved a wide reputation in both clinical medicine and pathology. The repu-

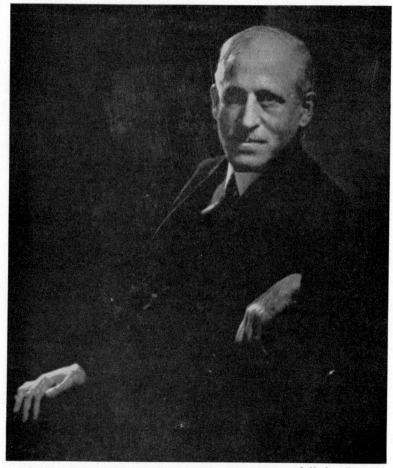

EMANUEL LIBMAN   *J. Mt. Sinai Hosp.*, 1947

tation of Mt. Sinai was further enhanced by two important additions
to its staff—Bela Schick of Vienna, who has achieved fame for his
work in allergy and infectious disease and whose name has become
lasting through his development of the Schick test; and I. Snapper,
formerly of Amsterdam and the Peking Union Medical College. In
ophthalmology Arnold Knapp was a leader.

American ingenuity and resourcefulness has nowhere been better
demonstrated than in the field of surgery, from the days of Ephraim
McDowell down to the present. In the early years of the twentieth
century, American surgeons were already the peers of surgeons else-

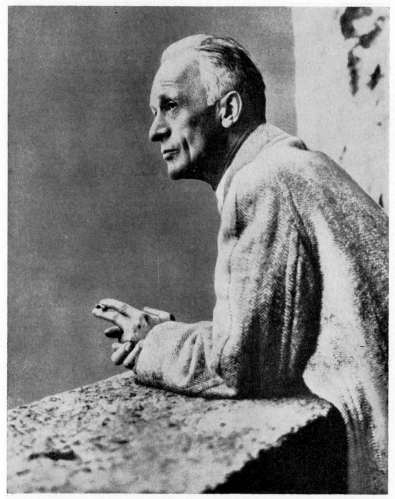

HARVEY CUSHING
A photograph by Arnold Klebs in 1929.

where in the world. In addition to the remarkable group in Chicago, there were many other groups who were not only skillful operators but scientific students intent on advancing the art of surgery. Halsted in Baltimore had an unusual group of pupils, Finney, Bloodgood, Young, and particularly Harvey Cushing, who became the international leader in neurological surgery.

Harvey Cushing, who was associated with Johns Hopkins from

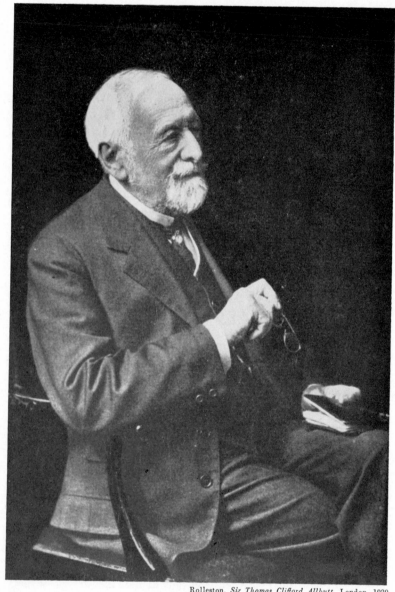

Rolleston, *Sir Thomas Clifford Allbutt*, London, 1929

CLIFFORD ALLBUTT

Photograph taken in 1920.

1896 until 1911, showed early an especial bent for research. Early in his career, he worked with Kronecker and Kocher in Bern, where he demonstrated the relationship between intracranial pressure and blood pressure, showing that "an increase in intracranial pressure occasions a rise in blood pressure." On his return to America, he introduced the new sphygmomanometer of Riva-Rocci into surgical practice and demonstrated the value of observing the blood pressure during operations. Turning his attention particularly to neurological surgery, Cushing soon attained a position of unquestioned leadership. In 1906, he described the relationship between pituitary tumors and sexual infantilism, an association he later demonstrated by experimental work. In 1912, he published a highly original monograph on the pituitary body and, in 1932, described hypophysial basophilism, since known as Cushing's disease. Cushing was a master of a lucid and charming style, and his *Life of Sir William Osler* is one of the masterpieces of medical biography and won a Pulitzer award for literature. He was deeply interested in medical history, assembled a notable private collection, and, at his death, left his nearly complete *Bio-bibliography of Andreas Vesalius,* which was published in 1943. Cushing left an impress on neurological surgery, not only through his individual contributions, but also through the assistants he trained. Dandy, Naffziger and Horrax, his former assistants, presently took their places as leaders in American neurosurgery.

Rudolph Matas of New Orleans, student, scholar and surgeon, did pioneer work on nerve-blocking, spinal anesthesia, and laryngeal intubation and, with his radical operation for aneurysm, aneurysmorrhaphy (1902), made the first advance in this type of surgery since the days of John Hunter. In Cleveland, George Crile carried out highly original experimental researches on surgical shock, blood pressure in surgery, hemorrhage and transfusion, and devised many new surgical operations. His famous "anoci-association," blocking of shock in operations by the combination of general and local anesthesia, reduced operative mortality to less than one per cent and is probably his most important contribution to surgery. This indomitable worker, on his retirement as professor of surgery at Western Reserve because of the age limit, organized the Cleveland Clinic, an important institution for the graduate training of physicians and surgeons. Lastly, at Rochester, Minnesota, a constantly increasing stream of surgeons from all over the world journeyed to that little town to watch the astounding surgical skill of William and Charles

Mayo and to study the reasons for their remarkable success. Surgically, at least, America had come of age.

Although the hospitals and clinics in England and France lacked the superb equipment and the generous financial support of the German institutions, many outstanding physicians, surgeons, pathologists and physiologists developed there. In England, Clifford Allbutt and Humphry Rolleston, master and pupil, both in turn Regius Professor at Cambridge, both skillful clinicians and men of broad culture, made important contributions to medicine. They also enriched the history of medicine with scholarly contributions, which were masterpieces of style.

Allbutt edited a *System of Medicine,* 1896-1899, which remains one of the best works of its kind in the English language; wrote his great work, *Diseases of the Arteries,* when nearly 80 years of age; and, six years later, published his scholarly *Greek Medicine in Rome,* to which every serious student of the subject is indebted. Rolleston developed the same cultural tastes and scientific interests as his teacher, became the undisputed dean of the English medical profession, was physician to King George V, and was created a baronet. His *Diseases of the Liver* was long an authoritative work, and his numerous articles and monographs on historical subjects have enduring worth.

In surgery, Berkeley Moynihan of Leeds had an international reputation, particularly in abdominal surgery, where his studies of duodenal ulcers were notable. Victor Horsley in London was a surgeon of unusual skill, gifted with great powers of imagination but tempered with an abundance of cool logic. Becoming interested early in his career in physiology, he began to study the localization of function in the brain, an investigation that presently led him into the field of neurosurgery, in which he was one of its most distinguished pioneers. In 1887, he performed the first operation for removal of a spinal cord tumor and, as early as 1890, made a report of 44 operations on the brain. In Liverpool, Robert Jones was making a lasting reputation as an orthopedic surgeon.

Sir Frederick Treves, whose chief activities were in the later years of the nineteenth century, was an acknowledged master of abdominal surgery and, in 1902, performed a successful operation for appendicitis on King Edward VII. Treves was one of the first to study carefully the surgical aspects of acute appendicitis, having written several early articles on the subject. His *Surgical Applied Anatomy* had phenomenal success and was widely used by medical students.

It was however, particularly in physiology that England excelled.

To quote the London *Times,* "The English School of Physiology is, by common consent, the most distinguished in the world. It had no more illustrious ornament than Starling."

Ernest Henry Starling (1866-1927) began his carrer as a physiologist and as a demonstrator of physiology at Guy's Hospital in 1889 and, from 1899 until 1923, was professor of physiology at University College, London. He made many important discoveries in physiology. In 1892, he demonstrated that the serum proteins produce the osmotic pressure which causes the absorption of fluid from the tissues. With William Bayliss, he discovered in 1902 secretin, which, excreted by the mucosa of the duodenum and ileum, is absorbed by the blood and causes the secretion of bile and pancreatic juice. For this and similar internal secretions, Starling introduced the term, "hormones." He studied the circulation with his well-known heart-lung preparation and found that the heart, to work at its maximum, must dilate and does so as the pressure in front of it increases—"Starling's law of the heart." In 1924 he demonstrated that the tubules of the kidney reabsorb water, chlorides, bicarbonates and glucose from the glomerular filtrate.

Starling was a brilliant lecturer and an inspiring chief, who attracted a large group of enthusiastic pupils and investigators. His laboratory became world-renowned as a center of physiologic research, reminiscent of the laboratory of Carl Ludwig in Leipzig some 60 years previously.

John Scott Haldane (1860-1936), a native of Edinburgh and a graduate of Edinburgh University, went to Oxford in 1887 as a demonstrator in physiology and remained there until his death. Becoming interested in the gases of coal mines, he studied their composition and their physiologic effects. He found "black damp" to be inert, "fire damp" to be methane, both inflammable and explosive, "after damp" to be carbon monoxide and responsible for most cases of asphyxiation after mine accidents. These discoveries were a great and lasting contribution to industrial hygiene. From 1905 until 1915, Haldane worked on respiration and demonstrated that the immediate stimulus to respiration is not oxygen but carbon dioxide—a discovery of fundamental importance to the physiology of respiration and of great practical application in anesthesia.

At Cambridge, the work of Joseph Barcroft (1872-1947) upheld the great traditions of the Cambridge school. Barcroft, a native of Newry, Ireland, studied at Cambridge, became a reader of physiology, and was professor from 1925 until 1937. His scientific reputation will endure and increase with the years.

His first striking piece of research was on the oxygen-carrying capacity of the blood, in which he classified the varieties of anoxia and demonstrated that the passage of gases through the alveolar epithelium is a physical process and that the lungs cannot take up oxygen unless the oxygen pressure in the air is higher than that of the blood. This demonstration disproved the theory of Haldane that, at high altitudes, oxygen was secreted in the lungs. While engaged in this investigation at high altitudes, Barcroft noted that the poly- cythemia which appears is associated with a decrease in the size of the spleen, a storehouse for blood. This led to his study of blood volume in terms of circulating blood and storage blood. His last work was on prenatal physiology, the effect of environment on the development of the nervous system. Fetal physiology is a young science, in which the name of Barcroft will be recorded as a notable pioneer.

Another outstanding physiologist of this period was Edward Sharpey-Schafer, who was born in London in 1850, the son of J. W. H. Schäfer, a native of Hamburg. Edward Schäfer studied medicine at University College, London, where he fell under the spell of the physiologist, William Sharpey, for whom he developed such a veneration that he named a son after him, and, when the boy was killed in the first World War, he himself took the name of Sharpey, becoming Edward Sharpey-Schafer.

Sharpey-Schafer was assistant professor of physiology at Univer- sity College from 1874 until 1883 and, from 1883 until 1899, was Jodrell professor of physiology. In 1899, he was called to Edinburgh as professor of physiology and held this position until his retirement, after teaching physiology half a century. He died in 1935.

His early interest lay in histology, and his *Essentials of Histology,* first published in 1885, was a standard textbook, which went through twelve editions. In 1889, he published, with Victor Horseley, who worked in his laboratory, a study of the functions of the cerebral cortex. With Oliver, he demonstrated in 1895 the pressor effects of extracts of the adrenal glands—one of the momentous discoveries in endocrinology. His method of resuscitation, or artificial respiration, was published in 1893 and became known as Schäfer's method. This remains the method most widely employed today. His *Text-Book of Physiology,* which appeared in 1898, immediately took its place among the best texts on the subject.

Sharpey-Schafer published many papers on physiological topics, including the absorption of fats, the functions of the spleen, pul- monary blood pressure and vagatomy. "Sharpey-Schafer is one of the greatest names in British physiology" (Garrison).

The roll of great British physiologists of this period includes the name of Charles Scott Sherrington, who has done some of the most important work of recent times on the nervous system. He was professor of physiology in Liverpool from 1895 until 1913, when he was called to the chair of the physiology at Oxford. Working objectively and avoiding speculation, he accumulated a large mass of observations which have been the basis of some most important generalizations. He has insisted that the essential function of the nervous system is the coordination of activities in various parts of the body. His investigations have covered "reciprocal innervation" and "reciprocal inhibition," by means of which antagonistic muscles, such as flexors and extensors, when stimulated by a reflex, have excitation of one center and inhibition of the other simultaneously. He taught that a reflex action is rarely an isolated phenomenon but one which involves several reflex arcs. He has studied the levels of nervous integration, the final common path, the proprioceptive system, the higher controlling centers, and central inhibitions, and has handled his very difficult and abstruse field with signal ability.

Henry Hallett Dale has been a leader in British pharmacological research. A native of London, he studied at Cambridge University and St. Bartholomew's Hospital in London, receiving his degree at Cambridge in 1903. He was lecturer at the University of London and, in 1928, became director of the National Institute for Medical Research. In 1906, Dale, with Barger and Carr, isolated ergotoxin, the active principal of ergot; in 1909, demonstrated the oxytoxic action of extracts from the pituitary gland; and, in 1910, began to study the effects of histamine on the circulation, work which led to the recognition of its role in certain pathological conditions. With Richards, he found in 1918 that the characteristic blood pressure-lowering effects of histamine were produced by peripheral dilatation of the capillaries and smaller arterioles. In 1919, he studied histamine shock and, in 1929, demonstrated the presence of histamine as well as of acetylcholine in the spleen. As early as 1914, he had shown the inhibitory effect of acetylcholine on the heart's action, and later investigations showed its role in transmission of nervous impulses at the neuro-muscular junction.

Dale was president of the Royal Society in 1940-1945, has been secretary of the Society for many years, was knighted in 1932, and received the Nobel prize for medicine in 1936. He is one of the most distinguished British scientists of the present era.

In France, there was a notable group of neurologists, Marie, Déjérine, Janet and Babinski. Pierre Marie, a native of Paris, was a

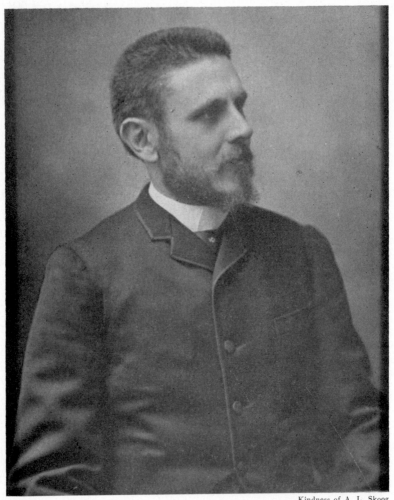

Kindness of A. L. Skoog

PIERRE MARIE

As he appeared during the period in which he described the perineal type of muscular atrophy, hypertrophic pulmonary osteo-arthropathy, hereditary cerebellar ataxis and delineated acromegaly pointing out the pituitary pathology.

pupil of Charcot, who, after his master's death, became the acknowledged leader of French neurologists. He described acromegaly in 1886, pulmonary osteo-arthropathy (Strümpell-Marie disease) in 1890, and hereditary cerebellar ataxia in 1893. In 1906, he attacked the prevailing Broca theory of aphasia, maintaining that Broca's area plays no role in spoken language, that there is only sensory aphasia, and that the motor aphasia of Broca is a combination of sensory aphasia with anarthria.

Jules Joseph Déjérine, a native of Geneva and for many years physician to the Salpêtrière, was a keen clinician and an excellent pathologist, with many important neurological contributions to his credit. With Landouzy, he described in 1886 the clinical picture now called the Landouzy-Déjérine type of progressive muscular atrophy and, in 1887, "Déjérine's neuro-tabes." In 1893, he gave the first description of hypertrophic progressive interstitial neuritis (Déjérine-Sotta's disease); and, in 1906, he described the thalamic syndrome. His *Anatomie des centres nerveux,* 1895-1901, in collaboration with his daughter, and his *Traité des maladies de la moelle épinière,* 1902, are characteristically meticulous and exact.

Pierre Janet, at first a student of philosophy, turned to medicine and, after receiving his M.D. at Paris in 1892, began practice as a specialist in neurology and psychiatry. He was appointed in 1903 professor of psychology at the Collège de France. In contrast to Marie and Déjérine, who were especially interested in organic nervous diseases and in studying their neuropathology, Janet was more interested in functional neuroses and in investigating their psychology. He developed the theory of psychologic automatism, studied the relations between neuroses and fixed ideas, investigated the mental states of hysterical patients, and described psychasthenia for the first time.

Another neurologist of international reputation was Joseph Jules Babinski, born in Paris of Polish parents in 1857. Babinski received his medical degree in Paris in 1885, was for several years chief of clinic under Charcot at the Salpêtrière and later *médecin des hôpitaux.* His first publications were on various medical problems; but, after 1890, he confined himself almost entirely to clinical neurology. In 1896, he stated, "In certain cases of paralysis, the toes on the affected side, instead of flexing when the sole is stimulated, execute an extensor movement on the metatarsal." This is the well-known Babinski sign or reflex, which has perpetuated his name in medical literature. Babinski's contributions to the study of cerebel-

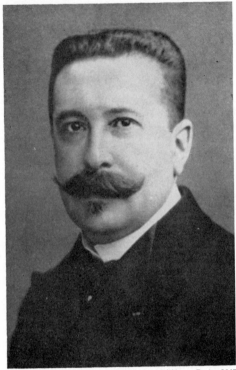

FERNAND WIDAL

lar function were noteworthy. He pointed out that, in cerebellar disease, muscles which normally contract and relax properly to produce
smoothly coordinated movements, or synergy, act in a haphazard
fashion to produce asynergia. This is demonstrated by another well-
known phenomenon, Babinski's sign of adiadokokinesia—the in-
ability to perform rapidly alternating movements.

Babinski's views on hysteria were provocative and caused much
controversy. Hysteria he maintained was produced by suggestion.
He called attention to many important points in the differential
diagnosis between hysteria and organic nervous diseases.

Among internists, Fernand Widal was one of the great names in
modern French medicine. Widal, the son of an army surgeon, was
born in Dellys, Algeria, in 1862 and studied in Paris, where he graduated and spent his entire professional life. His earlier work was

mainly on bacteriology, his most notable contribution being his discovery in 1896 of agglutinins for typhoid bacilli in the serum of patients suffering from typhoid fever—the well-known Widal test. His next important contributions were his demonstration of the increased fragility of the red blood cells in patients suffering from familial jaundice (1907) and his demonstration of the role played by sodium chloride in edema (1906)—one of the great physiological pathological discoveries of recent times.

Widal was a very logical and exact reasoner, a clear-seeing diagnostician, and a brilliant speaker and lecturer. He was a master of both the written and the spoken word, prepared his papers with great care, and was equally painstaking in the preparation of his lectures and addresses. An interesting and eloquent speaker himself, he never failed to be present when Viviani or Briand spoke at the *Chambre,* coming, as he remarked, to take lessons in eloquence.

Other prominent internists were Georges Henri Roger, who did excellent work in experimental pathology and physiology, notably on cholelithiasis and hepatic diseases, was dean of the Paris medical faculty, and, with F. Widal and P.-J. Teissier, was editor of the comprehensive *Nouveau Traité de Médecine,* in 22 volumes. Georges Hayem, professor of clinical medicine, who described and studied blood platelets in 1878, gave the first adequate description of acquired hemolytic jaundice (Hayem-Widal's disease) in 1898 and wrote the authoritative *Leçons sur les maladies du sang,* 1900. Hayem's solution for the dilution of the blood in blood-counts remains the standard diluent. Leon Ambard, a native of Marseilles, professor at Paris, carried out important studies on renal disease and devised the Ambard uremic constant.

Physiology was represented most ably by Charles Richet, whose experimental work covered a large field—the physiology of nerve and muscle, respiration, animal heat, liver function, dietetics, and serum therapy. In 1888, he had shown that animals, injected with bacteria, developed immune bodies; in 1890, had been the first to employ serum therapy; and, in 1902, had described anaphylaxis. One of the ablest physiologists and experimental pathologists of his time, he received the Nobel prize in 1913.

The Pasteur Institute was directed by Émile Roux, an old friend and colleague of Louis Pasteur, whom he assisted in his work on anthrax vaccination. Roux had worked on many phases of bacteriology, making discoveries of fundamental importance. He was a pioneer in the study of filtrable viruses, demonstrated with Yersin

the exotoxin of the diphtheria bacillus, the initial work which led
to Behring's discovery of diphtheria antitoxin, inaugurated therapy
with diphtheria antitoxin in France, and demonstrated with Metchnikoff the inoculability of syphilis in apes. He was one of the founders of modern serotherapy. Felix d'Hérelle, a Canadian, working
here discovered the bacteriophage in 1917.

Albert Calmette, another former pupil of Pasteur, was sent to
Saïgon in French Indo-China to take charge of the newly formed

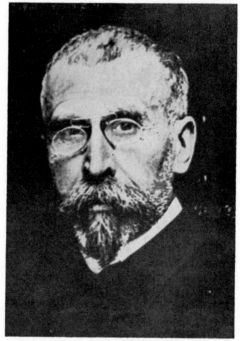

Les Médecins Célèbres, Paris, 1947

ÉMILE ROUX

Pasteur Institute. Finding that many deaths there were due to snake
bites, he prepared an effective serum to neutralize snake venom,
appying the same principle successfully employed in the preparation
of diphtheria antitoxin. Returning to France as director of the Pasteur Institute in Lille, he began to study tuberculosis, devised the
conjunctival test for tuberculosis—the Calmette test, and introduced
in 1924 preventive vaccination of children against tuberculosis, using
the vaccine B.C.G., prepared from living avirulent bovine tubercle
bacilli.

In nearby Brussels, the Pasteur Institute had as its chief, Jules Bordet, a quiet and modest but indefatigable worker. He opposed the somewhat complex theory of immunity as developed by Ehrlich in his side-chain theory. Comparing the processes of immunity to those of dyeing, Bordet assumed that toxin is neutralized by anti-toxin through absorption like that of a fabric taking up dyes. He also postulated the existence of a *substance sensibilisatrice* in anti-toxic sera, which sensitizes red blood cells or bacteria to the action of the *alexins* (complement), as a mordant does for a dyestuff. As Garrison points out, Bordet explained what he saw in terms of physical chemistry, Ehrlich in terms of structural chemistry. On the practical side, Bordet discovered bacterial hemolysis (1898), and, with Gengou, discovered the phenomenon of complement fixation, the underlying principle of the Wassermann reaction and of similar tests. Bordet received the Nobel prize in 1919.

Among French surgeons, Just Lucas-Champonnière, who had been one of Lister's pupils, was a commanding figure. It was he who had introduced antisepsis into France and had written the first authoritative work on antiseptic surgery. Marin-Théodore Tuffier, surgeon to the Pitié, Lariboisière and Beaujon hospitals, was a surgeon of international reputation. He spent much time in the experimental laboratory and was a pioneer in surgery of the kidneys and lungs, in pyelography, and in spinal anesthesia. He was the author of monographs on experimental surgery of the kidneys, on the surgical treatment of pulmonary tuberculosis, and on subarachnoid anesthesia. In 1913, he performed the first successful valvotomy for the relief of chronic aortic stenosis and was the first surgeon to transport a wounded soldier by airplane. Among the younger surgeons, Réné Leriche, of Lyon and later of Strassburg, achieved notable success, particularly in the field of neurological and vascular surgery.

Paris, at this time, had two outstanding urologists in Félix Guyon and Joaquin Albarran y Dominguez. Guyon, a native of the Island of Réunion, was professor of genito-urinary surgery at Paris and a brilliant teacher, whose clinics at the Necker hospital attracted students from all over the world. Albarran, his pupil and successor, was a native of Cuba, studied medicine at Madrid, where he graduated at the age of 19, came to Paris, and rapidly achieved a reputation, first as a bacteriologist and pathologist, later as a surgeon. After he succeeded Guyon, he raised the reputation of the Necker hospital even higher as a center of genito-urinary surgical activity. This *Traité des tumeurs de la vessie,* published in 1891, introduced a classification based on embryological origin. His *Médecine opéra-*

toire de voies urinaires, which was published in 1908, was the greatest book of its kind during this period.

Switzerland claimed one of the great masters of surgery. "At the
head of the surgical profession today," wrote Garrison in 1924,
"stands, by common consent, the honored name of Theodor Kocher
of Bern." Theodor Kocher was born in Bern in 1841, studied in

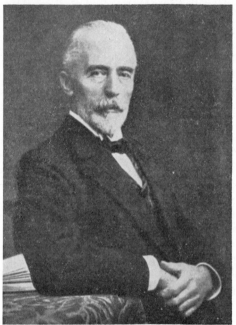

MacCollum and Taylor, *Nobel Prize-Winners,* Zurich, 1938

THEODOR KOCHER

Bern, graduated in Bern, was professor of surgery in Bern from
1872 until 1911, and died in Bern in 1917.

His life work centered on the problems of goitre—colloid and toxic,
for the achievements in which he received the Nobel prize in 1909.
He studied surgical problems in the operating room, in the physiological laboratory, and in the pathological laboratory. In addition
to his studies on goitre, he investigated intracranial pressure, lesions
of the spinal cord, and bullet wounds. Because of his skill and of
the perfect aseptic technique of his clinic, he was one of the first
surgeons successfully to resect and unite the intestines and to do
pioneer work in surgery of the abdomen. Calm, cool, imperturbable

and deliberate, he was complete master of every surgical condition he encountered. Kocher was a great favorite of Halsted, who resembled the Swiss surgeon in many ways. So it was natural that young Harvey Cushing, who "found Horsley preoccupied and everyone else in England on their holidays," (Fulton) left England and went to Bern to work with Kocher, whose interests were neurological. Cushing's first impressions were recorded in his diary for November 1, 1900:

> Kocher's clinic in A.M. . . . . But the operating!!—the J. H. H. outdone. It's easy to see why "the Professor" thought so highly of their work. Detailed technique, tedious operating, absolute hemostasis.

Hermann Sahli, the professor of internal medicine in Bern, was also a man of wide reputation. Like his colleague Kocher, Sahli was born in Bern, studied in Bern, graduated in Bern, and, after working with Cohnheim and Weigert in Leipzig, returned to Bern, where he became *Privatdozent* in 1882 and professor in 1888, holding this position until his retirement in 1929. He was an extremely active investigator and left his mark on many fields of internal medicine, particularly in diseases of the blood, of digestion, of the lungs, and in infectious diseases. He devised the well-known Sahli hemoglobinometer, still in use; described the anemia of ankylostomiasis, pseudo-chlorosis, and pseudo-anemia; introduced the methyl violet method for the estimation of free hydrochloric acid in the stomach; devised a micromethod for the estimation of blood sugar; and invented an arteriometer—an apparatus for measuring changes in the caliber of arteries, a pulsometer for measuring the rate of blood flow, and a blood pressure apparatus. He introduced salol, guaiacol and pantopon into therapeutics and was the author of a *Lehrbuch der klinischen Untersuchungsmethoden,* 1894, the most comprehensive work of its kind. It passed through seven German editions and was translated into English, Italian, Russian and Spanish. The English edition was long a favorite text in the United States.

In the nearby city of Zürich in 1911 the professor of surgery was a young man of 36, Ferdinand Sauerbruch, a native of Barmen. He was one of the pioneers in thoracic surgery and invented a low pressure cabinet, in which he placed his patients to prevent collapse of the lung. Later, he was professor of surgery at Munich and in Berlin and became an internationally known surgeon.

The outstanding Italian clinician of this period was Guido Baccelli (1832-1916), who, as Castiglioni remarks, "in many respects recalls the great Italian physicians of the Renaissance." Baccelli was eminent as a botanist, pathologist and clinician; as an educator, being at one time Minister of Public Education; as a hygienist who instituted measures for the sanitation of the Roman Campagna; and as a scholar who spoke Latin fluently and was active in promoting the excavations in the Roman Forum. He was an investigator in physical diagnosis, formulating the laws of the transmission of cardiac murmurs and describing aphonic pectoriloquy (Baccelli's sign). In therapeutics, he introduced the intravenous administration of quinine in malaria and treated aortic aneurysm by the introduction of a coiled wire into the aneurysmal sac. His best known publications were his *La patologia del cuore e dell'aorta* 1863-1867; and his *Di un nuovo metodo di cura gli aneurismi aortici,* 1856.

Edoardo Maragliano (1849-1940), professor of medicine at Genoa, is best remembered for his work on tuberculosis. In 1892, he prepared a vaccine for the treatment of tuberculosis. A senator of the realm, he was active in the promulgation of laws relating to public sanitation and to the health of workers. Pietro Grocco (1856-1916), professor at Berugia and Florence, gained a wide reputation as a student of pulmonary diseases and, in 1902, described "Grocco's sign." Guido Banti (1852-1925), professor of pathology at Florence, made important contributions on typhoid fever, pointing out that there was a blood stream infection in this disease. He is best remembered for his work on splenomegalic anemia, describing in 1898 the syndrome since known as Banti's disease.

Adelchi Negri (1876-1912), professor at Pavia, discovered in 1903 the "Negri bodies" in the brain of rabid animals, a discovery of great value in the diagnosis of rabies. Carlo Forlanini (1847-1918), professor of medicine at Pavia, introduced a new era in the treatment of pulmonary tuberculosis with the induction of artificial pneumothorax. Forlanini proposed this method in 1882 but did not carry it out until 1892. It gained universal acceptance in a few years and remains one of the great advances in the therapy of pulmonary tuberculosis.

Among surgeons, Edoardo Bassini (1844-1924), an old soldier in Garibaldi's army and later professor of surgery at Pavia, Genoa and Padua, enjoyed an international reputation. His reputation rests largely upon his operation for the radical cure of inguinal hernia, which, with some modifications, remains the operation employed today. Vittorio Putti, professor at Bologna, was a pioneer in kineplastic surgery.

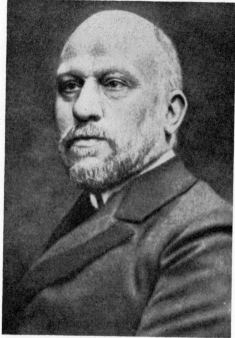

Biograph. Lex. Hervor. Ärzte, II, Berlin, 1933

ANGELO MOSSO

Aldo Castellani, a native of Florence, graduated at Florence in 1899 and went to London for three years to work at the School of Tropical Medicine. In 1903, while working in Uganda, he discovered *Trypanosoma gambiense* in the cerebrospinal fluid of patients suffering from sleeping sickness; in 1905, while in Ceylon, he discovered the spirochete of yaws (*Treponema pertenue*) and, in 1906, he discovered the spirochete of spirochetal bronchitis (Castellani's disease). He was successively professor of tropical medicine at Naples, lecturer at the London School of Tropical Medicine, professor of tropical medicine at Tulane University, and, during the Italo-Ethiopian War, was chief sanitary officer of the Italian Army. The remarkable health record of this army was largely the result of regulations initiated by Castellani. The *Manual of Tropical Medicine,* 1910, by Castellani and Chalmers is described by Garrison as "the standard text on tropical medicine in English."

Angelo Mosso (1846-1910) was one of the great physiologists of this period. Mosso graduated at Turin in 1870 and, after four years with Ludwig in Leipzig and with Claude Bernard, Ranvier and Marey in Paris, returned to Turin, where he became professor of physiology in 1879. A gifted investigator who was unusually skilled in technique, Mosso carried out many important investigations on fatigue, on circulation, and on respiration—investigations which brought him world wide fame and made his laboratory the greatest center for physiologic studies in Italy. He invented the ergograph, an instrument for measuring muscular work; the ponometer, an instrument for measuring pain; a sphygmomanometer for measuring the blood pressure in the finger; a plethysmograph, which measured the volume of organs; and many other useful types of apparatus. He studied intracranial and cerebral pressure, showed that fatigue is due to a toxin produced by muscular contraction, and studied respiration at high altitudes, believing the symptoms of distress to be due to a lack of carbon dioxide. He was the first physiologist to investigate apnea in man. During the last years of his life, he devoted himself to the study of archeology.

One of the great practical discoveries of this era was the introduction of an improved sphygmomanometer by Scipione Riva-Rocci, an assistant in the medical clinic of Carlo Forlanini in Pavia. The first accurate and practical instrument for the estimation of the blood pressure had been introduced by Samuel von Basch in 1880, 172

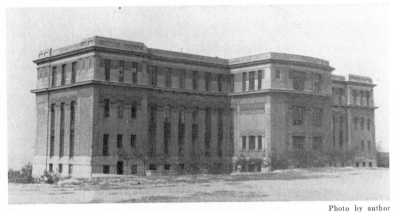

Photo by author

RAMÓN Y CAJAL INSTITUTE, MADRID

This institute, devoted to the study of the finer anatomy of the nervous system, was named in honor of the distinguished Spanish neurologist, who worked here the later years of his life.

years after Stephen Hales had discovered the blood pressure. The instrument consisted of a rubber ball filled with water, with a mercury manometer attached above it. The ball was pressed upon the pulse until the beat was obliterated, the point of disappearance registered by the manometer being considered the systolic pressure. Potain improved this instrument by attaching a rubber tube with an aneroid manometer to a compressible bulb filled with air. Neither instrument was widely used.

In 1896, Riva-Rocci introduced a new instrument consisting of a rubber bag, which was surrounded by a cuff of inelastic material connected with a mercury manometer, the cuff being placed about the arm. This instrument gradually made its way into medical practice and, in a few years, was used throughout the world. Sphygmomanometry was further advanced by the Russian, Nikolai Korotkoff, who introduced in 1905 the ausculation method of estimating the blood pressure. In a few years, the sphygmomanometer took its place, with the stethoscope and the clinical thermometer, as part of every physician's armamentarium.

In Spain, which had produced few medical men in the twentieth century with an international reputation, there appeared an outstanding anatomist—Santiago Ramón y Cajal (1852-1934). Employing the Golgi stain, with modifications of his own, Ramón y Cajal investigated the finer structure of the nervous system and made many extremely important fundamental discoveries in the field of neuropathology and neuroanatomy.

In Russia, there emerged Ivan Petrovich Pavlov, one of the greatest physiologists of modern times, who created two special fields of physiological endeavor—the relationship of psychic stimuli to digestion and the discovery of conditioned reflexes. Pavlov, the son of a poor village priest, was born in 1849 in Rjazan and studied at the University of St. Petersburg, where he received his degree and became instructor in physiology. After study with Heidenhain in Breslau and Ludwig in Leipzig, he returned to St. Petersburg, where he was successively associate professor and professor of physiology at the Army Medical Academy. In 1890, he became director of the Institute for Experimental Medicine.

Pavlov first studied the physiology of the circulation, but, as early as 1879, he published an article on digestion. During the following years, he worked on problems of digestion and summarized his investigations in his *Lectures on the Work of the Principal Digestive*

Glands, published in Russian in 1897 and translated into English in 1902. Pavlov's teacher, Heidenhain, had previously made a stomach pouch from which he could obtain pure gastric juice free from the admixture of food but, in the formation of his pouch, had destroyed the nerve supply. Pavlov, employing dogs with an improved technique, made a similar pouch or miniature stomach, with its nerve supply intact, and opening to the outside of the body. This pouch, the glands of which secreted gastric juice, was always referred

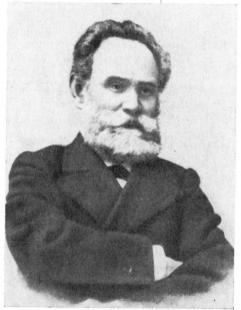

Les Médecins Célèbres, Paris, 1947

IVAN PAVLOV

to in Pavlov's laboratory, Babkin says, as the Heidenhain-Pavlov pouch. He next brought the esophagus to the surface of the body, where it was sutured, and then cut so that food taken by mouth would pass out of the upper end and food introduced into the lower end passed down into the stomach.

Pavlov found that the sight or smell of food caused copious secretion of both saliva and gastric juice, the secretion of gastric juice increasing as the animal was fed, even though the food never reached the stomach but passed out of the esophagus. The secretion, the result of this "sham feeding," he called the "psychic secretion." He also found that section of the vagus nerve abolished the secretion of gastric juice, proving that it is the secretory nerve of the gastric glands. When various foods, notably meat or meat extracts, were introduced into the stomach through the cut esophagus while the dog was inattentive or asleep, the mucosa of the pouch secreted gastric juice. Since this could not be the result of mechanical stimulation by the food, which some earlier observers had assumed to be the cause of gastric secretion, and as the quantity of the gastric juice, as well as its pepsin and hydrochloric acid content, varied with the different foods introduced, he considered this secretion the result of chemical stimulation and called it the "chemical secretion." For this most original work, Pavlov received the Nobel prize in 1904.

Impressed by the "psychic secretion" of the salivary and gastric glands, Pavlov next turned to a physiological study of this phenomenon, feeling that investigation of the psychic state of a dog was an unprofitable undertaking. The solution of this problem, to which he devoted 35 years, Pavlov, himself, considered his greatest achievement. Studying the secretion of the salivary glands by means of a fistula, he demonstrated two types of reflex actions—one inherited, the other developed from specific or psychic stimuli by training and association. This second type, the "conditioned reflex," was a physiological discovery of first rank and has had a profound influence not only on physiology but on psychology as well.

The outstanding work of Pavlov led to renewed interest in the problems of gastric digestion. These problems were intensively investigated by three American physiologists, who made important contributions to this field. Walter Cannon, while still a medical student at Harvard University, was impressed by the possibilities of employing an opaque material, impervious to x-rays, to study the processes of digestion in the intestinal tract and, in 1897, introduced bismuth to visualize the stomach. His paper on *The Movements of the Stomach studied by means of the Röntgen Rays,* published in 1898, was the first contribution to this most important field. Later, when professor of physiology at Harvard, he devoted himself mainly to the subject of the sympathetic nervous system, demonstrating the close relationship between the endocrine glands and the emotions, the role of the sympathetic-adrenal mechanism in the regulation of body functions, and the chemical mediation of nerve impulses.

Anton J. Carlson, a native of Bohuslän, Sweden, received his Ph.D. at Stanford University in 1902 and, afterwards, came to the University of Chicago, where he was appointed professor of physiology in

1914. Before coming to Chicago, Carlson had already achieved fame by the discovery that, in the Limulus crab, section of the cardiac nerve caused a cessation of the heart beat, proof of the neurogegic origin of the heart in this animal. In Chicago, he found, as Beaumont had in Alexis St. Martin, a patient who had a gastric fistula as the result of a gunshot wound. Carlson studied this patient with all the improved technical apparatus of a modern physiological laboratory and made many new and interesting discoveries. He registered the contractions of the stomach by inserting a bag connected with a kymograph and pointed out the importance of hunger pains and the contractions they produced. Carlson's *The Control of Hunger in Health and Disease,* published in 1916, contains a résumé of his most important work on gastric physiology.

Andrew C. Ivy, a graduate of Rush Medical College in 1922 and professor of physiology and pharmacology at Northwestern University, has studied especially the hormonal control of digestive processes. He has described cholecystokinin, which causes evacuation of the gallbladder; gastrin, which stimulates gastric secretion; enterogastrone, which inhibits gastric secretion; and urogastrone, which, likewise, produces an inhibition of gastric secretion.

Other American physiologists of this period made notable contributions to progress in other fields of physiology. Yandell Henderson, professor of applied physiology at Yale University, carried out important investigations upon the physiology of respiration and upon the volume output of the heart. He pointed out the importance of acapnia, showed that fatal apnoea could result from excessive forced breathing, and recommended the administration of carbon dioxide in conditions of shock, particularly in collapse due to anesthesia. Henderson also made important observations on the physiology of aviation and pointed out that high altitude flying could produce decompression sickness or caisson disease.

Lawrence Joseph Henderson, professor of biological chemistry at Harvard University, was gifted with an unusual capacity for abstract thinking and an ability to point out the common ground between the theoretical and the practical. In 1908, he formulated the theory of acid-base equilibrium, a discovery of far-reaching significance. After years of investigation, he demonstrated, for the first time, the quantitative relationship in eight variables in the blood. He adopted the teleological interpretation of vital functions and, in his well-known work, *The Fitness of the Environment,* set forth the relation of the properties of water in its various physical states to living phenomena. In his later years, Henderson turned his attention more and more towards sociology and became especially interested in the laws of social equilibria, a field in which he was particularly fascinated by the thinking of Pareto.

Another physiologist of distinction is John Farquhar Fulton, professor of physiology at Yale University since 1930. A graduate of Harvard Medical School, a Rhodes student at Oxford, and fellow of Magdalen College, Fulton has made important studies on cerebral function and on the physiological aspects of aviation and has contributed numerous scholarly papers to the history of medicine. After the death of W. H. Howell, he has edited Howell's well-known *Textbook of Physiology,* has written an authoritative *Physiology of the Nervous System,* an important work on *Muscular Contraction and the Reflex Control of Movement,* and is the author of *Readings in Physiology,* an anthology of the great physiological discoveries from the earliest times to the present. He has written many articles on physiological and historical subjects, and his *Harvey Cushing, A Biography* belongs to the best and lasting in medical biography. Fulton combines scientific originality with exact scholarship and a broad cultural background, giving a distinctive accuracy as well as charm to all his writings.

Howard W. Haggard, professor of applied physiology at Yale since 1938 and director of the laboratory, has made many contributions to physiology, particularly on noxious gases and respiration, and to the history of medicine. His *Devils, Drugs, and Doctors; The Lame, the Halt, and the Blind;* and *The Doctor in History* belong to the best books of their type, combining accurate scholarship with an unusually readable style. As editor of the *Quarterly Journal of Studies on Alcohol,* he is engaged in a scientific study of one of the most pressing problems of human society.

Medical education in North America, as we have seen, was deeply influenced by the example of the Johns Hopkins, which, according to Abraham Flexner, "was the first medical school in America of genuine university type." Johns Hopkins, however, exerted its influence only by example. A more powerful and somewhat acrid stimulus to improvement in medical education was supplied by Flexner's report on *Medical Education in the United States and Canada,* which was published in 1910.

The multiplication of medical schools in the United States during the nineteenth century was a striking phenomenon. Medical colleges "multiplied without restraint, now by fission, now by sheer spontaneous generation. . . . Wherever and whenever the roster of untitled practitioners rose above half a dozen, a medical school was likely at any moment to be precipitated" (Flexner). The distinction of being a "professor" had great powers of attraction for the practitioner.

Between 1810 and 1840, 26 new medical schools sprang up; between 1840 and 1876, an additional 47 appeared; between 1876 and 1910, the number existing in 1876 has more than doubled. Illinois gave birth to 39 medical colleges, 42 sprang up in Missouri, 43 in New York, 27 in Indiana, 20 in Pennsylvania, and 18 in Tennessee. The city of Cincinnati brought forth 20, the city of Louisville 18. The United States and Canada, in the course of a century, produced 457 medical schools, many of them short-lived and about 50 fraudulent. In 1910, the city of Chicago had 14 medical schools, Missouri 12, New York State 11, and Tennessee nine.

During the years 1909 and 1910, Flexner visited all the medical schools in the United States and Canada, 155 in number, and reported facts as he found them, the instruction given the students, the physical assets of the schools, their yearly budgets, and many other pertinent details. His report was a highly explosive document. Many medical schools castigated in his report closed their doors; others less harshly criticized set about to improve conditions. Flexner's report was ably seconded by the American Medical Association's Council on Medical Education, which carried on where Flexner left off. In 1949, instead of 143 medical schools, the *Journal of the American Medical Association* lists 72 "approved medical schools" in the United States and Canada.

Another event of significance in the scientific world was the foundation in 1901 of the Rockefeller Institute for Medical Research "to conduct, assist and encourage investigations in the sciences and arts of hygiene, medicine and surgery and allied subjects." This institution soon became to physicians and the public alike what the Pasteur Institute represented to France. In 1912, Alexis Carrel (1873-1944), a native of France and a worker at the Rockefeller Institute, received the Nobel prize in medicine, the first time this award had crossed the Atlantic. Under the direction of Simon Flexner, the Rockefeller Institute continued to make notable contributions in chemistry, infectious diseases, parasitology, tumor research, and virus diseases.

Here Noguchi, in 1913, demonstrated the *spirochaeta pallida* in the brain of paretics and ended all argument about the relationship of syphilis to paresis. In 1940, Landsteiner and Wiener at the Institute discovered a new blood group factor, the Rh factor, which plays

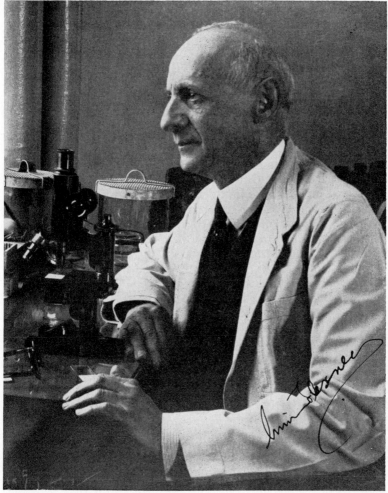

Kindness of Charles A. Doan

SIMON FLEXNER

an important role in causing reactions in blood transfusions and is responsible for Erythroblastosis fetalis.

In 1915, the department of animal pathology of the Rockefeller Institute was established at Princeton, New Jersey, under the direction of Theobald Smith. To quote J. Fischer, Smith "belongs among the most important investigators in the fields of bacteriology and epidemiology." He was the first to describe pleomorphism in bacteria (1886), to produce immunity in hog cholera with filtered extracts of the specific organisms (1884-1886), to discover the parasite of Texas fever (1889), to prove its transmission by the cattle tick, and to demonstrate anaphylaxis from the bacterial products of the diphtheria bacillus (1903), a discovery called by Ehrlich "the Theobald Smith phenomenon."

Increasing interest in the subject of tropical diseases and in the health problems facing a rapidly growing and expanding nation led to the establishment of schools of public health in the United States. Johns Hopkins, a pioneer in this field, founded in 1918 a school of public health with W. H. Howell as dean. This school soon achieved a great reputation, the work of McCollum on vitamins and of Raymond Pearl on biostatistics being especially noteworthy. Harvard established in 1922 a school of public health and tropical diseases, where important investigations were carried out by Rosenau, Strong, Wolbach, Sellards and others. In 1946, Tulane University established a department of tropical medicine and public health, which rapidly achieved distinction for the quality of its instruction and its research. Here the work of Bass, Faust and Craig was noteworthy. These schools, in addition to carrying out important investigations, have also trained many physicians who planned to devote themselves to careers in public health rather than to the private practice of medicine.

The Boer War, which began on October 11, 1899, and lasted two and one-half years, was a dark chapter in the history of sanitation. In this bitter struggle, the British Army lost 8,000 in battle while 14,000 died from preventable diseases. Typhoid fever attacked 57,684 soldiers, of whom 8,022 died. The typhoid bacillus had actually killed more than the bullets of the Boers.

Two years before the outbreak of the Boer War, Almoth E. Wright, professor of pathology in the Army School at Netley, had recommended the use of a vaccine prepared from killed typhoid bacilli as a preventive of typhoid fever. In 1899, this method was employed in the Indian Army with excellent results, and, with the outbreak of the Boer War, the British authorized the use of antityphoid vaccination in the army serving in South Africa.

Unfortunately, this vaccination was voluntary, instead of compulsory; the procedure was carried out in a haphazard fashion; the vaccine employed was often improperly prepared; records were carelessly kept and often lost. "No complete statistics of antityphoid vaccination in South Africa have ever been published, and they probably do not exist" (Russell). When typhoid fever showed an in-

creasing toll of victims, the army authorities decided that antityphoid inoculation was without value and ordered that antityphoid
vaccination cease.

For two years after the close of the war, the controversy over the
merits of antityphoid vaccination raged. Finally, a Royal Commission, after an exhaustive study of the question, made a favorable
report and rehabilitated the generally discredited procedure of antityphoid vaccination. In 1911, following a study of the subject by
Colonel Frederick F. Russell of the United States Army, the American Army, after a brief period of voluntary vaccination, introduced
"unequivocal compulsion." The results were startling. The typhoid
rate per 1000, which had been 2.43 in 1910, fell to 0.31 in 1912 and
to zero in 1913.

The first World War brought profound changes in the political,
social and economic structure of the world, changes which left their
impress also on medicine. Varied as the conclusions were regarding
the causes of the war, there is universal agreement with the statement of Hermann Sudermann that it was "the most gigantic imbe-
cility since the Crusades."

While the events leading up to the war caused many critics to as-
sert that the diplomats and statesmen at the helm in the various
states had learned little from history of the past and that certain
generals had learned nothing from the mistakes of previous wars,
the same criticism could scarcely be hurled at the medical services.

Typhoid fever, which had caused so many fatalities in the American Civil War, in the Spanish-American War, and in the Boer War,
played a minor role in the American Army during the first World
War. This was the result of careful inspection of the water supplies,
of proper disposal of sewage, and, especially, of compulsory antityphoid vaccination, which had been introduced into the American
Army in 1911. During World War I, 227 soldiers in the American
Army of 4,128,479 died of typhoid fever. If the death rate had been
that of the American Civil War, 51,133 soldiers would have died of
the disease; if the rate of the Spanish-American War had prevailed,
68,164 soldiers would have succumbed to the fever.

During the first few months of the war, tetanus exacted a heavy
toll of life in the British Army, the rate at one time being as high as
32 per 1000 wounded. By 1915, the British had learned their lesson
and had instituted prophylactic injections of tetanus antitoxin for
all wounded soldiers, a procedure which caused a sharp decrease in
the number of cases. The American Army profited by this experi-

ence and employed tetanus antitoxin in all wounded soldiers. The records of the Surgeon-General's Office in Washington show only four deaths from tetanus in the American Army from April 17, 1917, to December 31, 1919. During the American Civil War, two wounded soldiers out of each 1000 developed tetanus; whereas, during the first World War, less than two in 100,000 developed the disease.

The epidemic of typhus fever, which swept through Serbia in 1914, was reminiscent of the earlier ravages of this disease during the Thirty Years' War and in Napoleon's ill-fated invasion of Russia. Serbia had less than 400 doctors, most of whom contracted the disease and 126 of whom died. In six months, more than 150,000 people perished, and one-quarter of the Serbian Army died of typhus fever.

However, the disease did not spread widely outside Serbia. The Austrian and German army authorities, quite aware that lice spread the disease, introduced a rigid quarantine and deloused all prisoners of war as well as their clothing and baggage, with the result that the disease never became a menace, although there were isolated minor outbreaks, particularly in some prison camps. Typhus was never a problem in the United States Army during World War I. In 1917, there were only seven cases with no deaths; in 1918, there were 11 cases with two deaths; in 1919, no cases. Little typhus occurred in the armies of Britain, France, Italy and Germany, more in the armies of Russia and Austria, an eloquent bit of testimony as to which people were prone to harbor lice. At that time, Austria was in part a Balkan nation, and sanitation in the Balkans and in Russia stood at the bottom of the scale. After the withdrawal of Russia from the war, the Russian Revolution was followed by a chaos in hygienic as well as in political conditions, and typhus fever flourished again in Russia, as of old.

The pandemic of influenza in 1918 was truly global in character. Boston, New York, San Francisco, London, Paris, Berlin, Bombay and Calcutta all showed a sharp rise in their mortality rates. Such widely separated countries as Russia, Argentina, Australia, and the Philippines were attacked by the disease. Influenza entered the United States about the first of September, 1918, and spread with amazing rapidity, particularly in army camps, where large numbers of men were concentrated, training for overseas service. Influenza stalked through these camps, striking down victims right and left.

The Army Medical Corps had never seen such an appalling amount of illness. At Camp Devens, where 30,000 men were quartered, the base hospital, which had a maximum capacity of 2,500 beds, soon had 8,000 patients. In some army camps, 30 per cent of the soldiers became ill within a period of three weeks.

The disease was more severe among the recent recruits than among the seasoned troops. The figure for the last 17 weeks in 1918 show that the troops in the United States (1,493,000) showed an incidence of 22.6 per cent, whereas the American Expeditionary Force (1,745,000) had an incidence of only 4.5. Influenza took a staggering toll of life in the American Army—24,000 soldiers died of it, as compared with 34,000 killed in battle. In the wake of influenza came an epidemic of encephalitis lethargica, first clearly described by von Economo.

From the scientific standpoint, the experience of the Army Medical Department with influenza was most unsatisfactory. Here was an unparalleled opportunity to study a great epidemic, yet it came and went, leaving its etiological agent, mode of transmission, methods of control and prevention still shrouded in mystery. The influenza bacillus of Pfeiffer, which, at the beginning of the epidemic, was considered the specific agent, was found with such varying frequency that it was soon relegated to the role of a secondary invader. The opinion presently gained ground that influenza was caused by a filtrable virus, a viewpoint later proved correct when Smith, Andrews and Laidlaw, in 1933, produced the disease in ferrets by inoculating them intranasally with filtrates of throat washings obtained from patients early in the course of the disease. In 1940, Magill and Francis, working independently, discovered another virus of influenza, which has been called B virus to distinguish it from the first virus discovered, now known as A virus.

Empyema, a common complication of influenza, was, in the early period of the epidemic, treated by prompt surgical drainage, according to the accepted practice. The mortality rate was appalling, varying from 60 per cent to 85 per cent. Later, when necropsy showed that most of the victims still had an active pneumonia, repeated aspiration of the fluid was practiced and operation postponed. The death rate soon fell to nine per cent. This valuable wartime surgical lesson soon found its way into civilian surgery.

Many new and powerful antiseptics had been discovered prior to the first World War, so they were now employed in an attempt to sterilize the wounds. They failed to sterilize and, in most instances, were not only irritating, but actually harmful. The best results were obtained by using continuous irrigation with a neutral sodium hypochlorite solution—the Carrel-Dakin method.

A French Army surgeon, Georges Gross, who found the Carrel-Dakin method tedious and time-consuming, in 1915, began to experiment with a simpler method. He removed the bullet or shell fragment from the wound, together with any dead tissue, and then sewed the wound together. At the close of the war, Gross stated that he had sewn up nearly 80 per cent of the wounds he had seen and that 88.8 per cent of these had healed promptly.

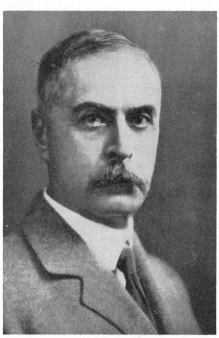

Biograph. Lex. Hervor. Ärzte, II, Berlin, 1933

CARL LANDSTEINER

Another radical departure was introduced by H. Winnett Orr, a lieutenant colonel in the American Medical Corps. Orr cleaned out the wound, packed it with petrolatum gauze and then applied a plaster cast, making no attempt to sterilize the wound. He found that most of his patients whose legs or arms were enclosed in plaster casts stood the trip from France to America with no difficulty and arrived home in excellent condition. Orr's method at the time gained no widespread approval, but it was trimphantly vindicated 15 years later in the Spanish Civil War.

The use of high explosives in the first World War produced mutilating wounds on a scale never before seen. This called for much ingenuity on the part of the plastic surgeons, who developed new skills and whose ingenuity wrote a new chapter in the progress of surgery. Many new procedures were employed in amputations, and greatly improved prosthetic devices were worked out.

Throughout the war, fighting was heavy and bloody, and the lives of many severely wounded soldiers were saved by blood transfusions. The subject of blood transfusion had been a hotly debated issue since the initial observations of Lower in the seventeenth century. In 1901, while studying blood agglutinins, Carl Landsteiner had shown that certain blood contained agglutinins for one specimen of blood but not for others. He succeeded in demonstrating that all blood can be classified into three definite groups, a discovery of great fundamental importance since it placed blood transfusion for the first time on a scientific as well as safe basis. It had previously been frequently observed that violent reactions, or even death, could follow a blood transfusion if the donor's blood was "incompatible." Landsteiner gave the explanation of this incompatibility. During the first World War, Captain Oswald H. Robertson, an American Army surgeon, found in 1918 that the blood of donors obtained under sterile precautions and mixed with a sodium citrate solution could be preserved in an ice-box for a month without deterioration and could be employed at any desired moment. This was the beginning of "blood banks," later established in many hospitals.

When the Armistice of November 11, 1918, brought the war to an end, the nations sat down soberly to study their losses. During World War I, more than 60,000,000 men had been mobilized, nearly 7,000,000 were killed in battle, and more than 19,000,000 were wounded. Appalling as these losses were, the number of civilians who died from direct or indirect causes was even greater. The Civil War in Russia led to a complete breakdown of even the most elementary sanitation and health regulations. There were more than 20,000,000 cases of typhus fever with more than 3,000,000 deaths. In 1921, there were more than 200,000 cases of cholera, 300,000 cases of typhoid fever, and 80,000 cases of smallpox. Syphilis assumed epidemic proportions. In 1922 in some parts of Russia, 80 per cent of the population were infected, and, in 1923, this percentage rose to 95 per cent. The number of civilians who died in Russia from disease, exposure and privation exceeded the combined battle losses of all the belligerents.

The subsequent triumph of the Bolshevik or Communist Party in Russia and the gradual rise of Russia as one of the dominant nations of the world is one of the most significant historical facts of the present century. Along with profound economic and social changes came equally profound changes in the scientific aims and methods in the fields of medical research and practice. Many observers have returned from tours or periods of observation in Russia quite enthusiastic about the advances of Russian medical science, the well-equipped hospitals and medical institutes and loud in their praise of the excellent medical care available to the sick. Others, while admitting the great improvement in medical care, have been less impressed by their medical discoveries and have pointed out that the Nobel prize in medicine has been given to only two Russians—Pavlov and Metchnikoff, both before Russia became a Communist nation. They also express grave doubts regarding the future of science in a nation that demands a Marxian approach to all matters of science and from time to time prescribes the proper

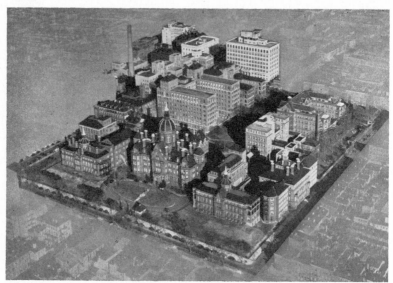

French, *History of the University founded by Johns Hopkins*, Baltimore, 1946

JOHNS HOPKINS HOSPITAL IN 1930

This aerial photograph shows the marked expansion of the Johns Hopkins Hospital in a period of forty years.

"party line" for scientists, musicians and artists as well as for political functionaries.

As we review the mortality and morbidity tables of the American, British, French and German Armies during the first World War, it is obvious that the medical departments of those armies had profited by the lessons of the past and from newer discoveries of medicine. The German official figures were 1,531,048 killed, while 155,013 died from disease, nearly 10 times as many killed as died from disease, a better health record than the previous record of the Japanese, who, in the Russo-Japanese War, had astonished the world by reporting four times as many deaths from battle as from disease. The record of the American Army was not so good. There were 47,940 killed in battle or dying later from wounds, and 50,714 died of disease. In comparison with the Civil War, where 61.04 per 1000 died of disease, the statistics of the first World War with 16.67 per 1000 dying of disease, showed marked improvement. The old diseases, smallpox, typhoid fever, tetanus and diphtheria, were kept to a minimum by preventive inoculation; yellow fever never appeared. Meningitis in the army camps took a heavy toll. "The sputum-borne infections, particularly the pneumonias, remained the insoluble problem of the war" (Garrison).

Germany, the loser in the war, faced a very uncertain future. Like the other belligerents, she had lost many of her brightest youth in the war and found at the end of it her country bankrupt, her political system a near chaos, and her famous universities badly shattered and in a precarious state. It seemed a vain hope that she could ever again play more than a very subordinate role in the world of science, where she had so recently ruled.

Yet, in 1924, six years after the close of the war, Flexner wrote in a survey of medical education in America, England, France and Germany:

There the German universities stand—still as a group the best organized, the best equipped, and the most soundly conceived that exist. Neither teaching nor research has stopped. With a tenacity that shows how deeply rooted in the natural consciousness is the respect for learning, scientists, young as well as old, are struggling to produce.

Again in 1930, Flexner wrote in a study of American, English and German universities, "Of the countries dealt with in this volume, Germany has in theory and practice come nearest to giving higher education its due."

Looking back through the perspective of two decades, it seems apparent now that this post-war period in Germany was an Indian summer, to be followed by the bleakest of winters.

In the United States and Canada, the post-war problems were small in comparison with those of the Old World. The United States had suffered no devastation, no famine, no widespread and prolonged epidemics of disease, no political upheavals, and the losses from battle were small in comparison to those of the other belligerents. The post-war period saw an unprecedented growth of medical schools and hospitals, marked improvement in the quality of medical instruction, and an increasing interest in medical research. An important role in this advance was played by the Rockefeller Foundation, founded in 1913 "to promote the well-being of mankind throughout the world." This Foundation was world-wide in its scope. It gave generous assistance both in money and in personnel to various countries in their battle against disease and aid in the development of medical, public health and nursing education in many countries, assisting them by providing new buildings with endowments as well as by establishing fellowships for study and research. These benefactions were given not only to our war-time allies but to defeated Germany and Austria as well. In the United States itself, the Foundation gave large sums to assist medical schools in providing new buildings and in improving the existing medical education as well as for raising the standards of medical practice.

In 1929, the Rockefeller Foundation, in addition to other benefactions, founded at Johns Hopkins an Institute of Medical History and established a professorship of medical history, whose first incumbent was William H. Welch. This Institute, in 1930, appointed Fielding H. Garrison as its librarian, a most auspicious beginning. Fielding H. Garrison, a graduate in arts at Johns Hopkins, entered the Surgeon-General's Library in Washington as a clerk, meanwhile studying medicine at Georgetown University. He received his M.D. in 1893, but the practice of medicine had little appeal for him, and

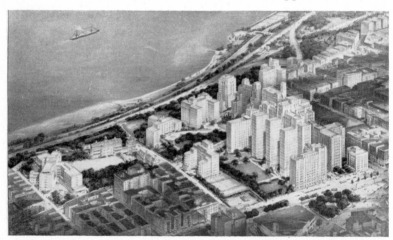

Sigerist, *Amerika und die Medizin*, Leipzig, 1933

THE COLUMBIA-PRESBYTERIAN MEDICAL CENTER IN NEW YORK, 1933

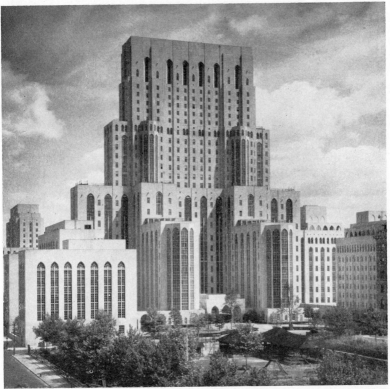

Sigerist, *Amerika und die Medizin*, Leipzig, 1933

THE NEW YORK HOSPITAL-CORNELL MEDICAL CENTER IN NEW YORK, 1933

he continued to work as assistant librarian for 40 years, with the exception of two years of military service in the Philippines.

During the years at the Surgeon-General's Library, much of his work was the preparation of the *Index Catalogue* and the *Index Medicus,* at first under the guidance of Billings and Fletcher. On the death of the latter, Garrison became editor of both publications. He gained an unrivalled familiarity with medical literature, both ancient and modern, working in a library unparalleled for its collection of medical books from the earliest times to the present. Gifted with an unusually retentive memory, a lover of literature as well as a gifted musician, he wrote with great accuracy and charm and enlivened his accounts of medical events with interesting allusions and anecdotes drawn from his wide cultural background.

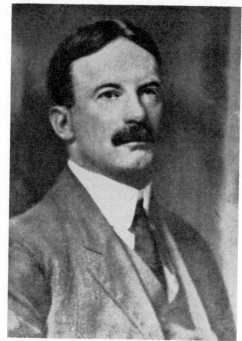

Bull. Inst. Hist. Med., 1937

FIELDING GARRISON

A photograph of Dr. Garrison about the time he published the first edition of his *Introduction to the History of Medicine,* 1913.

Garrison's chief claim to fame is his *Introduction to the History of Medicine,* which first appeared in 1913, subsequent editions appearing in 1917, 1921, 1924 and 1929. Despite its modest title, this work is a comprehensive history of medicine of some 900 pages, with reference to more than 3600 medical authors. Its wealth of references makes it the starting point for any student desiring to pursue investigations on any phase of medical history. Its success was instantaneous. "It probably has done more than any other work to foster and promote an interest in medical history" (Guthrie).

In addition to this work, Garrison wrote many articles dealing with various phases of medical history, and his *Revised Students' Check-List of Texts Illustrating the History of Medicine,* 1933, proved so valuable that it was revised and re-issued in 1943 by Leslie

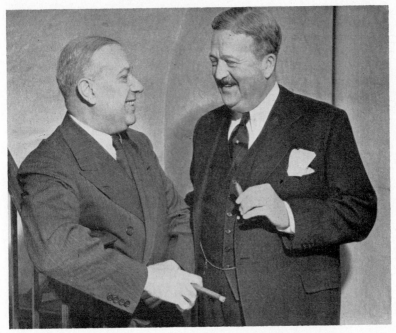

HENRY E. SIGERIST (LEFT) AND LOGAN CLENDENING (RIGHT)
Photograph taken in 1940.

T. Morton under the title, *A Medical Bibliography*. It is an invaluable reference book, containing a list of 5506 classics of medical literature with brief notes.

Welch resigned the professorship of medical history at the Institute in 1932, and Professor Henry E. Sigerist of Leipzig, favorite pupil and successor of Sudhoff, accepted the chair. Sigerist, born in Paris of Swiss parents, studied medicine at Munich and at Zürich, where he received his M.D. in 1917. He qualified as a *Privatdozent* for the history of medicine at Zürich. Later, he came to Leipzig to work with Sudhoff, whom he succeeded on the latter's retirement in 1925. Sigerist was an ideal choice for the position. An accomplished linguist, speaking four modern languages with equal fluency and reading Latin, Greek and Arabic with great ease, a careful and exact scholar trained by the master Sudhoff, a graceful and facile writer, a charming and polished speaker, he soon made the Institute the center of medical historical activity in the New World. He also founded the *Bulletin of the Institute of the History of Medicine,*

the first number of which appeared in January, 1933, and the November issue of which published Garrison's *Revised Students'*
Check-List. The Institute published 457 articles and monographs on
the history of medicine from 1929 to 1947. In 1947, Sigerist resigned
from his chair at Johns Hopkins and returned to his native Switzerland to devote his time entirely to writing *A History of Medicine,*
which he had planned for 25 years. The first volume of this monumental work, which he intends to complete in eight volumes, was
published early in 1951 and has been enthusiastically acclaimed by
reviewers and students of medical history.

The study of medical history received a great stimulus from the
foundation of the Institute of Medical History at Johns Hopkins in
1930, this subject thus being formally recognized as part of the
medical curriculum. However, it had by no means been entirely
neglected before that time. Osler, Welch, and other kindred spirits,
as early as 1890, had founded the Johns Hopkins Society of Medical
History, which met usually once a month and before the meetings
of which Osler, Welch, Cushing, McCrae, Steiner, MacCallum,
Hemmeter, Friedenwald and others read noteworthy papers on historical topics. In Chicago, a group of historically minded physicians
founded the Chicago Society of Medical History, and their *Bulletin,*
which has appeared continually since 1911, is a veritable mine of
information for the student of medical history. In Philadelphia,
David Riesman inaugurated a course in medical history and contributed himself many excellent articles on medical history. His
book, *The Story of Medicine in the Middle Ages,* remains today a
standard work on this subject.

At the University of Wisconsin, W. S. Miller, the anatomist,
founded a seminar in medical history, which stimulated great interest in this subject. Many papers of exceptional merit were read at
the meetings and subsequently published. Two of the active partici-
pants in the seminar, William S. Middleton and Chauncey D. Leake,
have since became well-known as active and gifted medical historians. At the University of Kansas, Logan Clendening, a brilliant
and unusual person, a colorful physician and scholar, established
a course in the history of medicine and wrote many interesting and
fascinating articles on historical medicine, in addition to several
books notable for their attractive style as well as their sound scholarship. He traveled widely and assembled an excellent collection of
books and a museum of medical history. In Philadelphia, Victor
Robinson created a department of medical history at Temple University and founded *Medical Life* (1920), the first American journal
in this field, which awakened a slumbering interest in medical his-

tory among wide circles of the medical profession. Robinson's *Story of Medicine* (1931), while written largely for the laity, has been called by competent critics one of the best one volume histories of medicine ever published.

The founding of the *Annals of Medical History* in 1917 was an outstanding factor in the promotion of interest in historical medicine. Under the able editorship of Francis R. Packard, this admirable journal published numerous articles of first rank and was noteworthy for its excellent illustrations and beautiful topography. Paul G. Hoeber, its publisher, spared neither pains nor expense in producing an artistic publication, and, in this respect, no historical or medical journal has ever equaled it. It ceased publication in 1942 to the great regret of its readers.

The American Association of the History of Medicine was founded in 1924 and became particularly active after the establishment of the Johns Hopkins Institute of Medical History, the *Bulletin* of which in 1939 became the official organ of the Association. The *Bulletin* has continued to be the mouthpiece of the Association and has constantly gained in prestige and reputation. A recent addition to this field, the *Journal of the History of Medicine and Allied Sciences,* Volume I bearing the date of 1946, has, under the editorship of George Rosen, immediately taken rank as an authoritative journal.

A powerful impetus to the study of medical history came from George Sarton, who became interested in the history and philosophy of science soon after his graduation from the University of Ghent. In 1912, he founded *Isis,* an international review devoted to the history of science, and, in 1927, published the first volume of his *Introduction to the History of Science,* two additional volumes of which have since appeared. This monumental work, which describes with accuracy and precision the progress of philosophy, religion, mathematics, astronomy, physics, chemistry, geography, natural history, medicine, historiography, law, sociology, education and philology, from the earliest times through the fourteenth century, is an imposing example of twentieth century scholarship. Sarton founded in 1936 *Osiris,* a journal of the history and philosophy of science and culture and, in 1940, was appointed professor of the history of science at Harvard.

A very important journal devoted to medical history and familiar to four generations of readers is *Janus, Zeitschrift für Geschichte und Literatur der Medicin,* as the title page of the first issue describes it. The first number appeared in Breslau in 1846 under the editorship of A. W. E. Th. Henschel, who had as associate editors such stalwarts as Bussemaker, Daremberg, Choulant, Haeser, Hecker and Wüstenfelt. After three years' struggle, *Janus* gave up the ghost but was revived in 1853 and, after two years' battling, once more disappeared. *Janus* was again revived in 1896, 50 years after its founding, under the editorship of H. F. A. Peypens and, for nearly a half century, published articles of lasting worth in English, French and German, numbering among its contributors and editors the leading medical historians of the period. It ceased publication in 1940, another victim of the Second World War.

A striking feature of medical practice during the early years of the twentieth century was the development of private clinics in various

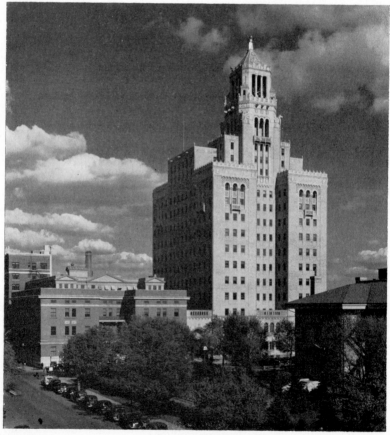

THE MAYO CLINIC

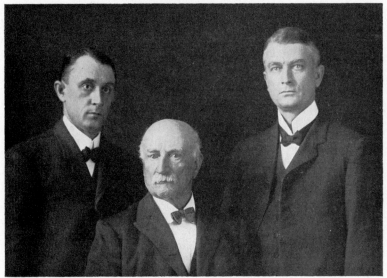

Wilder, *The Mayo Clinic, Rochester*, 1936

THE MAYOS

Dr. Charles Mayo, Dr. William W. Mayo, Dr. William J. Mayo.

parts of the United States. These clinics were consciously or unconsciously patterned after the Mayo Clinic at Rochester, Minnesota, which already, in the closing years of the nineteenth century, had attained a national reputation that became international.

The beginning of the Mayo Clinic dates from the opening of St. Mary's Hospital in Rochester in 1889 with 13 patients and a professional staff of three surgeons—William W. Mayo and his two sons, William J. and Charles H. Mayo. William W. Mayo was at that time 70 years of age, so the burden of the work fell upon his sons, on William J., who had been in general practice six years, and on Charles H., who had graduated the previous year. Neither brother had served as a hospital intern, and both were acutely conscious of their own limitations. In the beginning, the brothers did a general practice with emphasis on surgery but, as the years rolled on, devoted themselves exclusively to surgery, in which their remarkable skill and judgment presently raised them to the ranks of the great.

"In the years previous to 1900," wrote the Mayos, "the Clinic was essentially a well organized surgical practice." In 1901, a new era of organization began with the development of laboratories of pathology and experimental medicine. The completion of the Mayo Clinic building in 1914 provided additional space for medical research, and the establishment of the Mayo Foundation in affiliation with the University of Minnesota instituted a very extensive program of graduate medical education, making the Clinic one of the most important graduate medical institutions in the world. The fellows chosen by the Mayo Foundation study at the Clinic for three years, at the end of which period a certain number take advanced degrees. The alumni of the Mayo Foundation are now scattered throughout the world and hold responsible positions in medical centers in Great Britain, South Africa, Switzerland, Spain, Italy and China.

The growth of the Mayo Clinic has been phenomenal. In 1897, there were 915 surgical operations performed; in 1900, 1,823; in 1912, 9,168; in 1924, 23,628; and in 1949, 38,000. The number of patients registered in the Clinic in 1912 was 15,130; in 1924, 60,063; and in 1949, 141,772.

The members of the staff at the Mayo Clinic have made many important contributions to medicine. Noteworthy have been the introduction by Plummer in 1923 of iodine in the preoperative preparation of patients suffering from hyperthyroidism, a procedure which has saved countless lives; the isolation of thyroxin by Kendall in 1915; and the preparation of cortisone by Kendall and his co-workers in 1936. In addition to these noteworthy contributions, the staff of the Mayo Clinic has comprised a large number of outstanding specialists whose work is inextricably woven into the fabric of modern medicine. Edward C. Rosenow, bacteriologist; Walter C. Alvarez, Arley Barnes, Norman Keith, Philip Hench, Leonard Rowntree, Russell Wilder, Fredrik Willius, George Eusterman, H. Z. Giffin, J. Arnold Bargen and George Brown, internists; E. Starr Judd, Donald C. Balfour, Waltman Walters, Claude Dixon, William Braasch, and Fred Rankin, surgeons; Russell Carmen, radiologist; Paul O'Leary, syphilologist; and Henry F. Helmholtz, pediatrician, are but a few of the many well known to this generation.

Several other clinics were established in other parts of the United States, and their success has proved the correctness and vitality of the group practice idea when properly carried out. Outstanding among these are the Lahey Clinic in Boston, the Cleveland Clinic in Cleveland, and the Ochsner Clinic in New Orleans. A somewhat different approach was that of Arthur E. Hertzler, who, after an intensive medical education in the United States and Germany, returned to the town of Halstead, Kansas, a small hamlet ignored by the express trains, where he established a clinic. This clinic, under his skillful guidance, attained national fame. In addition to carrying on a large surgical practice, Hertzler was the author of 10 books on surgical pathology and found time to write several other books, among them his autobiography, *The Horse and Buggy Doctor,* which was a best seller.

One of the great achievements of the early years of the twentieth century was the discovery of insulin. The trail which led to this momentous discovery had been followed for several centuries. In 1674, Thomas Willis noted that the urine of diabetics "was wonderfully sweet as if it were imbued with Honey or Sugar," and Matthew Dobson, in 1776, proved by evaporating diabetic urine that it did contain sugar. In 1889, von Mering and Minkowsky made the enlightening discovery that extirpation of the pancreas in dogs produced diabetes; and, in 1900, Opie described lesions of the islands of Langerhans in fatal diabetes. The British physiologist, Edward Sharpey-Schafer, impressed by these observations, concluded that the islands of Langerhans must secrete a substance which controls carbohydrate metabolism. In 1916, he proposed the name of insulin for this hypothetical internal secretion of the pancreas.

In 1920, a young Canadian orthopedic surgeon, Frederick Banting, settled down in practice at London, Ontario, after service overseas in the Canadian Army. Obtaining a post as demonstrator of physiology in the University of Western Ontario, he became interested in diabetes and later went to the University of Toronto, where he worked on the problem with a young second-year medical student, Charles H. Best, in the laboratory of Professor J. J. R. Macleod. In 1922, eight months after they had begun their experiments, Banting, aged 30, and Best, aged 23, announced the discovery of insulin, a discovery which has revolutionized the treatment of diabetes mellitus.

The discovery of insulin gave a fresh and powerful impetus to the study of endocrinology. The concept of a hormone was suggested by Théophile Bordeu, the "vitalist," in 1775. He taught that each gland and organ of the body produced a specific secretion which passed into the blood and maintained the functions of the body in equilibrium. It was, however, only a theory, and he performed no confirmatory experiments. Claude Bernard, in 1855, introduced the term, "internal secretion," in describing his work on the glycogenetic function of the liver and later included the thyroid and the adrenals among the organs having an internal secretion. Edward Brown-Séquard studied from 1856 until 1893 the internal secretions of the thyroid, adrenals, testes, and pituitary

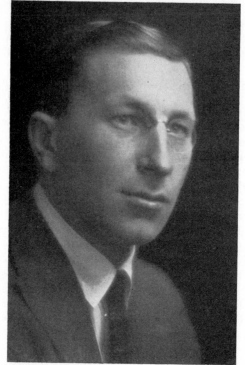

Photo Ashley and Crippen, Toronto

FREDERICK BANTING

gland and pursued the subject with an intensity that earned for him the appellation of "Father of Endocrinology." Harvey Cushing, recalling Brown-Séquard's somewhat naive attempts at rejuvenation with testicular extracts, called him the "Ponce de Leon of Endocrinology."

Before the close of the nineteenth century, Murray, in 1891, had successfully treated myxedema with thyroid extract. In 1891, Oliver and Schäfer demonstrated that adrenal extracts contained a substance which raised the blood pressure; and, eight years later, in 1899, Abel isolated this active principle—epinephrin or adrenalin. In 1902, Bayliss and Starling found in the mucosa of the duodenum and ileum "secretin," which stimulates the flow of bile and pancreatic juice. Three years later, Starling introduced the term, "hormone," to describe secretin and other internal secretions. In

1909, MacCallum and Voegtlin proved that the parathyroid glands control calcium metabolism and that post-parathyroidectomy tetany is due to the loss of calcium from the body and can be relieved by the administration of calcium. They pointed out that an animal deprived of the parathyroids developed a "calcium diabetes" with the loss of large amounts of calcium through the urine, just as de-pancreatized dogs suffered from diabetes mellitus with the loss of glucose. In 1912, Frank demonstrated the existence in the posterior lobe of the pituitary gland of an anti-diuretic hormone which controlled diabetes insipidus, a demonstration which also proved that diabetes insipidus was caused by insufficiency of the posterior lobe. In 1915, Kendall isolated and crystallized thyroxin, the active principle of thyroid extract; and, in 1921, Evans and Long demonstrated in the anterior lobe of the pituitary gland a growth hormone, an excess of which probably produces acromegaly and gigantism.

With the isolation of insulin in 1922, the pace of discovery was further accelerated. Allen and Doisy, in 1923, isolated an ovarian hormone, oestrin, which induces estrus and was subsequently crystallized by Doisy, Veler and Thayer in 1930. Collip, who had played an important role in the purification of insulin, isolated in 1925 parathormone, the active principle of the parathyroid glands, a deficiency of which produced tetany. Rogoff and Stewart, in 1927, obtained an active hormone from the cortex of the adrenal glands and, two years later, employed it in the treatment of Addison's disease. In 1929, Pfiffner and Swingle isolated and purified this cortical extract. In 1927, Zondek and Ascheim isolated the gonadotrophic hormone of the anterior pituitary, which controls the growth of the reproductive system, a discovery which led to their well-known test for pregnancy (1928). Corner and Allen, in 1929, isolated progestin, the corpus luteum hormone, which produces the characteristic changes in the uterine mucosa during pregnancy; and, in 1932, Evans and his colleagues produced diabetes mellitus in animals by the injection of anterior pituitary extracts, an observation confirmed by Young in 1937.

The isolation of the adreno-cortico-trophic hormone (ACTH) by Li, Evans and Simpson and by Sayers, White and Long in 1942 and of cortisone by Mason, Myers and Kendall in 1936 opened up a new field of research, the importance of which is still difficult to assess. The powerful effects of these hormones are the subject of intensive study at the present time.

These discoveries have clarified many hitherto obscure problems of normal and pathologic physiology. Their therapeutic and diag-

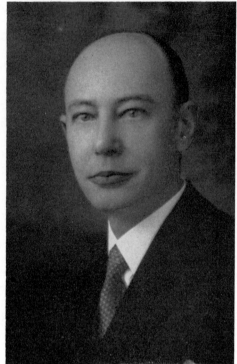

Photo Brown, Brookline, Mass.

GEORGE MINOT

nostic implications were obvious. Myxedema and adult hypothy-
roidism could now be treated with greater success than ever before.
Diabetes mellitus could be controlled with insulin, and diabetes
insipidus with pituitrin. Oestrin was found to be a valuable
palliative in the symptoms accompanying the menopause. Parathormone controls tetany, which occasionally results from injury to
the parathyroids during thyroidectomy, and the physician with
adrenal cortical extract at his command no longer regards Addison's
disease, as its discoverer called it, "an irremediable disease."

The other irremediable disease of Addison, Addisonian or pernicious anemia, became remediable at about the same time. George
Whipple began to study the liver while an assistant at Johns Hopkins and continued to investigate problems of liver physiology and
pathology during his later years at San Francisco and Rochester,

New York. In 1925, with the collaboration of Robscheit-Robbins, he pointed out the beneficial effect of raw beef liver upon blood regeneration in severe experimental anemia. George Minot and William P. Murphy of Boston, impressed by Whipple's work, began feeding patients suffering from pernicious anemia with raw liver and found that the anemia disappeared and the red blood count returned to normal. This treatment ranks as one of the greatest modern advances in therapy. In 1934, Whipple, Minot and Murphy joined the increasing numbers of American scientists who have received the Nobel prize.

Medical progress in the New World was by no means limited to the United States. Mexico, Central America, and South America, like their neighbor to the north, were powerfully influenced by the wave of scientific enthusiasm which swept over from Europe. These discoveries and modern methods Latin America was able to employ in the study of her indigenous diseases and of her own health problems.

In Oswaldo Cruz (1872-1917), Brazil had one of the outstanding sanitarians of this period. A native of Brazil and a graduate of the University of Rio de Janeiro, Cruz studied at the Pasteur Institute of Paris and, after his return to Brazil, became director of the National SerumTherapy Institute at Manquinhos in 1900. In the face of strong opposition, he proposed to eradicate yellow fever from Rio de Janeiro by combatting the mosquito and accomplished this task in less than three years. Through his influence, the public health service was reorganized, plague was intensively combatted, isolation hospitals founded, and smallpox vaccination intensified. His Institute, which was christened "The Oswaldo Cruz Institute" in 1908, became an active center of research, where important studies were carried out on plague, malaria, ankylostomiasis, serum therapy and hematology. Here a group of enthusiastic pupils were trained. Many prominent parasitologists of international reputation, such as Prowazek and Giemsa, worked at the Institute. Nicholas Senn wrote of Cruz—"A life-sized statue in pure solid gold to his memory would be put a feeble acknowledgment of the invaluable services he has rendered his country."

Another famous Brazilian scientist is Henrique da Rocha-Lima, a native of Rio de Janeiro. Da Rocha-Lima was a colleague of von Prowazek and worked with him on typhus fever in 1915. He gave the first adequate description of the organism of typhus fever, naming it *Rickettsia prowazeki*. In 1919, he was appointed professor of bacteriology at the Tropical Institute of Hamburg but later returned to Brazil.

Carlos Chagas (1879-1934), a favorite pupil of Oswaldo Cruz, worked for years in field campaigns against malaria, plague, influenza, leprosy, leishmaniasis, and other diseases. After the death of Cruz, he became director of the Oswaldo Cruz Institute and Director of Public Health. He described several new species of mosquitoes and trypanosomes but is best remembered for his work on a disease called South American trypanosomiasis, or "Chagas' disease." Chagas demonstrated that this disease was caused by a new species of trypanosome *(Schizotrypanosome cruzi)* and that it was transmitted by bugs of the *triatoma* genus, blood sucking insects, sometimes called cone-nosed bugs.

Carrión's disease was named after David Carrión, a Peruvian medical student, who, after inoculation with blood from a patient suffering from *verruga peruana,* died with symptoms of Oroya fever, thus proving the identity of the two diseases. The causative agent of this disease, the *Bartonella bacilliformis,* was discovered by Alberto Barton in 1909. Its vector is now thought to be the sandfly.

In 1915, Rodolfo Robler, a Guatemalian physician, proved that onchocerciasis, a disease common in his country, is caused by a species of filaria *(Onchocerca caecutiens).* In 1938, *mal del pinto,* or *pinto* mentioned by Cortés in 1520 and by Oviedo in 1535, was found to be caused by a treponema (spirochaete). These results were confirmed in 1940 in Mexico by Léon-Blanco, who studied a large number of cases.

Since much of Central and of South America is tropical or subtropical, most of their pressing health problems have been in the field of tropical diseases. The premier health institute of Latin America, the Oswaldo Cruz Institute, has now its counterparts in other Latin American countries.

Latin America, however, has shown outstanding progress in other fields of health. The new hospitals, notably those of Mexico City, Montevideo, Lima, Buenos Aires, and Rio de Janeiro, have few equals and no superiors either in America or in Europe. The scientific work published from the medical schools of Latin America is attracting world-wide attention. The physiological school of Bernardo A. Houssay and Braun-Menendez in Buenos Aires has been outstanding. Houssaye received the Nobel prize in 1947. In Mexico City, the National Institute of Cardiology, under the able direction of Ignacio Chavez, has become one of the most active centers for cardiological research on the American continent.

The hopes of optimists that nations had learned their lesson from the first World War and had decided upon a new era of peace were shattered by the outbreak of the Italo-Ethiopian War in 1935. In this unequal contest, the poorly equipped Ethiopian troops were no match for the mechanized legions of Mussolini. More striking even than the military superiority of the Italian Army was the superiority of its sanitary organization. One of the prime reasons for Italian success was the health of its armies due to the efficiency of its medical service.

Since louse-borne diseases were particularly prevalent in this part of the world, the Italian soldiers were watched carefully for any evidence of vermin infestation, and all prisoners of war were thoroughly deloused. With these precautions, the Italian Army had no cases of typhus fever, whereas the Ethiopian Army had some 20,000 cases. There were only 17 cases of relapsing fever, another louse-borne disease in the Italian Army while there were some 30,000 cases in the Ethiopian Army. The water and food supplies of the Italians were constantly inspected and tested, and flies and insects were kept from all food, with the result that this army of 500,000, living in a notoriously unsanitary country, had only 161 deaths from typhoid fever and only 453 cases of dysentery. Each Italian soldier received a lemon a day, and not a single case of

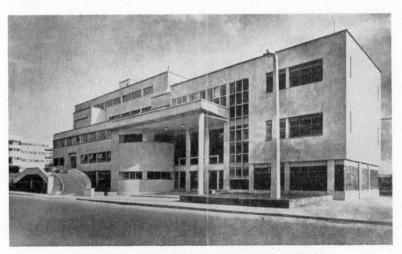

NATIONAL INSTITUTE OF CARDIOLOGY, MEXICO

The most complete and best equipped cardiological institute on the North American continent, founded and directed by Ignacio Chavez.

scurvy appeared, whereas the Ethiopian Red Cross reported 30,000 cases. The vaccinated Italian Army had no smallpox while this scourge ravaged the Ethiopian troops. Disease was a powerful ally of the Italians in their conquest of Ethiopia.

The bloody Spanish Civil War, which broke out in 1936, has been referred to as a preview of Armageddon. Many new instruments of destruction, created during the 18-year armistice following the first World War, found in Spain an excellent proving ground for the next trial of strength. Also, since these new instruments of warfare produced horrible wounds, the surgeons had abundant opportunity to test out new methods of treatment.

During the latter part of the war, Dr. Rudolph Matas of New Orleans visited the military hospitals in Catalonia and wrote a most interesting account of what he saw—

I must say that whatever preconceived notions I had of the treatment of war wounds—derived chiefly from the experience of the World War—they were completely upset by what I saw in the Catalonian war zone. . . . The Carrel-Dakin treatment had been tried unsuccessfully early in the war . . . the simplified technique based on the procedure of Winnett Orr of Lincoln, Nebraska, and Lorenz Böhler of Vienna . . . enormously simplified the care of the wounded and yielded better results. . . . When fresh wounds are relieved of all dead or devitalized tissues, they are, when put to complete rest, quite able to take care of themselves without the aid of antiseptics. . . . By the close of the war, plaster has risen to the level of an apotheosis in surgical esteem.

After the war, Dr. J. Trueta, chief surgeon of the military hospital in Barcelona, wrote that, in his first series of 1,073 cases of compound fractures of the limbs, there were only six deaths. In all, he treated 20,000 cases, with only 91 bad results and only four amputations. The great medical lesson learned from the Spanish Civil War was this improved treatment of compound fractures. The Carrel-Dakin treatment, so highly praised in the first World War, with its continuous irrigation, necessitating many nurses and doctors for its successful employment, had become a method mainly of historical interest.

The great unsolved problem of World War I was that of the sputum-borne infections, particularly the pneumonias. The first steps toward the solution of this problem were taken in Germany in 1935 by Gerhard Domagk, who found that prontosil, a dye stuff derived from sulfanilamide, protected mice against fatal doses of hemolytic streptococci. Several of his colleagues, testing the new compound on patients, found it to be very effective in the treatment of erysipelas and of streptococcic sore throat. One English physician, writing in the London *Lancet,* remarked, "The early reports might have indicated to anyone with a careful eye on the German literature that something new was brewing."

Tréfouël, at the Pasteur Institute, found that sulfanilamide, the parent compound of prontosil, was as effective as prontosil itself, so

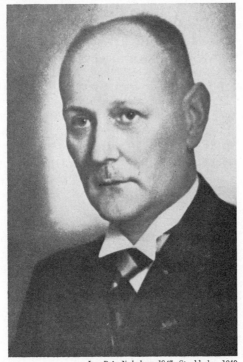

Les Prix Nobel en 1947, Stockholm, 1949

GERHARD DOMAGK

chemists in various countries began to study intensively the chemistry of sulfanilamide compounds. One year after prontosil was placed on the market, the I. G. Farbenindustrie announced that more than 1000 derivatives of sulfanilamide had been made. Later, more than 4000 such derivatives were described, although only a small fraction of these have ever been tested for their possible therapeutic effects.

Sulfanilamide itself was soon employed in the treatment of pneumonia with excellent results. In 1938, sulfapyridine, a derivative of sulfanilamide, was introduced by L. E. H. Whitby into the treatment of pneumonia and reduced the mortality to one-third of its former rate. Then, in 1940 came sulfathiazole, introduced by Perrin Long, which reduced the mortality from pneumonia in many clinics from its former rate of 20-30 per cent to three per cent. Another sulfonamide, sulfadiazine, introduced in 1940 by Richard Roblin, was found to be remarkably effective in epidemic cerebrospinal meningitis.

Surgeons were quick to recognize the great value of the sulfonamide compounds and immediately introduced them into surgical practice. Excellent results were obtained, especially in open wounds and in compound fractures. Surgeons no longer hesitated to sew up an infected wound after cleansing it, sprinkling it with a sulfonamide, or giving the patient the drug by mouth.

Sulfonamides have lowered the mortality in peritonitis, particularly when administered before operation. Such compounds as succinylsulfathiazole reduce markedly the intestinal flora and diminish the dangers of contamination during a surgical operation. In 1947, Balfour stated, "Operative mortality rates following surgery of the large intestine have decreased from 12 to three per cent since the advent of the use of sulfonamide drugs at the Mayo Clinic."

In dentistry, also, the sulfonamides have proved of great value. Extraction of infected teeth had often been followed by a complicating arthritis, and, in patients with chronic valvular disease, by the development of bacterial endocarditis. Bacteriological studies had shown that the extraction of infected teeth was commonly followed by a bacterial invasion of the blood stream. This great hazard was removed by giving the patient sulfonamides before and after operation, thus sterilizing the blood.

Germany, although constantly hampered by the repressive policy of the National Socialist regime, made a great contribution to the progress of medical science in the discovery of the therapeutic value of the sulfonamides. The world recognized the importance of this discovery, and Gerhard Domagk was awarded the Nobel prize in 1939. The government forbade the award, which was bestowed later.

Another noteworthy achievement in this twilight of German science was the development of the cathode ray, or electron microscope. The first electron microscope was constructed by Knoll and Ruska in 1931 at the *Technische Hochschule* of Berlin-Charlottenburg.

The first description of it was published by Knoll, Ruska and von Borries in 1932.

With this new instrument, magnification of 30,000 or even !00,000 diameters is possible. By means of it, viruses and bacteriophages are visible as well as the complex structure of many bacteria. Up to this time, bacteria had been regarded as simple unicellular structures dividing by simple cell division, or amitosis. With these new magnifications, some bacteria were found to divide by mitosis with the formation of chromosomes. The instrument has also found wide application in studying the finer structure of cells and tissues.

A third great achievement of German science during this period, one which at first attracted little attention, was the electroencephalograph. "Dr. Hans Berger's discovery of electroencephalography—one of the outstanding advances in recent medical research—was achieved singlehandedly and, as it were, almost in secret" (Ginzberg).

Hans Berger was born near Coburg in Bavaria in 1873. After graduating from the *Gymnasium,* he studied mathematics and physics, but later studied medicine, receiving his degree in medicine in 1897 at Jena, where he lived until his retirement after his sixty-first birthday. Although apparently more interested in physics, in physiology, and in organic nervous diseases, he was assistant to Binswanger in the psychiatric clinic until Binswanger went to Switzerland, when Berger succeeded him as professor and director of the psychiatric clinic in 1919.

Most physiologists, while not denying that brain tissue, like other tissue, produces electricity and that there is electrical activity in the cortex, felt it was not worth while to measure this activity. Berger, a physicist at heart, although a psychiatrist by profession, thought differently. He constructed an electroencephalograph and reported his results in 1929 in the *Archiv für Psychiatrie.* At first, psychiatrists were not impressed, but the firm of Carl Zeiss in Jena was interested and supplied him with funds to construct a new and expensive instrument. With his new instrument, Berger made many tracings on his assistants, members of his family, hospital attendants and patients, publishing additional articles in 1932, 1933 and 1934.

In 1938, having reached the age limit, Berger retired and became director of a private sanitarium at Bad Blankenburg, where he had neither funds nor equipment to go further with his researches. He had always been a quiet, shy and reticent man, singularly uncommunicative, and with none of the commonly accepted attributes of greatness. No one in Jena, least of all, his colleagues, had ever expected him to make a great discovery. He had worked alone and talked over his problems with no one except a few physicists and some assistants who had helped him with his experiments. He died in 1941. The electroencephalograph promises to be the important tool in the diagnosis of cerebral disease, as the electrocardiograph is to the diagnosis of heart disease.

The second World War, which began with the invasion of Poland on September 1, 1939, is contemporary history. Physicians and surgeons in all the nations responded to the call to arms and were active in the conquest of disease. The vast area of global conflict, the size of the contending armies, the huge toll of life dwarfed all previous wars.

In the early period of the war, the sulfonamides proved their great value in controlling and during the same diseases they had mastered in peace time. The sputum-borne infections, particularly the pneumonias, were no longer an insoluble problem; meningitis had lost most of its terror; gonorrhoea was usually cured in a few days. In the tropics, soldiers with bacillary dysentery showed a dramatic recovery when sulfaguanidine was administered early in the disease. But the most dramatic medical event of the war period was the development of antibiotics, with penicillin playing the leading role.

The early history of antibiotics has a certain resemblance to that of sulfanilamide. P. Gelmo, a German chemist, synthetized sulfamilamide in 1908, and from it were developed a series of dyes which were used in the textile industry. In 1914, it was observed that some of these dyes were highly bactericidal, but this research work was interrupted by the first World War and not resumed until 18 years later when Domagk investigated the subject again. The history of antibiotics stems even further back.

The antagonism of some growing organisms for other groups was noted by Louis Pasteur in 1877, and, in 1889, P. Vuillemin coined the term, "antibiosis." The first extensive therapeutic application of this principle was in 1898 by Rudolf Emmerich, professor of bacteriology and hygiene at the University of Munich. He extracted a substance from cultures of B. pyocyaneus, "pyocyanase," which destroyed the bacilli of anthrax, diphtheria, typhoid fever, and bubonic plague. Unfortunately, it proved to be a toxic substance and was soon abandoned as a therapeutic agent.

In 1928, 30 years later, Alexander Fleming, working at St. Mary's Hospital in London, noted that a mold with which a plate culture

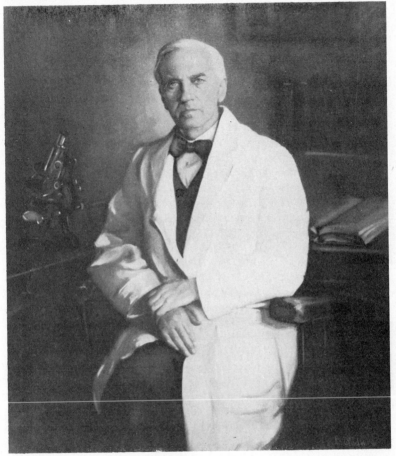

ALEXANDER FLEMING
Portrait by Bernard Godwin.

of staphylococci had been contaminated destroyed the bacteria. He
isolated the mold, grew it in pure culture, and showed that a filtrate
from the culture media in which it grew, killed in high dilutions, a
great variety of microorganisms and that the substance was not toxic
for small animals. Since the mold was a strain of penicillium, he
named the antibacterial substance penicillin.

Ten years passed before Florey, Chain, and their associates at
Oxford took up the study of penicillin. In the summer of 1941 at
the height of the war, they came to the United States and asked for

assistance in the manufacture of penicillin. After a tremendous co-operative effort, enough penicillin was available in the Spring of 1942 to treat a single patient. Plants for its production multiplied to such an extent that, a year later, the first wounded soldiers were treated, and the production of penicillin was gradually increased to the point where it was available, not only for soldiers, but for civilians as well. Dr. Chester Keefer states that, at first, the cost was $200 for 1,000,000 units; later, mass production reduced the price to $1.50.

Penicillin soon replaced to a great extent sulfonamides in the treatment of a variety of disease, notably streptococcic infections, pneumococcic pneumonia, and gonorrhoea. Ninety-eight per cent of the cases of gonorrhoea can be cured by a single injection of 300,000 units of penicillin in oil and wax. Even more startling are the results in the treatment of syphilis. Salvarsan, which Ehrlich introduced, had two great defects—the drug was toxic in large doses; and, if the dose were not sufficiently large, the spirochaete developed its own immunity against Salvarsan. Penicillin is practically non-toxic and can be administered in enormous doses. It may well be the *therapia magna sterilisans,* of which Ehrlich talked, and gives promise of being an actual cure for syphilis.

In 1944, Selman Waksman and his associates announced the discovery of streptomycin obtained from cultures of *Streptomyces griseus,* one of the higher bacteria found in heavily manured soil. Streptomycin also destroys a great variety of organisms, many of which are resistant to penicillin. It has proved particularly effective in tularemia, in infections with B. Coli, and in brucellosis, and has shown promising results in pulmonary tuberculosis.

Chloromycetin, or chloramphenicol, was first isolated from a strain of streptomyces, *Streptomyces venezuelae,* obtained from a sample of soil collected near Caracas, Venezuela, and studied by John Ehrlich in 1947. It has proved to be quite effective in typhus fever, in Japanese river fever (tsutsugamushi disease or scrub typhus), in Rocky Mountain spotted fever, in typhoid fever, and in brucellosis. Aureomycin, an antibiotic obtained from cultures of *Streptomyces aureofaciens,* was described by B. M. Duggar in 1948. This antibiotic is apparently effective in a variety of infections, including chronic urinary infections, lymphogranuloma venereum, Rocky Mountain spotted fever, Q fever, typhus fever, and virus pneumonias.

With the discovery of the sulfonamides and of the antibiotics, the first half of the twentieth century came to a dramatic close. It was, as

Dale remarked, "the period in which civilization first began to feel, for good or ill, the full impact of progress in the natural sciences." The second half of the nineteenth century was rich in major discoveries, many of which were not fully utilized until the twentieth century. The twentieth itself was also rich in great discoveries—in chemistry, in physics, and in biology as well as in medicine. Speaking generally, the nineteenth century was pre-eminently a century in which the firm foundations for pathogenesis and for diagnosis were laid; the first half of the twentieth, the period in which rational . therapeusis was built upon these foundations.

The discoveries in natural science have revolutionized our methods of transportation, our lighting and our communication systems, and have altered profoundly, though almost imperceptibly, our habits and ways of life. Equally profound have been the changes in the relative importance of diseases and the changes in the methods of treatment—the results of great improvements in sanitation as well as the discovery of powerful therapeutic agents. As a result, a physician today no longer looks on an approaching pestilence with helpless stoicism. Nor is he obliged to rely largely on *vis medicatrix naturae,* valuable as that precept still is, to cure his patients—with meningitis or pneumonia—for now he has a specific drug. Medical practice in the nineteenth century was largely empirical; in the twentieth, it is still empirical in a sense, but the empiricism today is based both on the experience obtained at the bedside and on that obtained in the laboratories of chemistry, of pharmacology, and of experimental medicine. Example of progress in the control and cure of disease are numerous. A few examples from health statistics, mainly of the United States, will suffice. The same pattern is repeated elsewhere.

Typhoid fever, once a dreaded menace to health and common in all localities, is rarely seen. This disease, which, in 1900, showed a death rate of approximately 31 per 100,000 population, caused in 1947 the death of only 0.2 per 100,000. This phenomenal decrease was the result of an improved water supply, rigid inspection of milk, proper disposal of sewage, careful inspection of food, and antityphoid vaccination. Occasional cases or small epidemics still ocur, but, for them, we now have a specific antibiotic—chloromycetin (chloramphenicol).

In 1900, tuberculosis had a death rate of 40.3 per 100,000; in 1947, 0.6. It has long ceased to be the "Captain of the Men of Death." This marked reduction in mortality is the result of advances in both public health and medical practice—the establishment of measures to check infection from tubercular patients, improvement in methods of diagnosis and of treatment, where diet and rest have been emphasized, a pioneer in this method being Edward L. Trudeau. Pneumonia, which, in 1900, showed a death rate of 202.2 per 100,000, caused in 1947 the death of 43.1 per 100,000. Here we see first the effect of sulfonamides, which, in 1937, had lowered the death rate to 114.9. The subsequent precipitous fall was due largely to the introduction of penicillin.

Diphtheria, which showed a death rate of 40.3 per 100,000 in 1900, fell to 0.6 in 1947. This marked decrease was due to improved techniques in diagnosis, more intelligent administration of diphtheria antitoxin, and, particularly, to widespread immunization of school children against diphtheria. This systematic immunization of school children against diphtheria by employing toxin-antitoxin mixtures or "toxoids," formed from toxins by chemical treatment, has been a notable advance. Toxin-antitoxin immunization and the newer toxoid immunization are given to children in whom the Schick test indicates susceptibility to diphtheritic infection. Anti-diphtheritic immunization was first used on a large scale by W. H. Park in New York City. The record of Hamilton, Ontario, is striking. The incidence of and the mortality from diphtheria in this city had remained constant for years with but minor fluctuations. In 1925, general immunization was instituted, with the result that, Hamilton, a city of 165,000, has had no deaths from diphtheria since 1930 and no cases of this disease since 1933.

Deaths incident to pregnancy, childbirth, and the puerperium dropped from 13.4 per 100,000 in 1900 to 3.5 in 1947. Deaths from diarrhoea and enteritis, which take a heavy toll among infants and young children, fell during the same period from 142.7 per 100,000 to 5.6. These figures are impressive. They reflect phenomenal improvement in the diagnosis and treatment of infectious diseases, great improvement in the fields of maternal care and child welfare. They also demonstrate that Pasteur, Koch and Behring built on solid foundation although they did not live to see the results that would have delighted and probably also have astounded them.

The lowered mortality from infectious diseases, while the most spectacular in the field of medicine, does not constitute the sole advance in this field. The notable contributions in diagnosis, particularly with the aid of x-rays, of the electrocardiograph, and of functional tests, marked a great advance. In 1900, most physicians used x-rays largely for the diagnosis of fractures and for the localization of foreign bodies. Today, thanks to great technical advances, the x-ray speaks almost the last word in the diagnosis of diseases of the heart and blood vessels, of the lungs, and of the stomach and intestines, and, since the discovery of cholecystography by Graham and Cole in 1924, of gall bladder disease as well. The widespread employment of the electrocardiograph has discovered facts of inestimable value in the diagnosis and treatment of cardiac disease.

In therapeutics, the discovery of insulin, of cortical adrenal extracts, and of many other hormones have revolutionized the treatment of diabetes, of Addison's disease, and of many other diseases regarded in the nineteenth century as having much pathologic interest but no therapeutic promise. Dietetics has progressed along with other branches of therapy. The institution of well balanced diets with the proper distribution of carbohydrate, protein and fat and with an adequate content of minerals, amino acids and vitamins have not only caused a powerful check on malnutrition, on rickets, and on scurvy but have also been a potent aid in the treatment of diseases of the gastro-intestinal tract, diseases of the heart, and diseases of metabolism.

Psychiatry made significant advances during the half century. In France, Pierre Janet deepened our knowledge of hysteria and psychasthenia by intense study of a great many patients. In Germanic lands, Krafft-Ebing investigated psychoneuroses, explored new fields in psychiatry, and definitely established the relationship of general paralysis to syphilis even before the Wassermann reaction was discovered. Emil Kraepelin, in Heidelberg and in Munich, strongly influenced the psychiatry of the period, his classification of psychoses with clear-cut clinical descriptions having brought much clarity and precision to psychiatric thinking. The work of Sigmund Freud, with his contributions on sexual impulses, on the interpretation of dreams, and on the technique of psychoanalysis, has wrought a revolution in psychiatry. This psychiatric progress, particularly in the field of neuroses, has made a deep impress on all fields of medicine. The importance of the psychic element in disease, the influence of environment, heredity, and childhood impressions, and psychosomatic trauma as etiological factors in disease have been accepted by all. The practicing physician has long recognized that the majority of his patients consult him for functional complaints; often his psychotherapy helps them more than his pills.

The development of electroencephalography was a great achievement, particularly in the diagnosis of organic brain disease and of border-line states as well. The introduction of several types of "shock" treatment for psychotic conditions represents a significant therapeutic advance. Sudden and dramatic improvement occurs in a considerable percentage of patients although the psychosis may recur. A "shock," or series of epileptiform convulsions, produced by an overdose of insulin, was first employed in schizophrenia by Sakel in 1934. Injections of metrazol were introduced by Meduna in 1935, and later faradic electrical stimulation applied to the forehead was used. The mechanism of this improvement, when it occurs, is, however, not yet well understood.

In some respects, surgery shows a less spectacular advance than medicinal therapeutics. Most of the spectacular operations of surgery had been performed before the advent of the twentieth century. The first successful gastrostomy had been performed by Sédillot in 1849; the first successful resection of the esophagus by Billroth in 1872; the first successful resection of the stomach, likewise, by Billroth in 1881. Lawson Tait had done the first successful cholecystotomy in 1879, although preceded by Jean Louis Petit in 1743; Mikulicz had

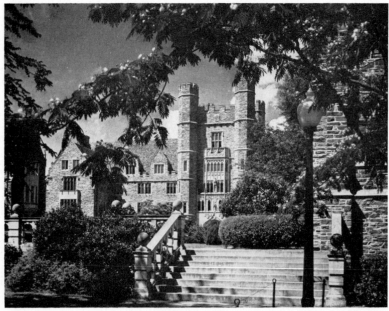

Kindness of Bureau of Public Information, Duke University

DUKE UNIVERSITY MEDICAL SCHOOL

The buildings are an interesting example of Gothic architecture adapted to modern uses.

first sutured a perforated gastric ulcer in 1885; and Wölfler had perfected the operation of gastroenterostomy in 1881. The fields of neurosurgery, of lung surgery, and of cardiac surgery had not, however, been extensively invaded until after Schloffer, in 1906, first successfully removed a pituitary tumor. Graham and Singer, in 1932, first successfully removed an entire lung for carcinoma of the bronchus; and Gross and Hubbard, in 1939, carried out the first successful ligation of a patent ductus arteriosus.

"These great men of the past," writes Jefferson,

—Moynihan, Murphy, the Mayo brothers, and George Crile, and some of the Continental leaders, about whom it is impossible to write without almost Dickensian hints of caricature in spite of the intense seriousness of their purpose—have few if any counterparts among the more serious and less flamboyant figures of today.

One great reason for this is undoubtedly the fact that the brilliant techniques initiated by these great pioneers, the careful preparations for operation, and the painstaking postoperative treatment, which they carried out with such meticulous care, have been so widely followed that they have become almost routine. Surgery, too, has become much safer since the advent of the sulfonamides and the antibiotics. Moynihan's oft-repeated dictum, "We have made surgery safe for the patient, we must now make the patient safe for surgery,' describes aptly one of the most fundamental advances in twentieth century surgery.

Neurosurgery has made phenomenal advances in the twentieth century, much of it stemming from the work of Cushing and his pupils. Shortly before his death, Walter Dandy remarked, "When I was Dr. Cushing's resident during the years 1911 and 1912, two intracranial tumors were removed, one survived." In 1932, Cushing wrote a monograph describing 2,000 verified cases of intracranial tumors with an operative mortality of 13.9 per cent. Dandy, Cushing's most brilliant pupil, introduced in 1918 a new and revolutionary method for the diagnosis of cerebral tumors, which was announced in his paper, "Ventrilography following the injection of air into the cerebral ventricles," published in the *Annals of Surgery*. This new method rapidly found world-wide acceptance and remains one of the epochal advances in neurosurgery. Dandy made other notable contributions to this field. In 1917, he produced hydrocephalus experimentally, explained the various types of hydrocephalus as due to strictures of the aqueduct of Silvius, obstruction of the foramina of Magendie and Luschka, and devised surgical operations for the amelioration of the different varieties. He also devised an operation for the relief of Ménière's disease (1928) and was a pioneer in the operation of lobectomy.

Extensive surgical operations on the lungs, involving often resection of an entire lung, are being performed with increasing frequency and success. This success is due to three factors—increased skill and knowledge of the operator, greatly improved anesthesia by the endotracheal method, and complete asepsis obtained by sulfonamides or antibiotics.

Surgery of the great vessels of the heart and of congenital heart lesions, with which the names of Gross, Blalock, Bailey and others are associated, forms one of the most amazingly interesting and hopeful chapters in the history of modern surgery. The same factors that made surgery of the lungs possible have performed the same service for surgery of the heart.

The specialty of anesthesia, born with the discovery of Morton, made more spectacular advances during the second half of the nineteenth century than in the first half of the twentieth. According to the *British Medical Journal,* "Since 1900, advances in anesthesia have been largely in the nature of consolidation of the work of its pioneers and perfection of techniques already in existence." This statement, while undoubtedly correct, may create the impression of an understatement when we consider the perfection of these techniques, which has led to greater comfort, almost to the point of pleasure, for the patient, a greater precision in the choice and administration of the type of anesthetic particularly adapted to certain operations, and, lastly, a greater reduction in mortality rates from operation.

There is little similarity between the anesthetist of 1900, who dropped ether or chloroform upon a towel or bit of gauze held over the face of the patient, and the anesthetist of today, who sits beside a delicate anesthesia apparatus with which he can administer several anesthetics, either successively or simultaneously, regulating accurately the flow of each, registering the patient's blood pressure and heart rate throughout the operation, and giving the patient either oxygen or carbon dioxide whenever his condition demands it.

Several new and important anesthetics have been added to the anesthetist's armamentarium. Ethylene was introduced by Luckhardt in 1918, cyclopropane by Waters in 1930, divinyl oxide by Leake in 1933, and cyprome ether by Krantz and his colleagues in 1940.

New methods of inducing anesthesia have also been studied. Rectal anesthesia was advocated by Pirogoff, who produced anesthesia in 1847 by instilling ether into the rectum. In the subsequent years, many observers worked with this method, obtaining only moderate success until 1913, when Gwathmey introduced oil-ether colonic anesthesia. Later, in 1926, Butzengeiger introduced avertin as a rectal anesthetic, a method which had definite advantages over that of Gwathmey.

The greatest advance in anesthesia since the discovery of ether anesthesia by inhalation is, by common consent, the development of intravenous anesthesia. This idea has been adumbrated by many investigators since Sir Christopher Wren, in 1656, made intravenous injections of opium, beer and wine into the veins of a dog and studied their effects. Chloral hydrate, paraldehyde, chloroform, ether and morphine have been investigated for their suitability as intravenous anesthetics. After barbital (veronal) was synthesized by Emil Fischer in 1902, the effects of various barbituric acid compounds, when injected intravenously, were investigated. Evipan (evipal), which was introduced by Weese and Scharpff in 1932, was found to produce very safe anesthesia for operations of short duration. In 1941, Geyer stated that more than 4,000,000 patients had been operated upon under evipan anesthesia. Pentothal sodium, introduced by Lundy in 1934, has similar anesthetic properties and, at the end of December, 1941, had been employed in 31,931 operations at the Mayo Clinic. The advantages of intravenous anesthesia for operations on the mouth, head and neck are obvious.

Endotracheal anesthesia, like intravenous anesthesia, had forerunners in Vesalius, Robert Hook, and John Snow and was actually used as early as 1869 by Friedrich Trendelenburg. The present methods of endotracheal anesthesia were developed mainly by Rudolph Matas (1898), Franz Kühn (1900), S. J. Meltzer and John Auer (1909), who demonstrated that, if air were blown into the trachea of an animal whose respiration was paralyzed, full oxygenation of the blood could be maintained. Elsberg, in 1910, made the clinical application of the principle discovered by Meltzer and Auer. The value of endotracheal anesthesia for operations involving incisions through the chest wall, with the ensuing temporary pneumothorax, is obvious. It has done away completely with the low pressure cabinets, under which Sauerbruch, at the beginning of the century, performed operations on the lungs.

Spinal anesthesia, first carried out on dogs in 1885 by J. Leonard Corning employing cocaine, received its clinical trial at the hands of Rudolph Matas in 1899. He was, according to Keys, "the first

American to report on true spinal anesthesia." The employment of cocaine for this purpose was associated with danger because of the toxicity of the drug. The discovery by Einhorn in 1904 of novocaine (procaine hydrochloride), a drug having the anesthetic properties of cocaine but much less toxicity, added much to the safety and the increased popularity of spinal anesthesia.

Infiltration anesthesia was first demonstrated before the German Congress of Surgeons by Carl Schleich in 1892. He employed dilute solutions of cocaine intracutaneously. This new method of anesthesia gradually made its way into surgical practice; and, five years later, Crile amputated a patient's leg without causing pain after injecting the sciatic and anterior crural nerves. The substitution of novocaine for cocaine increased the safety and stimulated a more widespread employment of infiltration anesthesia, just as it had in the case of spinal anesthesia.

One of the most striking changes in anesthesiology has been the advances since 1900 in the status, training and ability of the anesthetist. This change is registered in the lessened mortality from anesthesia. In 1948, Sington stated that he had administered 100,000 anesthetics in the London hospital with only three deaths.

The anesthetist is no longer, to employ a term long current in England, simply a "chloroformist" who does the bidding of his surgical master. He is a very important member of the surgical team, a pharmacologist as well as a physiologist, familiar with the effects produced by the anesthetic he administers and alert to the changes in his patient from a normal physiological condition to an abnormal pathological state. Asklepiades of Bithynia took as his motto: "To heal *tuto, cito, jucunde*"—safely, speedily, pleasantly. The modern anesthetist has achieved this ideal as nearly as any disciple of the healing art.

Ophthalmology, a separate branch of medicine since the days of ancient Egypt, has kept step with its sister sciences throughout the centuries and has also registered notable advances during the first half of the twentieth century. The discovery of the ophthalmoscope by Helmholtz in 1850 was a sufficiently powerful stimulus to set ophthalmology apart as the first great medical specialty. During the twentieth century, it has acquired new knowledge of ocular physiology, a better understanding through biochemical research of the metabolism of the eye, and a new conception of visual optics, largely from the labors of Gullstrand, who was awarded the Nobel prize in 1911. Ophthalmology has profited, as every other branch of medicine, through the discovery of the sulfonamides and antibiotics.

Otolaryngology owes one of its greatest advances to the invention of the laryngoscope by Manuel Garcia, a Spanish singing teacher in London. In 1855, Garcia sent an account of his instrument to the Royal Society, and, three years later, the laryngoscope was routinely employed by Czermak and Türck in Vienna. In 1902, Killian of Freiburg introduced peroral endoscopy, and, two years later, Chevalier Jackson in America, with an improved bronchoscope, began his remarkable career as a bronchoscopist and, in 1907, published the first textbook on bronchoscopy. Today the removal of a foreign body from the bronchus is an operation rather commonplace than spectacular. In otology, Robert Bárány added greatly to our knowledge of the vestibular system, work which earned for him the Nobel prize in 1915. The fenestration operation for deafness, developed by Holmgren of Stockholm, Sourdille of Nantes, and Lempert of New York, has been successful in a large number of cases.

The rapid growth of industrial plants, notably in the United States, has posed new problems unknown to the previous generation of physicians. The problems of installing proper safeguards for health, of proper lighting, of supervision of diets, of correct sanitation, and of the prevention as well as the care of the increasing number of industrial accidents have led to the creation of a new medical specialty—that of industrial medicine. The modern industrial plants maintain on their staffs sanitary engineers, trained dieticians and are equipped with excellent hospitals, furnished with the latest x-ray and surgical equipment under the direction of skilled physicians and surgeons as well as competent well-trained nurses. The rapid development of aviation, both in peace time and in war, has led to similar advances in this field and to the creation of a totally new branch of medicine—aviation medicine.

Physical therapy, well-known to the ancient Greeks, after centuries of neglect as well as of suspicion on the part of physicians because of its frequent association with quackery, has, in the twentieth century, earned recognition as an important branch of medical therapeutics. This new development, spurred particularly by the experiences of the First and Second World Wars, has shown notable advances in the United States, where Coulter, Kovacs, Kessler, Hans Kraus, and Howard Rusk have, by their skillful guidance, firmly established the great importance of physical therapy and rehabilitation. The achievement of returning the maimed and injured to their useful places in human society has a moral and economic value that can scarcely be exaggerated.

The advances in tropical medicine have been notable, and the inhabitant of the tropics in 1950 faces a very different future from that of his predecessor in 1900. The discovery of the causative organism in several important tropical diseases, the demonstration of the vectors in certain diseases, the development of powerful insecticides, notably D.D.T., which destroy the insect vector, and the discovery of the sulfonamides and antibiotics have all played their role in this advance. With all these advances, however, the problem of malaria still looms.

Malaria has been eradicated in many localities by the drainage of swampy land and by the destruction of mosquitoes. Yet, it remains the greatest problem of tropical medicine and one of the greatest killers of the human race, causing the death of some 2,000,000 persons annually. In 1932, health reports to the League of Nations showed that 17,750,760 cases of malaria had been treated that year. India, the largest of all the malarial countries, had an estimated 100,000,000 cases that year, of which only from 8,000,000 to 10,000,000 were treated. In 1935, more than 6,500,000 cases of malaria were treated in the British colonies, which had a population of 61,000,000.

While rarely seen in the United States north of the latitude of the Ohio River, malaria is a serious menace in the many southern states. In 1935, the Metropolitan Life Insurance Company estimated that there were 900,000 cases of malaria in the United States. In 1935, there were 4,435 deaths from malaria in 13 southern states.

In 1900, Manson, discussing the therapy of malaria, wrote, "All drugs sink into insignificance in comparison with quinine." However, during World War I, quinine was unsuccessful as a prophylactic and proved totally inadequate to check the massive infection with malaria which raged in Macedonia. During the past 25 years, four powerful anti-malarial drugs have been synthetized which will do what quinine fails to do—Plasmoquine, introduced by Roehl in 1926; Atebrin, described by Kikuth in 1932; Paludrine, studied by Curd, Davy and Rose in 1945; and Chloroquine, first produced in Germany, "captured" in North Africa, re-synthetized in the United States, and extensively investigated in 1946.

The present status of malarial therapy has been summarized by Boyd:

It can be claimed that ways and means have been discovered by which, in favorable circumstances, mosquitoes—and hence malaria—can be eradicated; by which infection can be suppressed where eradication is impossible or impracticable; and by which attacks of malaria can be cured where suppression has been faulty or when suppressive drugs are withdrawn. The major problems of malaria are now administrative rather than medical.

Leishmaniasis, or kala-azar, the causative agent of which was discovered in 1903, was shown in 1942 to be transmitted by a sandfly (*Phlebotomus argentipes*). Antimony was found to have a powerful action on the parasites, and, by employing some of the compounds of antimony, a high percentage of cures can be obtained. Trypanosomiasis has been treated successfully with suramin (Bayer 205). But, as this compound does not pass the blood-brain barrier and was of little value in advanced cases, pentamidine has also been used with encouraging results.

In the treatment of bacillary dysentery, sulfaguanidine has proved its value, and streptomycin has given promising results in the therapy of plague. Leprosy has been controlled with the ethyl esters of chaulmoogra oil, and marked clinical improvement has been noted although permanent cures are seldom produced. More promising results have been obtained with promin.

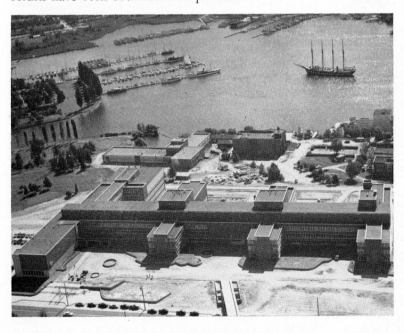

UNIVERSITY OF WASHINGTON MEDICAL SCHOOL
These buildings demonstrate the adaptability of modern architecture for hospital and laboratory purposes.

These therapeutic advances have been mainly the legacy of chemo-therapy, the results of painstaking studies on the pharmacologic effects produced by changes in the chemical structure of certain drugs, the anti-parasitic nature of which had been demonstrated. These brilliant achievements were obtained by following the path blazed by the pioneer—Paul Ehrlich.

There is, however, a shady side to this sunny picture. Cancer, which showed a death rate of 64 per 100,000 in 1900, had a mortality of 132.4 in 1947, according to the vital statistics of the United States. During this same period, the death rate from diabetes mellitus rose from 11.0 to 26.2; from diseases of the heart, from 137.4 to 321.2. These sombre figures will not be accepted as the inevitable, immutable result of an aging population but as a fresh challenge to be met, a new menace to be conquered.

Medical research in the last quarter of the first half century advanced at an accelerated tempo, particularly in the United States. This accelerated tempo was accompanied by a tremendous increase in laboratory facilities and in the number of investigators devoting themselves to medical research. The investigator today no longer ekes out his scientific life in a dim, poorly lighted basement with make-shift equipment and a niggardly budget. He has usually an adequately appointed laboratory, supplied with all the equipment he desires and has at his disposal a budget, the size of which would have caused his predecessor of half a century ago to rub his eyes in incredulous astonishment. The large pharmaceutical houses, which, at the beginning of the century, seemed chiefly concerned in the manufacture and sale of tinctures, pills and powders and carried on a hit-and-run fight with the American Medical Association, have now, without exception, well-appointed research laboratories, manned by competent investigators who have made some of the note-worthy contributions to medical science. They are important members of the great team that is struggling to conquer disease.

This team spirit in investigation has its counterpart in medical practice. The growth of medical science has been so great that the day of the universal specialist has passed. The concept of the clinic, consisting of a group of men, each skilled in a certain field, has taken firm root and continues to grow. Specialization, with an inherent tendency to narrow the broad medical outlook a physician should have, has its obvious dangers for both physician and patient. A large clinic brings divided responsibility, which has a certain weakness, as well as a tendency to regard the patient as a clinic number with an interesting pathological condition instead of a suffering human being. Such possible defects are, however, not defects in the idea of a clinic but defects in the manner of carrying out this fruitful idea.

There is also the danger that the clinician or the investigator may become more interested in his technical apparatus than in the results obtained. Such individuals should be reminded that Jenner made his epochal discovery while a country doctor at Berkeley and that Claude Bernard laid the foundation of modern physiology, to quote Pasteur, in a "sepulchre-like cellar."

Medicine, during the past half century, has enjoyed increasing esteem for its scientific discoveries. The public no longer doubts the great progress it has made, no longer regards its followers as adherents of a particular sect, chiefly interested in proving the truth of its tenets. Its criticism is more valid, more fundamental—the complaint that its great discoveries are not available to all who have need of them. The solution of this problem will be a discovery taking its place among the great discoveries of medicine. This discovery, like all the great ones, may be at the end of a long trail strewn with false hypotheses and inconclusive experiments.

Biographical Addenda

THE TWENTIETH CENTURY

1877-1950—Emil Abderhalden was born in Ober-Uzwil, St. Gallen, Switzerland, and received his M.D. at the University of Basel in 1902. He was at first *Privatdozent* in Berlin and, in 1911, became professor of physiology in Halle. Most of his scientific work was in the field of physiological chemistry. He was the author of *Lehrbuch der physiologischen Chemie,* Berlin and Vienna, 1906; and, *Lehrbuch der Physiologie,* Berlin and Vienna, 1925/1927. He is remembered especially as the editor of the monumental *Handbuch der biologischen Arbeitsmethoden.*

1836-1925—Clifford Allbutt was born in Dewsbury, Yorkshire and studied at Cambridge and St. George's Hospital in London, receiving his M.B. from Cambridge in 1861. He settled down to practice at Leeds and, from 1864 to 1884 was physician to the Leeds Infirmary. In 1871, he published an important monograph on the *Use of the Ophthalmoscope* and, in 1873, published several papers on cardiac disease. He moved to London in 1889 and was appointed in 1892 Regius Professor of Physic in Cambridge University.

In 1893, Allbutt began to plan a *System of Medicine,* which appeared in eight volumes between 1896 and 1899. A second edition of 11 volumes was published in 1905-1911. In 1921 appeared his scholarly *Greek Medicine in Rome,* and his great work, *Diseases of the Arteries, including Angina Pectoris,* was published in 1915 when he was 80 years of age. He was created a knight in 1907. He was a man of great erudition, scholarly in his tastes, a master of English prose.

1866-1942—Ludwig Aschoff was a native of Berlin and studied medicine at Bonn, Berlin and Strassburg, receiving his M.D. at Bonn in 1889. After serving under von Recklinghausen at Strassburg, he went to Marburg as professor of pathology in 1903, and three years later, was called to Freiburg, where he remained until his retirement.

Aschoff was one of the greatest pathologists of his time and drew students from all over the world to his laboratory. His pathological investigations cover a wide field and include important investigations on cholelithiasis, thrombosis, scurvy, appendicitis, and rheumatic fever, in which he described the "Aschoff bodies." His *Lehrbuch der pathologischen Anatomie,* 1909, went through seven editions and was an outstanding text. Aschoff also wrote many excellent papers on historical topics.

1857-1932—Joseph Jules Babinski was born in Paris of Polish parents, received his medical degree in Paris in 1885, and was for five years Charcot's chief of clinic at the Salpêtrière. His first notable work was his description of the reflex now known as Babinski's sign (1896). In

1899, he turned his attention to the study of cerebellar disease, pointed out the characteristic asynergy, and described the test for diadokokinesia. He also made extended studies of the psychoses, maintaining that hysteria was caused by suggestion. "During the Great War, Babinski was probably more successful in dealing with the war neuroses than any practitioner in France, or perhaps in any other country" (Fulton).

1891-1944—Frederick Grant Banting was born in Alliston, Ontario, Canada, received his M.D. degree at Toronto, and, after service in the first World War, practiced surgery in London, Ontario, and, from 1920 to 1921, was demonstrator of physiology at Western University. In 1921, he went to Toronto with an idea that obsessed him—to isolate from the pancreas a hormone that would control diabetes mellitus. With the assistance of Charles H. Best, of J. B. Collip, the biological chemist, and of J. J. R. Macleod, professor of physiology, he isolated insulin, the discovery of which was published the following year. The Nobel prize for medicine in 1923 was divided between Banting and Macleod. In 1924, Banting received the honor of knighthood. He was killed in 1944 in an airplane accident.

1876-1936—Robert Bárány was a native of Vienna, where he received his degree in 1900. He served as assistant to von Noorden in the medical clinic at Frankfurt-am-Main, in the psychiatric clinic of Kraepelin in Freiburg, and in the surgical clinic of Gussenbauer in Vienna. In 1905, he became assistant in the otological clinic in Vienna and, the following year, discovered the well-known Bárány tests for disturbances of the labyrinth, work which won him the Nobel prize in 1914. He went to Uppsala in 1917 as *Privatdozent* and became professor in 1926.

1872-1947—Joseph Barcroft was born in Newry, Ireland, of Quaker parents and was educated at Cambridge, becoming a fellow of King's College and later a reader in physiology. He was elected F. R. S. in 1910 and, in 1925, became professor of physiology, holding this chair until 1937. He was knighted in 1935.

Barcroft's scientific reputation is one that will endure and grow. His first striking piece of research was on the oxygen carrying capacity of the blood, in which he devised a blood-gas apparatus, worked out oxygen-dissociation curves, classified the varieties of anoxia, and disproved the theory of oxygen secretion in the lungs advocated by Haldane. Barcroft demonstrated that the passage of gases through the alveolar epithelium is a physical process and that the lungs cannot take up oxygen unless the oxygen pressure in the air is higher than that in the blood. In the course of this work, he went to the Andes to study the effects of high altitudes on the blood and found that the polycythemia of high altitudes was accompanied by a diminution in the size of the spleen. This led him to study blood volume in terms of circulatory blood and storage blood. His last work was on pre-natal physiology, in which he studied the effect of environment on the development of the nervous system.

1867-1943—Lewellys Franklin Barker was born in Milldale, Ontario, Canada, and received his medical degree at Toronto in 1890. After serving an internship in the Toronto General Hospital, he went to Baltimore as assistant physician to the Johns Hopkins Hospital. From 1897 to 1899, he was associate professor of anatomy and, from 1899 to 1900, associate professor of pathology. In 1900, he was called to the University of Chicago as professor of anatomy, a position he held until 1905, when he returned to Johns Hopkins as Osler's successor in the chair of medicine. In 1921, he became professor emeritus but continued teaching until his death.

Barker's talents were "in the compilation and exposition of knowledge, rather than in the domain of original research" (Chesney). A man of great personal charm, distinguished in appearance and endowed with the gift of clear and systematic exposition, he was a forceful and inspiring teacher. His *Nervous System and Its Constituent Neurones*, 1899, written while he was associate professor of anatomy, remains a standard treatise. In 1916, he published with Pincoffs *The Clinical Diagnosis of Internal Diseases* and, in 1922, edited a five volume work on *Endocrinology and Metabolism*. He was generous with his associates and assistants and beloved by his students.

1860-1924—William Maddock Bayliss was born in Wednesbury, Staffordshire, and entered University College, London, in 1881, where he became a pupil of Sharpey-Schafer and of Sanderson. He followed the latter to Oxford but returned to London as professor of general physiology in University College. He collaborated with Starling in the work on secretin and peristalsis and wrote three noteworthy books —*The Nature of Enzyme Action,* 1908; *The Principles of General Physiology,* 1914; and the *Physiology of Food and Economy in Diet,* 1917. His *Principles* is written from the viewpoint of physical chemistry and was a very important contribution to this field.

1861-1949—August Bier, a native of Helsen in Waldeck, studied medicine at Berlin, Leipzig and Kiel. At Kiel, he was a pupil of Esmarch, and, after receiving his degree there in 1888, he became a *Privatdozent* and was later professor of Greifswald, Bonn and Berlin. He was a pioneer in the introduction of lumbar anesthesia and in the employment of hyperemia for therapeutic purposes.

1854-1932—Frank Billings, a native of Wisconsin, graduated at the Chicago Medical College in 1881 and, after study abroad and teaching at his Alma Mater, went to Rush Medical College in 1898 and was soon dean. "His genius for leadership was so marked, that had he chosen business or any other profession than medicine, he would have been a leader—a distinguished member of the bar, head of a railway system, a great captain of industry, an outstanding political figure, or a statesman of national proportions. . . . He was trying to better medical education, to further research, to improve facilities for the care of the unfortunate cripple, the needy invalid. . . . At the (University of Chicago) it may be said: 'If you seek his monument, look about you' " (Herrick).

1867-1935—Joseph Colt Bloodgood was born in Milwaukee, Wisconsin, and received his M.D. degree from the University of Pennsylvania in 1891. He became resident surgeon at the Johns Hopkins Hospital in 1893 and was connected with the medical school until his death. He organized the surgical pathological laboratory at the hospital and amassed a large collection of pathological specimens. He became greatly interested in the study of cancer and spent much of his time in his later years in making the medical profession and the lay public aware of the importance of early diagnosis and prompt operation in cases of malignant tumors.

1868-1939—Richard Clarke Cabot was born in Brookline, Massachusetts, graduated at Harvard in 1892, and was associated with the Harvard Medical School from 1899 until 1920, when he became professor of social ethics at Harvard University. His first book, *Clinical Examination of the Blood,* appeared in 1896 and went through five editions. In 1901 his *Physical Diagnosis* was published which went through 10 editions and was the most widely used text on that subject. He introduced the idea of teaching medicine by case histories, and his *Differential Diagnosis,* 1911-1915, had a wide appeal. He inaugurated and developed the hospital social service at the Massachusetts General Hospital, and this new departure was rapidly taken up by a large number of hospitals.

Richard Cabot engaged in many controversies with members of his own profession. "His talents and vital interests did not fit within the orthodox boundaries of the practice of medicine. . . . One does not classify Richard Cabot as a great clinician. He was too versatile for that" (Roger I. Lee).

1871-1945—Walter Bradford Cannon was a native of Prairie du Chien, Wisconsin, and studied at Harvard University, where he received his arts degree in 1896 and his medical degree in 1900. In 1897, while still a medical student, he employed bismuth to visualize the stomach and, in 1898, published the first comprehensive study of the stomach's movements during digestion. He published in 1911 a monograph, *Mechanical Factors of Digestion,* which summarized his work on digestion up to that time. During the next few years, he studied the sympathetic nervous system and, in his monograph, *Bodily Changes in Fear, Hunger and Pain,* 1915, pointed out the close relationship between the endocrine glands and the emotions. His later researches established that the peripheral sympathetic nerve endings are activated by a substance resembling adrenalin, which he called "sympathin" (1931) and considered a hormone. He was professor of physiology at Harvard from 1906 until his retirement in 1942.

1873-1944—Alexis Carrel was born in Sainte-Foy near Lyon, France, received his M.D. at Lyon in 1900, and, in 1904, went to the University of Chicago, where he worked in the department of physiology. In 1906, he went to the Rockefeller Institute as an associate member, becoming a full member six years later. In 1902, he perfected the technique of end-to-end anastomoses of blood vessels. In 1908, he successfully transplanted organs; in 1910, he showed that blood vessels could be preserved in cold storage for long periods before employing them for transplantions; and, in 1910 with Burrows, he grew cultures of sarcoma in culture media, using the technique of Harrison. In 1912, Carrel received the Nobel prize. In 1914 working with Tuffier, he carried out a series of successful experimental valvotomies. During the first World War, he devised with Dakin the well-known Carrel-Dakin treatment for wounds, which was widely employed.

1876-1951—Henry Asbury Christian was a native of Virginia, graduated from Randolph-Macon College in 1895. He received his M.D. at Johns Hopkins in 1900 and soon thereafter worked in pathology under Dr. Frank B. Mallory at the Boston City Hospital. In 1908, when only 32 years of age, he was appointed Hersey Professor of Theory and Practice and became first physician-in-chief to the Peter Bent Brigham Hospital. He held this position until he retired in 1939. During World War II, he was recalled to active teaching.

Dr. Christian was a master clinician, an interesting and forceful teacher, a clear, at times pungent writer. He was the author of *Diagnosis and Treatment of Diseases of the Heart,* revised Osler's *Principles and Practice of Medicine,* and was editor of *The Oxford Medicine* and *Oxford Monographs on Diagnosis and Treatment.* He was much revered by the younger group of physicians, who admired his clinical skill and respected his fairness and integrity.

1884-1945—Logan Clendening was born in Kansas City, Missouri, studied at the University of Michigan, and received his M.D. degree from the University of Kansas in 1907. After study and travel abroad, he began the practice of medicine in Kansas City, leaving his practice to serve in the Medical Corps of the U. S. Army during the First World War. On his return from the war, he became instructor in medicine in the University of Kansas and was connected intimately with this institution until his death. His first medical book, *Modern Methods of Treatment,* appeared in 1924 and was quite successful. Three years later, his *The Human Body,* a book for the general public, was published and was an instantaneous success, more than 500,000 copies having been sold. Following this, Clendening began a daily column on health advice, gave up his private practice, and devoted himself entirely to teaching medical students and to literary pursuits. His column, informative, sparkling with wit and anecdote, was also quite successful, appearing in 383 daily newspapers with a combined circulation of 25,000,000.

Clendening became early interested in medical history, collected a noteworthy library, and wrote many articles on medical history. His *Source Book of Medical History,* published in 1942, is a stimulating and valuable work. At the time of his death, he was working on a book of diagnosis, which was completed by his colleague, Edward H. Hashinger, and appeared in 1947 with the title, *Methods of Diagnosis.* Clendening was the author of

15 books and of more than 80 medical and historical papers.

1872-1950—Charles Franklin Craig was born in Danbury, Connecticut, and received his M.D. at Yale in 1894. He entered the United States Army in 1898, where he had a distinguished career and was at one time professor of bacteriology at the Army Medical School. He retired from the army in 1931 and became professor of tropical diseases at Tulane University, holding this position until his retirement in 1938. Craig was particularly known for his work on malarial parasites.

1864-1943—George Washington Crile was born in Chili, Ohio, received his medical degree at the medical school of Wooster University in Cleveland in 1887, and then studied in Vienna, London and Paris. Returning to Cleveland, he was successively demonstrator of histology, professor of physiology, and, in 1900, clinical professor of surgery at Western Reserve University, holding this position until 1924, when he retired, not to rest but to found and head the Cleveland Clinic.

Crile was a man of prodigious energy and of wide medical and cultural interests, gifted with an unusual imagination and an infectious enthusiasm—all of these qualities combining to make him one of the outstanding surgeons of his generation. He was a skillful operator and a man deeply interested in physiological problems. His studies on shock, blood transfusion, anoci-association, and the surgical treatment of arterial hypertension, as well as the numerous surgical techniques he devised, are lasting contributions to the development of modern surgery. A man of great tact, personal charm, and deep sympathies, combined with innate modesty, he was a beloved figure among his contemporaries.

1869-1939—Harvey Cushing, the outstanding neurological surgeon of the present century, was born in Cleveland, Ohio, and received his medical degree at Harvard in 1895. After a year at the Massachusetts General Hospital, he went to Johns Hopkins in 1896, and his professional life was closely connected with Johns Hopkins, where he became associate professor in 1902 and where he worked until 1911, when he was called to Harvard as professor of surgery. After his retirement at Harvard in 1932, he went to New Haven, where he was active until his death.

Cushing's achievements in neurosurgery were phenomenal, and his position of leadership unquestioned. In 1906, he described the relationship between pituitary tumors and sexual infantilism, an association which he demonstrated by experimental work in 1910. In 1912, he published a surgical and physiological classic, *The Pituitary Body and Its Disorders,* and, in 1917, *Tumors of the Nervus Acusticus.* His *Life of Sir William Osler,* 1925, is one of the select number of great medical biographies. A man of broad culture and the master of a very lucid and interesting style, Cushing wrote many charming essays, some of which were collected and published under the title, *Consecratio medici,* 1928. He was an avid collector of medical masterpieces and bequeathed his valuable library to Yale University. In addition to numerous papers on medical history, Cushing wrote *A Bio-bibliography of Andreas Vesalius,* which was unfinished at his death but was completed and published in 1943 by his friend and colleague, John F. Fulton, whose *Harvey Cushing—A Biography,* 1946, is a worthy rival of Cushing's own biography of Osler.

1852-1935—Charles Loomis Dana was born in Woodstock, Vermont, and received his degree at Columbia University in 1877, was professor of physiology at the Woman's Medical College from 1880 until 1888 and professor of psychiatry and neurology at the Post Graduate Medical School of New York from 1886 until 1898, and, in 1902, became professor of neurology at Cornell University. One of the most prominent neurologists of his time, he was among the first to differentiate the primary combined scleroses, described acute transverse myelitis and serous meningitis, and proposed resection of the posterior spinal roots within the dura for pain, athetosis, and spastic paralysis, an operation which was performed by Robert Abbe in 1888. Dana's *Textbook of Nervous Diseases,* first published in 1892, went through nine editions. An ardent student of medical history, he contributed many articles to this subject, and, in 1926, published his *Peaks of Medical History,* a most valuable and interesting work.

1886-1946—Walter Edward Dandy was born in Sedalia, Missouri, and graduated from the Johns Hopkins Medical School in 1910. He subsequently served for eight years at the Johns Hopkins Hospital as a surgical house officer, part of the time on Cushing's service. He became a member of the medical faculty during this period and was later clinical professor of surgery. In 1913, three years after his graduation, Dandy reported his fundamental studies on hydrocephalus, which added greatly to the knowledge of the pathogenesis of this condition and its treatment. In 1918, he introduced ventrilography, one of the greatest advances ever made in neurosurgery. In 1925, he described a new operation for trigeminal neuralgia and, in 1928, devised an operation for the relief of Ménière's disease, which many consider his second greatest achievement. Dandy "possessed a fortunate combination of qualities: character, a clear thinking brain, industry, an intuitive imagination, independence of thought and action, fearlessness and daring, manual dexterity and a colorful personality" (Blalock).

1849-1917—Jules Joseph Déjérine was a native of Geneva and received his medical degree at Paris in 1879. He was successively physician at the Charité, Bicêtre, and the Salpêtrière. One of the leading French neurologists of his period, he made many contributions to the pathology of aphasia, encephalitis, poliomyelitis, syringomyelia and neuritis.

1854-1915—Paul Ehrlich.

1858-1930—Christian Eijkman was born in Nijkerk, Holland, received his doctor's degree at Amsterdam in 1883, and studied later with Robert Koch in Berlin. He went to the Netherlands East Indies in 1886 and, a year later, became director of the laboratory at Batavia, where he carried out fundamental investigations on the etiology of beriberi. He returned to Holland in 1896 and, two years later, became professor of hygiene at the University of Utrecht, holding this position until his retirement in 1898. In 1899, he received the Nobel prize in medicine, sharing this honor with Hopkins.

1860-1927—Willem Einthoven was born in Samarang, East Indies, and studied medicine at Utrecht, where he received his doctor's degree in 1885. The same year, he was appointed professor of physiology at Leyden, where he worked until his death. His fame rests on his construction of a string galvanometer and the first practical electrocardiograph. He received the Nobel prize in 1924.

1860-1939—Anton Freiherr von Eiselsberg was born in Steinhaus, Austria, and studied medicine at Vienna, Würzburg, Zürich and Paris, receiving his doctor's degree at Vienna in 1884. He became an assistant to Billroth, went to Utrecht as professor in 1893 and to Königsberg in 1896 and, in 1901, returned to Vienna as professor of surgery. He achieved a great reputation as a skillful surgeon, a stimulating teacher, and a man of wide culture. He carried out many important bacteriological investigations and was a pioneer in brain surgery.

1852-1914—Rudolf Emmerich, a native of Mütterstadt, Rhineland, studied in Munich and became Hoffmann's assistant at the Hygienic Institute of Leipzig in 1877. He went to Munich in 1881 as assistant to Pettenkofer, was appointed associate professor of bacteriology and hygiene in 1888, and became professor in 1902. He was an active investigator and the discoverer of pyocyanase.

1866-1943—James Ewing was born in Pittsburgh, graduated at Amherst College in 1888, and received his medical degree at Columbia University in 1891. After serving a year's internship, he entered the pathological laboratory of Dr. T. Mitchell Prudden at Columbia and worked there until 1899, when he was called to the chair of pathology at Cornell University. He taught at Cornell 33 years. "Perhaps no teacher in the history of the school has left so deep an imprint of his personality upon both students and teachers" (Conner). Ewing was a frequent contributor to scientific journals, was one of the founders of the *Journal of Cancer Research* and the author of *Neoplastic Diseases,* which appeared in 1919 after 10 years of unremitting work.

1840-1902—Christian Fenger was a native of Copenhagen, where he received his medical degree in 1867. He was deeply interested in pathology, became a *Privatdozent,* but, being discouraged at his prospects of obtaining professional rank, emigrated first to Egypt and then to North America, settling in Chicago in 1877. He was a master of several languages, exceptionally well educated, had had surgical experience during the Schleswig-Holstein War and the Franco-Prussion War, and was familiar with the work of Virchow, Rokitansky, and the rising new generation of bacteriologists.

After working for a time as a pathologist, Fenger gravitated to surgery and soon became one of the outstanding surgeons of Chicago, a careful and meticulous operator with an unrivaled knowledge and familiarity with pathological conditions. As a man, he was greatly respected and beloved. He taught surgery for many years at Rush Medical College.

1863-1942—John Miller Turpin Finney was born in Natchez, Mississippi, and graduated from Harvard Medical School in 1889. He came to Baltimore soon afterwards and joined the staff of the Johns Hopkins Hospital, with which he was connected until his death. He was successively associate in surgery, professor of clinical surgery, and, from 1922 until 1925, head of the department. He was a most genial and lovable person, an excellent teacher, an unusually able surgeon and made many solid contributions to abdominal surgery.

1836-1946—Simon Flexner was born in Louisville, Kentucky, and graduated in medicine at the University of Louisville in 1889. He came to Baltimore in 1890 as a graduate student in pathology, was appointed associate professor of pathology in Johns Hopkins in 1895 and professor of pathological anatomy in 1898. The next year, he accepted the chair of pathology at the University of Pennsylvania, resigning in 1903 to head the Rockefeller Institute in New York, holding this post until his retirement in 1935.

Flexner published many papers in the fields of pathology and bacteriology dealing particularly with snake-venom, the transmission of poliomyelitis to monkeys, fat necrosis in pancreatitis, and cerebrospinal meningitis, for which he prepared a specific anti-serum. In 1900, he isolated a specific type of *B. dysenteriae,* since known by his name. Flexner also wrote the biography of his old chief, Dr. Welch—*William Henry Welch and the Heroic Age of American Medicine,* 1941. Much of the success of the Rockefeller Institute in its early years was the result of his inspiration and guidance.

1871-1938—Thomas Barnes Futcher was a native of St. Thomas, Ontario, graduated in medicine in Toronto, and, in 1894, came to Baltimore as assistant resident physician on Osler's service. His subsequent medical career was associated with Baltimore and the Johns Hopkins Hospital, where he rapidly acquired a reputation as a brilliant diagnostician and excellent teacher. He was active as a practitioner and teacher for 45 years and was at work in the hospital when he died suddenly from a coronary occlusion.

1860-1936—John Scott Haldane was born in Edinburgh, where he studied medicine and graduated in 1884. After graduation, he went to Dundee, where he worked with Professor Carnelly, studying the bacterial and chemical contamination of the air in stores and schools. This work, published in 1887, overthrew the erroneous idea that "sewer gas was the cause of diphtheria, scarlet and typhoid fevers." Following this work, he went to Oxford as demonstrator in physiology and was henceforth associated with that university.

Haldane became interested in the gases of coal mines and determined their composition before and after explosions and their physiological effects. "Black damp" was found to be air diluted with some inert gas and so depleted of oxygen as to be incapable of supporting life or a candle flame. "Fire damp" he discovered to be methane and both inflammable and explosive. "After damp" is carbon monoxide. He found carbon monoxide to be the cause of most cases of asphyxiation after mine accidents. The investigations were a great contribution to industrial hygiene.

From 1905 until 1915, Haldane worked on respiration, making one of the great contributions to this subject—the demonstration that the immediate cause of respiration is not oxygen but carbon dioxide.

1841-1933—Georges Hayem.

1878-1942—Lawrence Joseph Henderson was a native of Lynn, Massachusetts, and received both his A.B. and his M.D. degrees at Harvard in 1898 and 1902. After two years spent at the University of Strassburg, he returned to Harvard, where he was successively lecturer, instructor, and assistant professor of biochemistry, becoming full professor in 1919. He was the author of *The Fitness of the Environment*, 1913; *The Order of Nature*, 1917; and *Blood*, 1928.

1873-1944—Yandell Henderson was born in Louisville, Kentucky, and received his B.A. degree in 1895 and his Ph.D. degree in 1898, both from Yale University. After two years' study in Marburg and Munich, he became instructor in physiology at Yale and, in 1921 he was made professor of applied physiology.

Henderson's important physiological work was largely on respiration and circulation. He made studies on the volume output of the heart, pointed out the stimulating effect of carbon-dioxide on respiration, and drew attention to the dangers of caisson disease in high altitude flying.

1865-1927—Charles Franklin Hoover was born in Miamisburg, Ohio, and received his A.B. from Harvard in 1887 and his M.D. in 1892. From 1890 until 1894, he worked in Vienna with Neusser and in Strassburg with Friedrich Kraus. On his return to America, he settled in Cleveland, Ohio, where he lived until his death.

In 1907, he was appointed professor of medicine at Western Reserve and became a very prominent medical consultant, especially skilled in the diagnosis of pulmonary, cardiac and hepatic diseases.

1861-1947—Frederick Gowland Hopkins was born in Eastbourne, England, studied at Guy's Hospital, and received his Ph.D. degree from the University of London in 1894. He went to Cambridge in 1898 to teach chemistry, was appointed Reader in chemical physiology in 1902, and was made in 1914 professor of biochemistry, the first professor in this subject. In 1906, he began the study of "accessory food factors" and was one of the pioneers in the study of vitamins. He was knighted in 1925, received the Nobel prize in 1929, and was president of the Royal Society in 1930.

1857-1916—Victor Horsley was born in Kensington, London, the son of an artist and the nephew of Sir Frances Seymour Haden, notable as a surgeon and famous as an etcher. He studied medicine at London University College and Hospital and, in 1880, passed his examinations for membership in the Royal College of Surgeons. From 1884 to 1890, he was professor-superintendent of the Brown Institution, an institute for the study of diseases of animals. In 1886, he became surgeon to the National Hospital for the Paralysed and Epileptic.

His first work was on myxedema, for which he suggested implantation of normal thyroid tissue. In 1885, he was active in introducing Pasteur's method for the treatment of rabies. He began in 1887 to study localization of function in the brain, a work which, by degrees, led him into the field of brain surgery, in which he was one of the most distinguished pioneers. The same year, he performed the first operation for removal of a spinal cord tumor. In 1890, he reported 44 operations on the brain and, in 1909, 149 operations for removal of the Gasserian ganglion.

Horsley was quite active in politics and an implacable foe of alcohol. He served in the British Army during the first World War and died at Amarah on the Tigris in 1916 following a heat stroke.

1873-1926—John Howland was a native of New York and received his M.D. from New York University in 1897. After serving an internship, he spent a year studying in Berlin and Vienna and, on his return from Europe, became assistant to Dr. L. Emmett Holt. In 1910, he spent a year with Czerny at Strassburg and,

from 1911 until 1912, was professor of pediatrics at Washington University, St. Louis. In 1912, he was called to Johns Hopkins as professor of pediatrics, holding this position until his death.

In addition to being an excellent clinician and teacher, Howland was deeply interested in chemical problems of pediatrics and carried out important investigations on dysentery, liver necrosis, tetany and rickets.

1870-1948—Reid Hunt was born in Martinsville, Ohio, received his B.A. at Johns Hopkins in 1891, and, in 1896, received the degree of Ph.D. at Johns Hopkins and M.D. at the University of Maryland. He worked with Binz, Nussbaum and Ehrlich in Germany and with Abel at Johns Hopkins. In 1904, he was appointed head of the Pharmacological Division of the Hygienic Laboratory of the United States Public Health Service, holding this position until he was called to Harvard as professor of pharmacology in 1913. He retired in 1936.

Hunt carried out fundamental research on the accelerator nerves of the heart and on the toxicity of methyl and ethyl alcohol, demonstrated that the potency of thyroid extracts depended upon their iodine content, showed the detoxifying action of thyroid extract on acetonitrile, and discovered the activity of acetylcholine in the body.

1830-1919—Abraham Jacobi, a native of Hartum, Westphalia, received his doctor's degree from the University of Bonn in 1851. Forced to leave Germany because of his political activities, he came to New York, where he became professor of pediatrics in New York Medical College in 1861, and, in 1870, was appointed professor at the College of Physicians and Surgeons in New York. He was a tireless writer and speaker, the acknowledged dean of American pediatricians, and, at the age of 82, was elected president of the American Medical Association.

1859-1947—Pierre Marie Felix Janet was born in Paris, studied at first philosophy, received his Dr. ès lettres in 1889, then turned to medicine, took his M.D. in 1892, and began practice as a specialist in neurology and psychiatry. He was appointed professor of psychology at the Collège de France in 1903 and, in 1913, became a member of the Institute de France.

Janet made important observations on hypnotism and, in 1903, was the first to describe psychasthenia. Among his numerous works, the best known are *L'automatisme psychologique,* 1889; *État mental des hystériques,* 1893; *Nevroses et idées fixes,* 1898; *Les obsessions et la psychasthénie,* 1903; *Les médications psychologiques,* 1925-1928; and *L'amour et la haine,* 1930.

1857-1940—Julius Wagner von Jauregg was born in Wels, Upper Austria, and studied medicine in Vienna, where he graduated in 1880. After working for six years in the department of pathology and another six in the psychiatric clinic, he became *Privatdozent* for neurology and psychiatry. From 1889 until 1903, he was professor in Graz but returned to Vienna as professor, holding this position until his retirement in 1928. He received the Nobel prize in 1927.

His earliest work was on the func-

tion of the accelerator nerves and on the effects of the vagus on respiration. In 1887, he studied the effects of fevers on psychoses and suggested the inoculation of paretics with malaria. As this method seemed at the time impractical, he produced fever with tuberculin and vaccines. Thirty years later, in 1917, he returned to this subject and introduced the malarial treatment of paresis. He was the author of an important treatise on goitre, *Myxödem und Kretinismus,* 1912.

1837-1932—William Williams Keen was a native of Philadelphia and graduated from Jefferson Medical College in 1862. He served as a surgeon during the Civil War and published with Mitchell and Morehouse a notable monograph on nerve injuries. After the war, he went to Europe, returning to Philadelphia in 1866 to practice. In 1889, he was elected professor of surgery at Jefferson Medical College and soon gained an international reputation as a surgeon, teacher and writer. He was America's first "brain surgeon." He wrote many articles, and his *System of Surgery,* 1906-1921, in eight volumes, was an event in surgical literature. He was universally respected and honored and received honorary degrees from Brown, Northwestern, Toronto, Edinburgh, Yale, St. Andrew's, Pennsylvania, Upsala and Harvard.

1852-1931—Shibasaburo Kitasato was born in Kumamoto, Japan, and studied medicine first in Kumamoto, then in Tokio, where he received his degree in 1883. Two years later, he went to Berlin, where he worked in Koch's Institute. Here in 1889, he was the first to grow the tetanus

~~bacillus and, in 1890, discovered~~ with Behring the tetanus antitoxin. He returned to Japan in 1892 and established a private laboratory near Tokio, where, in 1894, he discovered the plague bacillus. His laboratory was taken over by the government and combined with the university, upon which action Kitasato resigned and established the Kitasato Institute in 1897. He trained a large number of prominent bacteriologists and founded in 1917 the *Kitasato Archives of Experimental Medicine,* of which he was editor until 1925. He was created a baron in 1924.

1841-1917—Theodor Kocher was born in Bern, where he studied medicine and received his doctor's degree in 1865. In 1872, he was appointed professor of surgery at Bern and held this position until 1911. Kocher was one of the great surgeons of his time, being noted for his scientific approach to all operative problems, his meticulous technique, and his wide knowledge of surgical literature. He trained many of the outstanding surgeons of Europe and was especially noted for his work on the thyroid gland. He received the Nobel prize in 1909.

1857-1944—Carl Koller graduated at Vienna in 1882 and, two years later in 1884, introduced the use of cocaine as a local anesthetic in operations on the eye. In 1888, he began the practice of ophthalmology in New York, where he lived from that time until his death. He was very successful as an ophthalmologist and the recipient of numerous honors.

1856-1926—Emil Kraepelin was born in Neu-Strelitz, Mecklenburg, and studied at Leipzig and Würzburg. While a student, he decided to become a psychiatrist and, after receiving his doctor's degree in 1878, was assistant to Gudden in Munich and to Flechsig in Leipzig. In 1886, he was appointed professor of psychiatry at Dorpat, went to Heidelberg as professor in 1890, and returned to Munich in 1904 as professor and director of the psychiatric institute.

Kraepelin was one of the great psychiatrists of his period and exercised a deep influence on the development of psychiatry. His greatest service was his classification and systematizing of mental diseases. Before his time, there had been no clear differentiation of the endogenous and the organic psychoses.

1866-1944—Alexander Korányi was born in Budapest, received his doctor's degree there, and studied further at Strassburg. In 1893, he became a *Privatdozent* at Budapest, in 1900 associate professor, and in 1907 full professor. He was a close student of renal disease, devised several functional tests including cryoscopy of the urine and was one of the first observers to point out the retention of chlorides in edema.

1840-1903—Richard Freiherr von Krafft-Ebing was born in Mannheim, graduated at Heidelberg in 1863, and, in 1872, became professor of psychiatry in Strassburg. In 1889, he was called to Vienna as director of the First Psychiatric Clinic and, in 1892, became professor in the Second Psychiatric Clinic in the Allgemeines Krankenhaus, holding this position until his retirement in 1902.

Krafft-Ebing was a brilliant lecturer and an excellent teacher and introduced many reforms in teaching and in the treatment of patients. His *Lehrbuch der gerichtlichen Medizin*, 1875, was the best German work on forensic psychiatry, and his *Psychopathia sexualis*, 1886, was an exhaustive treatise on sexual inversions and perversions.

1858-1936—Friedrich Kraus was a native of Bodenbach, Bohemia, and graduated M.D. at Prague in 1882. In 1894, he was appointed professor of medicine at Graz and, in 1902, became professor and director of the II University Clinic at the Charité in Berlin, where he worked until his retirement in 1927.

Kraus was a very popular and inspiring teacher and, in addition to publishing a large number of original articles on diseases of the blood, metabolism, heart and lungs, was editor of a system of medicine, *Spezielle Pathologie und Therapie*, in nineteen volumes, published in 1919-1925.

1881-1941—Allen Kramer Krause was born in Lebanon, Pennsylvania, received his bachelor's degree from Brown University in 1901 and his M.D. from Johns Hopkins in 1907. While a patient at Saranac Lake in 1909, he developed a great interest in tuberculosis and worked there until 1916, when he was called to Johns Hopkins as associate professor of medicine and physician in charge of the Phipps Tuberculosis Dispensary and, the same year, became managing editor of the *American Review of Tuberculosis*. "Krause was soon recognized as the leading American in the formulation of concepts on the pathogenesis of tuberculosis. A brilliant writer, facile

speaker and imaginative investigator, he stimulated all workers in the field" (Esmond Long). He wrote numerous authoritative articles on tuberculosis in several textbooks and systems of medicine.

1874-1950—August Krogh was born in Grenaa, Jütland, studied zoology and physiology at Copenhagen, where he received his master's degree in 1899 and his doctor's degree in 1903. From 1899 until 1908, he was assistant in the physiological laboratory, and, in 1916, he became professor of physiology.

In 1908, he spent much time in Greenland investigating the diet and metabolism of the Eskimos. In the following years, he carried out important investigations on respiration, on the capillary circulation, and on the oxygen consumption of the muscles. In 1920, he received the Nobel prize in medicine.

1868-1943—Karl Landsteiner was a native of Vienna, where he received his doctor's degree in 1891. After graduation, he studied chemistry with Emil Fischer for several years, then returned to Vienna, and, in 1898, became assistant in the pathological institute. In 1900, he discovered iso-agglutinins in the human blood and demonstrated the existence of specific blood groups, a discovery that made blood transfusions safe. In 1909 with Poppen, he showed that poliomyelitis could be transmitted to monkeys by intraspinal injections. After World War I, he left Vienna for The Hague, where he worked until 1922, when he went to New York as a member of the Rockefeller Institute. In 1940 with Wiener, he discovered the Rh factor in human blood. Landsteiner made many important discoveries in immuno chemistry, and his scientific activity may be judged by the fact that, from 1892 to 1943, he published 346 scientific articles. He received the Nobel prize in 1930.

1849-1907—Oskar Lassar, a native of Hamburg, after studying at Heidelberg, Göttingen, Strassburg and Berlin, received his M.D. at Würzburg in 1872. He spent several years working in physiology and pathology and then became *Privatdozent* for dermatology in Berlin in 1880. He was one of the best known German dermatologists of his time.

1874-1941—Dean Lewis, a native of Kewanee, Illinois, received his medical degree in 1899 at Rush Medical College, where he became professor of surgery and was an acknowledged leader of his profession in Chicago. An excellent surgeon and an inspiring teacher, he was called to Johns Hopkins in 1925 as professor of surgery and surgeon-in-chief to the Johns Hopkins Hospital. He made many contributions to surgical literature, notably on the hypophysis and on surgery of the nerves, and edited a well-known *Practice of Surgery*.

1881-1945—Thomas Lewis was born in Wales and received his medical education in London at the University College Hospital, where he spent his entire professional life. Through the influence of Sir James Mackenzie, he was drawn into the field of cardiology, particularly electrocardiography. In 1909, he described with the aid of the electrocardiograph auricular fibrillation in man. Two years later, at the age of 29, he published the *Mechanism of the Heart Beat,* a classic in cardiology, which was greatly enlarged in later editions. He was also the author of two very popular smaller works—*Clinical Disorders of the Heart Beat,* 1912; and *Clinical Electrocardiography,* 1913, both of which went through six editions. Lewis also did important work in other fields of vascular pathology and noted the similarity between urticaria and the physiological response to histamine. He was knighted in 1921.

1872-1946—Emanuel Libman was born in New York City, graduated from the College of the City of New York in 1891, and received his M.D. from the College of Physicians and Surgeons, Columbia University, in 1894. After serving as house physician to Mt. Sinai Hospital, he went abroad, where work in Escherich's laboratory determined his future interests in clinical bacteriology. On his return to New York, he became associate pathologist to Mt. Sinai Hospital, the institution with which his subsequent professional career was associated.

Libman combined almost phenomenal powers of clinical observation with a thorough knowledge of pathology. His greatest scientific achievements were his studies of subacute endocarditis and of blood stream infections. His work on atypical verrucous endocarditis is perpetuated by the eponym, Libman-Sacks disease.

1854-1946—Adolf Lorenz, a native of Weidenau, Austria, studied in Vienna, where he received his medical degree in 1880. In 1889, he was appointed professor and director of the orthopedic clinic, holding this position until his retirement in 1924. He was an orthopedic surgeon of international reputation, well known for his methods of treating flatfoot, clubfoot, and congenital dislocation of the hip.

1874-1944—William George MacCallum was born in Dunnville, Ontario, and graduated in the first class of the Johns Hopkins Medical School in 1897. From 1900 until 1908, he was associate professor of pathology at Johns Hopkins, professor of pathological physiology in 1908, and, from 1909 until 1917, professor of pathology at Columbia University, New York. He returned to Johns Hopkins in 1917 as professor of pathology and held this position until his death.

MacCallum made many important contributions to medical science. Outstanding was his discovery in 1897 that the so-called flagella of the malarial parasite were sexual forms, the proof in 1909 that the parathyroid glands control calcium metabolism, and his demonstration of the relationship between the islands of Langerhans and carbohydrate metabolism. His *Text-book of Pathology,* which appeared first in 1916, was a valuable and widely used text.

1853-1925—James Mackenzie.

1876-1935—John James Richard Macleod was born in Dunkeld, Scotland, studied medicine at Aberdeen and Leipzig, and received his medical degree at Aberdeen in 1898. In 1903, he went to the Western Reserve University as professor of physiology and held this position until 1918, when he accepted the chair of physiology in Toronto. In 1928, he was called to Aberdeen as regius professor of physiology. He died in 1935.

Macleod's physiological investigations were mostly in the field of carbohydrate metabolism, and, in 1923, he shared with Banting the Nobel prize for the discovery of insulin.

1853-1940—Pierre Marie was born in Paris, where he received his M.D. in 1883. Two years later, he became physician at the Salpêtrière under Charcot and, after Charcot's death, was the acknowledged leader in French neurology. His doctor's dissertation on Basedow's disease, 1883, was an important monograph, in which he pointed out that tremor was a cardinal sign. He described acromegaly in 1886, pulmonary osteoarthropathy (Strümpell-Marie disease) in 1890, and hereditary cerebellar ataxis in 1893. He also made important observations on aphasia and in many other diseases of the nervous system. In 1907, he was appointed professor of neurology in the Paris faculty.

1870-1935—Thomas McCrae was born in Guelph, Ontario, graduated in medicine at the University of Toronto and, in 1896, came to the Johns Hopkins Hospital on the staff of William Osler. He began practice in Baltimore in 1904 but continued quite active in the teaching of medicine at Johns Hopkins. In 1912, he was called to Jefferson Medical College as professor of medicine, holding this position until his death.

McCrae was eminent in medical teaching and practice and collaborated with Osler as editor of the well-known *System of Medicine*. After Osler's death, he edited the eleventh and twelfth editions of Osler's *Principles and Practice of Medicine*.

1851-1920—Samuel James Meltzer was born in Courland, was trained for the rabbinate, but became a merchant in Königsberg. Later, he took up the study of medicine and received his M.D. in Berlin in 1882. The following year, he emigrated to America and began practice in New York, working at the same time in the pathological laboratory of Bellevue Hospital and in the physiological laboratory of Columbia University. In 1904, he gave up private practice and became associated with the Rockefeller Institute. He carried out many important investigations in physiology and pharmacology on deglutition, adrenalin, insufflation, shock, anaphylaxis, hemolysis, and other subjects.

1866-1950—Adolf Meyer was born in Niederweiningen near Zürich, Switzerland. After passing his *Staatsexamen* for the practice of medicine in 1899, he did postgraduate work in Paris, London, Edinburgh, Zürich, Vienna and Berlin and received his M.D. degree from the University of Zürich in 1892. He came to the United States in 1892, and, after holding various teaching positions as pathologist and psychiatrist, he was appointed professor of psychiatry at Cornell in 1904. In 1910, he was called to Johns Hopkins as professor of psychiatry and director of the Phipps Psychiatric Clinic, holding these positions until his retirement in 1941.

Meyer was the author of numerous articles on neurology, psychiatry, pathology, and mental hygiene and, at the time of his retirement, was regarded as the dean of American psychiatrists.

1867-1937—Joseph Leggett Miller was born in Kewanee, Illinois, and received the B.S. degree from the University of Michigan in 1893 and the degree of M.D. from Northwestern University in 1895. After serving an internship, he began a life-long association with Dr. Frank Billings. He was successively associate professor at Rush Medical College and clinical professor at the University of Chicago. He was the author of numerous articles on arteriosclerosis, typhoid fever, foreign protein therapy, arthritis and thyrotoxicosis. He was for 22 years editor-in-chief of the *Archives of Internal Medicine*.

1885-1950—George Richards Minot, who came of a long line of distinguished New England physicians, was born in Boston and received his medical degree at Harvard in 1912. In 1927, he became director of the Thorndike Memorial Laboratory of the Boston City Hospital and professor of medicine at Harvard University, holding these positions until his death.

In 1926, in collaboration with William P. Murphy, he announced the discovery of liver therapy for pernicious anemia. He was a stimulating and inspiring teacher and leader, the Thorndike Memorial Laboratory under his direction becoming one of the outstanding centers of medical research in North America.

1853-1907—Paul Julius Moebius was born in Leipzig, studied first theology and philosophy, receiving his doctor's degree in philosophy, then began the study of medicine, receiving his M.D. in 1877. After working in the policlinic under Strümpell, he became *Privatdozent* in 1883 but gave up teaching 10 years later. He was an excellent neurologist and wrote several books on nervous diseases. His literary interests are obvious in his pathological studies of Rousseau, Nietzsche and Goethe. He wrote on Basedow's disease for Nothnagel's *Handbuch* and described the well-known Moebius's sign in this condition.

1865-1936—Berkeley George Andrew Moynihan was born in Malta and studied in Leeds, London and Berlin, graduating in medicine at the University of London in 1887. His professional life was spent in Leeds, where, after 16 years of service at the Leeds General Infirmary, he was appointed professor of surgery. Moynihan was one of the outstanding English surgeons of his time and won international fame as an abdominal surgeon, his work on duodenal ulcer being especially noteworthy. In recognition of his great services to surgery and to his country, he was created a baronet in 1922 and elevated in 1929 to the peerage with the title of Lord Moynihan of Leeds.

1858-1941—Friedrich von Müller, one of the greatest German clinicians of his period, was born in Augsburg and received his M.D. in Munich in 1882. In 1888, he was appointed professor at Bonn and subsequently held chairs in Breslau, Marburg and Basel. He went to Munich in 1902 as professor, holding this chair until his retirement.

Müller did original work in many fields of medicine. In 1893, he demonstrated the increased metabolism in Graves' disease and, the same year, described eosinophilia in asthma. He devoted much time to the study of percussion and auscultation, employing exact methods in these investigations. He was a very inspiring teacher and trained a large number of prominent internists. Garrison, in 1924, described him as "perhaps the most scientific teacher of internal medicine today."

1857-1916—John Benjamin Murphy was born in Appleton, Wisconsin, graduated at Rush Medical College in 1879, and, after two years of study abroad, chiefly in Vienna, returned to Chicago and began the practice of surgery. He was, at different times, professor of surgery at Rush Medical College, the College of Physicians and Surgeons in Chicago, and Northwestern University. From 1895 until his death, he was chief surgeon to Mercy Hospital, Chicago.

He gained international reputation as an abdominal surgeon, devised the well-known "Murphy button," and was a pioneer in vascular surgery. An inspiring teacher, an excellent speaker, and a dominating personality, he was a towering figure in Chicago medical circles for a generation.

1866-1936—Charles Nicolle was a native of Rouen, received his medical degree in 1894 and, from 1895 until 1903, taught in the medical school of Rouen. In 1903, he was appointed director of the Pasteur Institute of Tunis and soon raised this institution to the rank of a leading center for bacteriological research. Nicolle's contributions to medical science were both numerous and important. He demonstrated the protective power of convalescent serum in measles, typhus fever, and undulant fever. He found that grippe is due to a filterable virus and proved that leishmaniasis is transmitted by the dog flea. In 1909, he demonstrated that typhus fever could be transmitted from monkey to monkey by the bite of the body louse. He celebrated in 1928 the twenty-fifth anniversary of his appointment as director of the Pasteur Institute of Tunis and, the same year, received the Nobel prize.

1876-1928—Hideyo Noguchi was born at Inawashiro, Japan, studied medicine at Tokio from 1893 to 1897, and received a license to practice medicine in 1897. From 1898 to 1900, he worked at the Institute for Infectious Diseases in Tokio and, in 1900, came to Philadelphia, where he worked in pathology under Dr. Simon Flexner at the University of Pennsylvania. In 1904, when the Rockefeller Institute was founded, he joined the staff as a member, a position he held until his death.

Noguchi was the first to demonstrate *Spirochaete pallida* in the brain of paretics and to transmit syphilis to rabbits from the brain tissue of patients dying of paresis (1913). He cultivated several varieties of spirochaete outside the body and, in 1915, cultivated a bacteria-free vaccine virus in the tissues of rabbits. He was a most distinguished bacteriologist and investigator. He died of yellow fever in Africa while studying this disease.

1858-1925—Albert John Ochsner was a native of Baraboo, Wisconsin, graduated at Rush Medical College in 1886, and, after postgraduate study in Vienna, Berlin and London, began practice in Chicago. He was soon one of the most skillful and best known surgeons there. His *Clinical Surgery*, 1902, *A Handbook of Appendicitis*, 1902, and *Treatise on Surgical Diagnosis and Treatment*, four volumes, were widely read and deservedly popular.

1871-1946—Erwin Payr was a native of Innsbruck, where he graduated in 1894. After working in Vienna and Graz, he became professor of surgery at Graz, Greifswald, Königsberg, and then at Leipzig in 1911. He was an excellent and learned surgeon, making contributions to many surgical subjects, notably on diseases of the joints, surgery of the abdominal organs, breast, and thyroid gland. He was a contributor to several systems of surgery and one of the editors of the *Ergebnisse der Chirurgie und Orthopädie*.

1879-1940—Raymond Pearl was born in Farmington, New Hampshire, graduated at Dartmouth College in 1899, and received the Ph.D. degree at the University of Michigan in 1902. He was instructor in biology at the University of Michigan for four years and then studied in Leipzig, London and Naples. On his return to the United States, Pearl was instructor in zoology at the University of Pennsylvania, then professor of biology at the Maine

Agricultural Experiment Station, and went in 1918 to Johns Hopkins as professor of biometry and vital statistics.

While a graduate student in London, Pearl worked with Karl Pearson, who greatly influenced his scientific interests and future. Pearl was the author of some eight authoritative books on biometry, beginning with *The Biology of Death,* 1922, and closing with *The Natural History of Population,* 1939.

1868-1927—Karl Petrén, a native of Halmstad, Sweden, received his medical degree at Lund in 1895. After graduation, he worked in Paris with Déjérine and in Strassburg with Naunyn. In 1902, he was appointed professor of medicine in Uppsala and, in 1910, at Lund. He published many articles on physiology, on diseases of the spinal cord and of the joints, and on metabolic diseases, particularly on diabetes mellitus. He introduced the Petrén diet in the treatment of diabetes—a low-protein, high-fat diet—and considered protein as the chief ketogenic factor.

1874-1929—Clemens Freiherr von Pirquet was born in Aspern, Lower Austria, and received his medical education at Graz, where he graduated in 1900. Soon afterwards, he went to Vienna, worked in Escherich's clinic, and, in 1908, received the appointment of professor of pediatrics at Johns Hopkins. Two years later, he went to Breslau and, in 1911, was called to Vienna as Escherich's successor in the chair of pediatrics. Von Pirquet is well known as the originator of the skin test (Pirquet test) for tuberculosis

and for his fundamental work on allergy.

1875-1915—Stanislaus von Prowazek was born in Neuhaus, Bohemia, studied first at Prague and then at Vienna, where he graduated Ph.D. in 1899. After studying with Ehrlich at Frankfurt and with Hertwig at Munich, he went to the *Kaiserliches Gesundheitsamt* in Berlin and, in 1907, succeeded Schaudinn as director of the zoological department at the Institute of Tropical Medicine in Hamburg. In 1913-1914, he went to Belgrade and Constantinople to study typhus fever and, in 1915, died of this disease at Kottbus. Von Prowazek found in typhus fever the same organisms Ricketts had previously described, which are now known as *Rickettsia prowazeki.*

1852-1934—Santiago Ramón y Cajal was born in Petilla de Aragon, Spain, studied at Saragossa, where he received his licentiate, and, after service in the Spanish Army in Cuba, was assistant in the medical clinic at Saragossa. He obtained his doctor's degree at Madrid in 1877 and was successively professor of anatomy and histology in Saragossa, Valencia, Barcelona and Madrid. In 1920, a new institute, the Institute Cajal, was built for him by King Alfonso XIII, and here he worked until his death.

Employing the Golgi stain with improvements of his own, Ramón y Cajal made fundamental discoveries on the anatomy of the nervous system, demonstrating cells and structures never seen before. He was a tireless worker and published more than 200 scientific papers and, in addition, a *Textura del sistema nervioso del hombre y de los vertebrados,* 1897-1904, in three volumes, and *Estudios sobre la degeneración y regeneración del sistema nervioso,* 1913-1914, as well as 11 other books. He shared the Nobel prize of 1906 with Camillo Golgi.

1850-1935—Charles Richet was born in Paris, the son of a surgeon, and was himself destined for a surgical career. While still a medical student, however, he became interested in physiology and decided to devote himself to this field. He received his M.D. at Paris in 1877 and, from 1887 until 1927, was professor of physiology in the Paris faculty. His experimental work covered a large field, the physiology of nerve and muscle, respiration, animal heat, liver function, dietetics, and serum therapy. In 1888, he demonstrated that animals, when injected with bacteria, developed immune bodies and, in 1890, was the first to employ serum therapy. The same year, he described anaphylaxis. In addition to being the author of numerous scientific articles, he wrote several works on physiology, psychology and philosophy. He received the Nobel prize in 1913.

1871-1910—Howard Taylor Ricketts was born in Findlay, Ohio, and studied medicine at Northwestern University, Chicago, where he graduated in 1897. After two years' service at the Cook County Hospital, he decided to devote himself to the study of pathology and, in 1902, was appointed associate professor of pathology at the University of Chicago. In 1906, he demonstrated the transmission of Rocky Mountain fever by the bite of infected ticks

and described the causative agent in the eggs of infected ticks. Four years later, he went to Mexico to study *tabardillo* and found in this disease small organisms similar to those in Rocky Mountain spotted fever. He contracted *tabardillo* (Mexican typhus) and died at the early age of 39. The organisms he described for the first time have been named *Rickettsia* in his honor.

1886-1947—Victor Robinson was born in the Ukraine and, when a child, was brought to the United States. He studied law at New York University but, finding it uncongenial, turned to pharmacy and received the degree of Ph.C. from Columbia University in 1911. From pharmacy, he turned to medicine, receiving his doctor's degree from the Chicago College of Medicine in 1917. On his return to New York, he soon gave up the practice of medicine and devoted himself entirely to the study of medical history.

Robinson's *Pathfinders in Medicine,* which first appeared in 1912, was quite successful and was followed by subsequent works, some 13 in all. In 1920, he founded *Medical Life,* the first, and for many years the only, monthly journal written in English devoted to the history of medicine. It ceased publication in 1938. A chair of the history of medicine was created for him in 1929 at Temple University. Robinson wrote easily and well and did much to stimulate interest in medical history.

1860-1946—Georges Henri Roger, a native of Paris, received his medical degree at Paris. He was successively professor of experimental pathology and of physiology and was from 1917 until 1930 dean of the medical faculty. His investigations were largely in the fields of pathology, experimental bacteriology, and physiology. His *Introduction a l'étude de la médecine* went through eight editions and was translated into English. He was also the author of monographs on diseases of the liver, of the spinal cord, and of the digestive organs. With Binet, he was the editor of a *Traité de physiologie normale et pathologique,* in 12 volumes, and, with Widal and Teissier, of the *Nouveau Traité de médecine,* in 22 volumes.

1862-1944—Humphrey Davy Rolleston was born in Oxford, England, where his father, George Rolleston, was physician to the Radcliffe Infirmary and later professor of anatomy and physiology. He studied at Cambridge, where he received the degrees of M.B. in 1888 and M.D. in 1892. Soon after graduation, he became assistant physician at St. George's Hospital as well as demonstrator of anatomy, physiology and pathology at Cambridge. At Cambridge, he became a close friend of Sir Clifford Allbutt, whom he aided in preparing the first edition of his successful *System of Medicine,* the second edition of which carried Rolleston's name as co-editor.

In 1925, Rolleston succeeded Allbutt as regius professor of physic at Cambridge, retiring at the age of 70. From 1928 until the year of his death, he was editor of *The Practitioner.* He was the only physician since Francis Glisson to be both president of the Royal College of

Physicians and professor of physic at Cambridge. He was physician to George V and was created a baronet in 1924. It is said that no English physician received so many honorary degrees as he.

Rolleston's *Diseases of the Liver, Gallbladder and Bile Ducts,* 1905, was an authoritative work and went through three editions. His *Endocrine Organs in Health and Disease,* 1936, as a history of the subject, is unsurpassed for accuracy. A great student of medical history, he was the author of *Clifford Allbutt, A Memoir,* 1929; *Internal Medicine,* 1930, in the *Clio Medica* series; and *The Cambridge Medical School,* 1932. He wrote charming and authoritative articles on many medico-historical subjects.

1865-1934—Ernst von Romberg.

1859-1917—Sir Marc Armand Ruffer was born in Lyon, France, received his B.A. at Brasenose College, Oxford, and his M.D. at the University College, London, in 1889. After study with Pasteur and Metchnikoff, he became in 1891 the first director of the British Institute of Preventive Medicine, but, following a severe infection with diphtheria, he went to Egypt for his health. In 1896, he was appointed professor of bacteriology in the Cairo Medical School, became president of the Sanitary Maritime and Quarantine Council of Egypt in 1901, and was soon recognized as one of the great sanitarians of his time. He rid Egypt of the cholera, reorganized the sanitation of Greece, and was of great assistance to the Indian Plague Commission. During the World War, he was head of the Red

Cross in Egypt. His studies on the pathology of mummies, which appeared in several medical journals, were collected and published by Roy L. Moodie in 1921 with the title, *Studies in the Paleopathology of Egypt.*

1871-1906—Fritz Schaudinn.

1844-1908—Nicholas Senn was born in Buchs, St. Gallen, Switzerland, emigrated to the United States at eight years of age, and studied medicine at Northwestern University in Chicago, graduating from there in 1868. In 1873, he began to practice in Milwaukee, and, in 1877, he entered the University of Munich and received an M.D. in 1878. In 1888, he became professor of surgery at Rush Medical College and practiced in Chicago until his death.

Senn was a highly trained, scientific surgeon and made important contributions to the study of air embolism (1885), surgery of the pancreas (1886), and gunshot wounds. He was active as an army surgeon during the Spanish-American War, was the first to employ x-rays in the treatment of leukemia, devised a method of detecting intestinal perforation by inflation with hydrogen gas, and founded the Association of Military Surgeons of the United States.

1850-1935—Edward Sharpey-Schafer was born in London, the son of J. W. H. Schäfer, a native of Hamburg. Edward Schäfer was educated at University College, London, where he came under the influence of William Sharpey, whom he admired greatly and whose name he later added to his own. Sharpey-Schafer was appointed professor of physiology at University College in 1883 and held this chair until 1899, when he was called to Edinburgh as professor. He retired from this post in 1933, after teaching for half a century.

Sharpey-Schafer's first work was in the field of histology, and his *Essentials of Histology,* which was first published in 1885, went through 12 editions and was widely used by English-speaking medical students. In 1888, he carried out an investigation of the functions of the cerebral cortex with Victor Horsley and, in 1895 with Oliver, first demonstrated the pressor effects of adrenal extracts. His *Text-Book of Physiology* appeared in 1898, and, during the years at London and at Edinburgh, he had coming from his pen a steady flow of scientific articles on ciliary and amboid movement, the function of the spleen, fat absorption, pulmonary blood pressure, and vagotomy. In 1904, he described a method of resuscitation, since known by his name.

1860-1927—Ernest Henry Starling was born in Bombay, India, the son of a British official, and studied medicine at Guy's Hospital. He was early attracted to physiology and, after two years' intensive study, went in 1886 to Heidelberg, where he worked with the physiologist Willy Kühne, a former pupil of Claude Bernard. On his return to London, he decided definitely to devote his life to physiology. In 1889, he became a demonstrator of physiology at Guy's and, in 1893, worked with Heidenhain in Breslau and with Metchnikoff in Paris. On his return to London, he worked with Bayliss in Schäfer's laboratory at University College. In 1899, when Schäfer left for Edinburgh, he was appointed Jodrell professor of physiology at University College, holding this chair until 1923. He died on board ship off Kingston, Jamaica, in 1927.

Starling's first important scientific research, carried out with Bayliss in 1891, was on the electromotive phenomena of the mammalian heart, finding that the rate of transmission of the contraction wave was about five metres per second and that it was slowed at the auricular ventricular groove. In 1892, he turned his attention to the study of lymph flow and, by a series of brilliant experiments, demonstrated the functional significance of the osmotic pressure of the blood proteins. He showed that, since the capillaries are permeable to the blood crystalloids, the effective osmotic pressure is exerted by the serum proteins and this pressure causes the absorption of fluid from the tissues. In 1902 with Bayliss, he discovered secretin, a substance secreted by the mucosa of the duodenum and ileum, which, when introduced into the blood stream, causes a secretion of bile and pancreatic juice. For such internal secretions, Starling proposed the name, "hormone." Turning back to the study of circulation, he devised his well-known heart-lung preparation, with which he discovered several fundamental facts, among them the "Starling's law of the heart"— that, to work at its greatest efficiency, the heart must dilate, which it does when the pressure in front of it increases. His last important work,

carried out with the perfused isolated kidney, was his demonstration that water, chlorides, bicarbonates and glucose are reabsorbed by the tubule cells from the glomerular filtrate.

1872-1948—Richard Pearson Strong was born at Fortress Monroe, Virginia, received his bachelor's degree at Yale in 1893 and his doctor's degree at Johns Hopkins in 1897. He served as assistant surgeon in the United States Army from 1898 until 1902 and was director of the laboratory and professor of tropical diseases in the University of the Philippines until 1913, when he went to Harvard as professor of tropical medicine, holding this position until his retirement in 1938.

Under his leadership, many scientific expeditions were sent out to study disease in the tropics. During the First World War, Strong headed the Red Cross Commission which went to Serbia to combat typhus fever and, after the entry of the United States into the war, was placed in charge of the division of infectious diseases in the A.E.F. He was the author of *Diagnosis, Prevention and Treatment of Tropical Diseases,* which passed through seven editions, and wrote numerous important scientific papers and monographs on typhus fever, oroyo fever, plague, beriberi and onchocerciasis.

1853-1925—Adolf Strümpell was born in Courland and studied at Dorpat and Leipzig, receiving his doctor's degree in 1875. He was appointed associate professor at Leipzig in 1883, was called as full professor to Erlangen in 1886, to Breslau in

1903, and to Vienna in 1909, but returned to Leipzig in 1910, where he remained until his death.

Most of his investigations were in diseases of the nervous system. His textbook of medicine, *Lehrbuch der speziellen Pathologie und Therapie,* which first appeared in 1884, went through 30 editions.

1864-1932—William Sydney Thayer was born in Milton, Massachusetts, and received his M.D. at Harvard in 1889. The following year, he became assistant resident at the Johns Hopkins Hospital and, after eight years in the hospital, began practice in Baltimore in 1898. He was made clinical professor of medicine in 1905 and professor in 1918. He retired from active duties with the Johns Hopkins Hospital in 1921 after 31 years' continuous service.

Thayer was a highly cultured man, a great lover of books, extremely well read, and an almost uncanny clinician. He did excellent research on malaria fever and on endocarditis and was one of the first to point out the occurrence of eosinophilia in trichinosis.

1853-1923—Robert Tigerstedt, one of the outstanding physiologists of the twentieth century, was born in Helsingfors, where he studied medicine and received his degree in 1881. He worked for a time with Ludwig in Leipzig, was professor at the *Karolinska Institut* in Stockholm from 1886 until 1900, and was professor of physiology at the University of Helsingfors from 1900 until 1919.

Tigerstedt did important work on the mechanical stimulation of nerves, on the circulation, on the organs of special sense, and on metabolism, and, in 1898, discovered renin, a pressor substance isolated from the kidney. He was the author of a noteworthy text on physiology of the circulation, *Lehrbuch der Physiologie des Kreislaufes,* Leipzig, 1893, and his *Lehrbuch der Physiologie des Menschen,* 1898, belongs to the best general texts on general physiology.

1840-1920—Carl Toldt was born in Bruneck, in Tyrol, received his medical degree in Vienna in 1864, became a *Privatdozent* for microscopic anatomy, and in 1876, was called to Prague as professor. In 1884, he returned to Vienna as professor of anatomy, serving in this capacity for 24 years until his retirement in 1908. During this period, he directed the construction of the new Anatomical Institute, assembled a large museum of anatomy, and built up a large library for his institute.

Toldt was at first interested mainly in histology and embryology and published in 1877 a noteworthy book, *Lehrbuch der Gewebelehre.* Later, he devoted himself largely to gross anatomy and anthropology. His *Anatomischer Atlas,* 1896-1900, the result of seven years' intensive labor, was an extremely popular text and widely used by American students.

1844-1924—Friedrich Trendelenburg was born in Berlin and studied in Glasgow and Berlin, receiving his M.D. at Berlin in 1866. He was assistant to Langenbeck from 1868 until 1874, went to Rostock in 1875 as professor of surgery, was called to Bonn in 1882, and became professor at Leipzig in 1895, holding this chair until his retirement in 1911.

Trendelenburg was a scientific surgeon of much originality, and his name is perpetuated in medical literature by Trendelenburg's cannula, Trendelenburg's operation for the excision of varicose veins, Trendelenburg's gait due to paralysis of the gluteal muscles, Trendelenburg's test for incompetency of the venous valves, and Trendelenburg's position. In 1886, he described a plastic operation for hydronephrosis and, in 1908, attempted the surgical removal of a pulmonary embolism, an operation first successfully performed by Kirschner in 1924.

1853-1923—Sir Frederick Treves was born in Dorchester, England, studied in London, and, after serving for several years as assistant surgeon and lecturer on anatomy at the London Hospital, became surgeon in 1883. In 1885, he was appointed Hunterian professor of anatomy at the Royal College of Surgeons. He was a brilliant lecturer, a man of great ability as a surgeon, and achieved a wide reputation as a teacher of anatomy and as a pioneer in abdominal surgery, especially as an advocate of appendectomy. His *Surgical Applied Anatomy* was a popular work among English-speaking surgeons and medical students, went through many editions, and was translated into French.

1848-1915—Edward Livingston Trudeau, one of the pioneer American scientific students of tuberculosis, was born in New York City and graduated from the College of Physicians and Surgeons in 1871.

Himself a victim of tuberculosis, he became convinced of the need for adequate sanitaria and established a small cottage sanitarium in the Adirondacks, equipped with a clinical laboratory. From these small beginnings, he developed the Trudeau Sanitarium, which achieved a worldwide reputation as an institution for the study and treatment of tuberculosis.

1857-1929—Théodore Tuffier was a native of Bellême, France, and studied medicine in Paris, where he received his M.D. degree in 1885. He was an excellent surgeon, active in experimental surgery, and was a pioneer in surgery of the chest. He was a prolific writer and made many contributions to surgical literature.

1866-1925—August von Wassermann.

1875-1943—Harry Gideon Wells was a native of New Haven, Connecticut, and received the degree of M.D. at Rush Medical College in 1898 and the degree of Ph.D. at the University of Chicago in 1903. He became interested in pathology, joined the staff of the pathological department, and became professor of pathology in 1913. His *Chemical Pathology*, 1907, went through five editions and was followed by *Chemistry of Tuberculosis*, 1923, with DeWitt and Long; and *Chemical Aspects of Immunity*, 1925, which was translated into French and German. Wells was a most active investigator, a stimulating teacher, and a pioneer in the chemistry of pathologic processes.

1864-1940—Karel Frederik Wenckebach was born in The Hague, received his M.D. at Utrecht in 1888, was appointed professor of medicine at Groningen in 1901 and at Strassburg in 1911, and was called to Vienna in 1914 as professor of medicine, holding this post until his retirement in 1929.

Wenckebach made a great reputation as a cardiologist and is remembered by Wenckebach's sign in adhesive pericarditis and Wenckebach's phenomenon in cardiac arrhythmia. He was the first to demonstrate the value of quinine in paroxysmal fibrillation (1914) and wrote an important monograph on the heart in beriberi (1934).

1862-1929—Fernand Widal, the son of a French Army surgeon, was born in Delbys, Algeria, and studied medicine in Paris, where he received his M.D. in 1889. In 1894, he became *agrégé* and, in 1911, professor. His first scientific work was his doctor's dissertation, in which he described streptococci in *phlegmasia alba dolens*. In 1889, he began to work on preventive vaccination against typhoid fever and, in 1896, announced the agglutinin reaction for typhoid fever—Widal reaction.

In 1900, he worked on cyto-diagnosis of body fluids and, in 1907, on hemolytic anemia, demonstrating the increased fragility of the red blood cells in this condition. He pointed out in 1906 the role played by sodium chloride in the production of edema.

1866-1931—John Whitridge Williams was a native of Baltimore, received his M.D. at the University of Maryland in 1888, and, after postgraduate study in Berlin, returned to Baltimore and became a voluntary assistant in the department of gynecology at the Johns Hopkins Hospital in 1891. He was a member of the hospital staff until his death. In 1899, he was appointed professor of obstetrics and was dean of the medical school from 1911 until 1923.

Williams was deeply interested in pathology and made important studies on the pathology and bacteriology of the genital organs, the physiology of pregnancy, the etiology of eclampsia, and on cystoma papillare. His *Obstetrics,* first published in 1903, was the most popular text in its field and went through seven editions before his death. He was an excellent speaker, a gifted teacher, and the outstanding American obstetrician of his time.

1863-1936—William Holland Wilmer was born near Richmond, Virginia, and received his M.D. from the University of Virginia in 1885. He began practice in Washington, D.C., in 1889 and, in 1906, became professor of ophthalmology in Georgetown University. In 1927, Wilmer gave up his practice in Washington and went to Baltimore to direct the new Wilmer Ophthalmological Institute of the Johns Hopkins Hospital, an institute which soon took high rank among similar institutions. Wilmer retired in 1935.

1861-1947—Almoth Edward Wright was born in Coolcarrigan, Ireland, and studied in Leipzig, Strassburg, Marburg and Dublin, receiving his degree in Dublin in 1883. After teaching pathology at Cambridge and physiology in Sydney, Australia, he held the chair of pathology in the Army Medical School at Netley from 1892 to 1902 and, in 1904, became professor of experimental pathology in the University of London.

Wright made many important contributions to medical science. He is the father of anti-typhoid vaccination, the great value of which he demonstrated in 1896. He introduced in 1897 the agglutination test for undulant fever. In 1903, he discovered opsonins, and his work on the "opsonic index" was a fundamental contribution to the science of immunology.

1870-1945—Hugh Hampton Young was a native of San Antonio, Texas, graduated in medicine at the University of Virginia in 1894, and, the following year, went to Johns Hopkins Hospital, with which he was associated until his death. In 1897, he became interested especially in urology and, in a long career in that specialty, became one of its most prominent leaders. He was a skillful

and original surgeon, a person of many tastes and interests, a man of boundless drive and dynamic enthusiasm. He founded the *Journal of Urology* in 1917, was its editor until his death, and was a prolific contributor to the literature of urology.

1870-1949—Georg Zuelzer was born in Berlin and studied medicine in Freiburg and in Berlin, where he received his doctor's degree in 1893. He began practice in Berlin in 1900 and devoted much time to research on hormones. He was the first to obtain an active pancreatic extract, called by him "Acomatol," which contained insulin. Serious reactions followed its use, and it was abandoned. He also claimed the discovery of a peristaltic hormone, "Hormonal," effective in chronic constipation, and a heart hormone, which he named "Eutonon."

Nobel Prize Winners in Medicine and Physiology

1901—**Emil von Behring,** German, the discoverer of diphtheria and tetanus antitoxin.

1902—**Sir Ronald Ross,** British, the discoverer of the transmission of malaria by mosquitoes.

1903—**Neil Finsen,** Danish, pioneer in heliotherapy.

1904—**Ivan Pavlov,** Russian, physiologist, who made epochal studies on digestion.

1905—**Robert Koch,** German, a founder of modern bacteriology and discoverer of the tubercle bacillus.

1906—**Camillo Golgi,** Italian, outstanding anatomist, discoverer of the Golgi stain.

Santiago Ramón y Cajal, Spanish, pioneer in the study of the finer anatomy of the nervous system.

1907—**Charles Laveran,** French, discoverer of the malarial parasite.

1908—**Paul Ehrlich,** German, father of modern chemotherapy and hematology.

Elie Metchnikoff, Russian, discoverer of phagocytosis.

1909—**Theodor Kocher,** Swiss, surgeon, well-known for his investigations on goitre.

1910—**Albrecht Kossel,** German, physiologist, who made outstanding discoveries in the chemistry of the cell and the cell nucleus.

1911—**Allvar Gullstrand,** Swedish, who discovered the intracapsular mechanism of accommodation.

1912—**Alexis Carrel,** French by birth, worked in America, studied extra vital cultivation and rejuvenation of tissues as well as the transplantation of organs.

1913—**Charles Richet,** French, physiologist, discoverer of anaphylaxis.

1915—**Robert Bárány,** Austrian, oto-rhino-laryngologist, discoverer of the tests for vestibular function.

1919—**Jules Bordet,** Belgian, bacteriologist, discoverer of complement fixation and pioneer student of bacterial hemolysins and bacteriolysis.

1920—**August Krogh,** Danish, made important discoveries on the anatomy and physiology of the capillaries.

1922—**A. V. Hill,** English, for studies on the physiology of muscular contraction.

Otto Meyerhof, German, pioneer in the study of tissue respiration, for his research on the oxidation and utilization of lactic acid in muscle.

1923—**Frederick G. Banting, J. J. R. Macleod,** Canadians, discoverers of insulin.

1924—Wilem Einthoven, Dutch, inventor of the electrocardiograph.

1926—Johan Fibiger, Danish, pathologist, made important studies on cancer.

1927—Julius Wagner von Jauregg, Austrian, discoverer of fever therapy for paresis.

1928—Charles Nicolle, French, discovered the transmission of typhus fever by lice.

1929—Frederick Gowland Hopkins, English, and **Christian Eijkman,** Dutch, pioneers in the study of avitaminosis.

1930—Karl Landsteiner, Austrian, demonstrated different groups of red blood cells.

1931—Otto Warburg, German, made important observations on ferments.

1932—Sir Charles S. Sherrington, English, neurologist, carried out fundamental investigations on the physiology of the nervous system.

Edgar Douglas Adrian, English, physiologist, who studied the physiology of the nervous system.

1933—Thomas Hunt Morgan, American, biologist, for his work on genetics and experimental embryology.

1934—George R. Minot, William P. Murphy, George H. Whipple, Americans, discovered the therapeutic value of liver in pernicious anemia.

1935—Hans Spemann, German, in recognition of his investigations on embryonic evolution, particularly on the causes of organ development.

1936—Sir Henry H. Dale, English, physiologist, demonstrated the pharmacologic action of histamine and acetyl choline, and chemical transmission of nerve impulses.

Otto Loewi, Austrian, physiologist, discovered the presence of chemical intermediaries in nervous reactions and the role of choline esterase.

1937—Albert Szent-Györgyi, Hungarian, isolated Vitamin C (ascorbic acid) and Vitamin P.

1938—Corneille Heymans, Belgian, pharmacologist and physiologist, whose work on the functions of the carotid sinus was noteworthy.

1939—Gerhard Domagk, German, bacteriologist, discovered the therapeutic value of sulfonamides.

1940—Henrik Dam, Danish, biochemist, discovered and isolated Vitamin K.

Edward Alexander Doisy, American, biochemist, isolated the active principle of the ovarian hormone (estrin).

1944—Joseph Erlanger, Herbert Spencer Gasser, Americans, physiologists, for their work on the action current of nerves.

1945—Sir Alexander Fleming, Ernest B. Chain, Sir Howard Walter Florey, British, bacteriologists, discovered penicillin.

1946—Herman J. Muller, American, biologist, produced mutations by the employment of x-rays.

1947—Carl F. Cori, Gerty Cori, Americans, for their discovery of the process in the catalytic metabolism of glycogen.

Bernardo Houssay, Argentinian, physiologist, for his work on the role of the anterior pituitary hor-

mone in the distribution of glycogen in the body and in the control
of diabetes.

1948—Paul Müller, Swiss, discovered that DDT was an effective in-
secticide.

1949—Walter B. Hess, Swiss, for his
studies on the reaction of animals to
electric shock.

Antonio Moniz, Portuguese, devised
and perfected prefrontal lobotomy.

**1950—Edward C. Kendall, Philip S.
Hench,** Americans, and **Tadeus
Reichstein,** of Polish birth, working
at Basel, Switzerland, for their
work on pituitary adreno-cortico-
tropic hormone (ACTH) and cortisone (compound E).

General Bibliography

Artelt, Walter: Einführung in die Medizinhistorik. Stuttgart, Enke, 1949.

Baas, Johann Hermann: Grundriss der Geschichte der Medicin und des heilenden Standes. Stuttgart, Enke, 1876.

Biographisches Lexikon der hervorragenden Aertze aller Zeiten and Völker, unter Mitwirkung der Herren prof. E. Albert . . . prof. A. Anagnostakis . . . u. a. und unter Spezial-redaktion von Dr. E. Gurlt . . . und Dr. A. Wernich herausgegeben von Dr. August Hirsch . . . 2. aufl. durchgesehen und ergänzt von prof. F. Hübotter . . . und prof. H. Vierordt . . . Berlin, Urban, 1929-34. 5 v.

————: Ergänzungsband. Nachträge zu den Bänden I-V, bearbeitet von prof. W. Haberling . . . und prof. H. Vierordt . . . Berlin, Urban, 1935.

Biographisches Lexikon der hervorragenden Aerzte der letzten fünfzig Jahre, hrsg. und bearb. von Dr. I. Fischer . . . Zugleich fortsetzung des Biographisches Lexikons der hervorragenden Aertze aller Zeiten und Völker . . . Berlin, Urban, 1932-33. 2 v.

Bishop, W. J.: Some medical bibliophiles and their libraries. J. Hist. Med., 3:229, 1948.

Buck, Albert Henry: The growth of medicine from the earliest times to about 1800. New Haven, Yale, 1917.

Cabanès, Augustin: Chirurgiens et Blessés à travers l'histoire. Paris, Michel, 1918.

Camac, C. N. B.: Imhotep to Harvey; backgrounds of medical history. New York, Hoeber, 1931.

Castiglioni, Arturo: Storia della medicina . . . Nuova edizione, ampliata e aggiornata. Verona, Arnoldo Mondadori Editore, 1948. 2 v.

————: A history of medicine. Translated from the Italian and edited by E. B. Krumbhaar. New York, Knopf, 1941.

Clendening, Logan: Source book of medical history. New York, London, Hoeber, 1942.

Cumston, Charles Greene: An introduction to the history of medicine, from the time of the pharaohs to the end of the XVIIIth century. New York, Knopf, 1926.

Dana, Charles L.: The peaks of medical history; an outline of the evolution of medicine for the use of medical students & practitioners. New York, Hoeber, 1926.

Davis, Nathan Smith: History of medicine, with code of medical ethics. Chicago, Cleveland Press, 1903.

Diepgen, Paul: Geschichte der Medizin. Berlin und Leipzig, G. J. Göschen, 1914-23. 3 v.

————: Geschichte der Medizin. Berlin, de Gruyter, 1949.

Fasbender, Heinrich: Geschichte der Geburtshülfe. Jena, Fischer, 1906.

Fulton, John Farquhar: Selected readings in the history of physiology. Springfield, Ill., Thomas, 1930.

Galdston, Iago: Progress in Medicine. New York, Knopf, 1940.

Garrison, Fielding H.: An introduction to the history of medicine, with medical chronology, suggestions for study and bibliographic data. Philadelphia and London, Saunders, 1929.

Graham, Harvey: The story of surgery. New York, Doubleday, Doran, 1939.

Gurlt, E.: Geschichte der Chirurgie und ihrer Ausübung. Volkschirurgie—Alterthum—Mittelalter—Renaissance, Berlin, Hirschwald, 1898. 3 v.

Guthrie, Douglas: A history of medicine. Philadelphia, London, Lippincott, 1946.

Haeser, Heinrich: Lehrbuch der Geschichte der Medicin und der epidemischen Krankheiten. Jena, Hermann Dufft, 1875-82. 3 v.

Harvey-Gibson, R. J.: Outlines of the history of botany. London, Black, 1919.

Hawks, Ellison: Pioneers of plant study. London, Sheldon Press; New York and Toronto, Macmillan, 1928.

Hoefer, Ferdinand: Histoire de la chimie, Paris, Firmin Didot, 1866-69. 2 v.

Holländer, Eugene: Anekdoten aus der medizinischen Weltgeschichte. Stuttgart, Enke, 1931.

————: Äskulap und Venus eine Kultur- und Sittengeschichte im Spiegel des Arztes. Berlin, Im Propylaen, 1927.

————: Die Karikature and Satire in der Medizin. Stuttgart, Enke, 1921.

————: Die Medizin in der klassischen Malerei. Stuttgart, Enke, 1923.

————: Wunder, Wundergeburt und Wundergestalt in einblattdrucken des fünfzehnten bis achtzehnten Jahrhunderts . . . Stuttgart, Enke, 1921.

Laignel-Lavastine, Maxine: Histoire générale de la médecine, de la pharmacie, de l'art dentaire et de l'art vétérinaire. Paris, Michel, 1936-38-49. 3 v.

Leonardo, Richard A.: History of surgery. New York, Froben, 1943.

Long, Esmond R.: A history of pathology. Baltimore, Williams & Wilkins, 1928.

————: Selected readings in pathology from Hippocrates to Virchow. Springfield, Ill., Thomas, 1929.

Major, Ralph H.: Classic descriptions of disease, with biographical sketches of the authors. Springfield, Ill., Thomas, 1945.

Mettler, Cecilia C.: History of medicine; a correlative text, arranged according to subjects. Philadelphia, Blakiston, 1947.

Meyer, Ernst S. C. von: A history of chemistry from earliest times to the present day; being also an introduction to the study of the science. Tr. with the author's sanction by George M'Gowan. London and New York, Macmillan. 1891.

Meyer-Steineg, Theodor, and Sudhoff, Karl: Geschichte der Medizin im Überblick mit Abbildungen. Jena, Fischer, 1921.

Neuburger, Max, and Pagel, Julius: Handbuch der Geschichte der Medizin. Begründet von Dr. med. Th. Puschmann . . . Bearb. von . . . Arndt . . . Bartels u. z. Hrsg. von Dr. med. Max Neuburger . . . und Dr. med. Julius Pagel, Jena, Fischer, 1902-05. 3 v.

Neuburger, Max: History of Medicine. Translated by Ernest Playfair. London, Frowde, 1910-25. 2 v.

Nordenskiöld, Erik: The history of biology; a survey. New York, Tudor, 1936.

Osler, Sir William: The evolution of modern medicine; a series of lectures delivered at Yale university on the Silliman foundation, in April, 1913. New Haven, Yale, 1921.

Pagel, Julius L.: Einführung in die Geschichte der Medicin. Berlin, Karger, 1898.

Pazzini, A.: Storia della medicina. Milano, Società Editrice Libraria, 1947. 2 v.

Power, Sir D'Arcy, and Thompson, C. J. S.: Chronologia medica; a handlist of persons, periods and events in the history of medicine. London, Bale, Daniels, 1923.

Puccinotti, Francesco: Storia della medicina. Livorno, Massimiliano Wagner, 1850-66. 3 v. in 4.

Ruhräh, John: Pediatrics of the past; an anthology. New York, Hoeber, 1925.

Sarton, George: Introduction to the history of science, Baltimore, Pub. for the Carnegie institution of Washington by Williams & Wilkins, 1927-47. 3 v. in 5.

Shryock, Richard Harrison: The development of modern medicine; an interpretation of the social and scientific factors involved. Philadelphia, Univ. Penn. Press; London, H. Milford, Oxford, 1936.

Siebold, Ed. Casp. Jac. von: Versuch einer Geschichte der Geburtschilfe. Tübingen, F. Pietzcker, 1901-04. 3 v. in 4.

Sigerist, Henry E.: The great doctors; a biographical history of medicine. Translated by Eden and Cedar Paul. New York, Norton, 1933.

Singer, Charles J.: The evolution of anatomy; a short history of anatomical and physiological discovery to Harvey; being the substance of the Fitzpatrick lectures delivered at the Royal college of physicians of London in the years 1923 and 1924. London, Paul, 1925.

———: A short history of medicine, introducing medical principles to students and non-medical readers. New York, Oxford, 1928.

Sprengel, Kurt: Versuch einer pragmatischen Geschichte der Arzneikunde. Halle, J. J. Gebauer, 1821-40. 6 v. in 8.

Still, George Frederic: The history of paediatrics; the progress of the study of diseases of children up to the end of the XVIIIth century. London, H. Milford, Oxford, 1931.

Sudhoff, Karl: Beiträge zur Geschichte der Chirurgie im Mittelalter; graphische und textliche Untersuchungen in mittelalterlichen Handschriften. Leipzig, Barth, 1914-18. 2 v.

———: Geschichte der Zahnheilkunde. Leipzig, Barth, 1926.

Thorndike, Lynn: A history of Magic and Experimental Science. New York, Macmillan, 1923-41. 6 v.

Weinberger, Bernhard Wolf: An introduction to the history of dentistry, with medical & dental chronology & bibliographic data. St. Louis, Mosby, 1948. 2 v.

———: Orthodontics; an historical review of its origin and evolution, including an extensive bibliography of orthodontic literature up to the time of specialization. St. Louis, Mosby, 1926. 2 v.

Withington, Edward Theodore: Medical history from the earliest times, a popular history of the healing art. London, Scientific Press, 1894.

Wunderlich, C. A.: Geschichte der Medicin. Vorlesungen gehalten zu Leipzig im Sommersemester 1858. Stuttgart, Ebner & Seubert, 1859.

PRIMITIVE MEDICINE

Ashburn, P. M.: The Ranks of Death. New York, Coward-McCann, 1947.

Badianus manuscript . . . , The. Introduction, translation and annotations by Emily Walcott Emmart. Baltimore, Johns Hopkins Press, 1940.

————: The de la Cruz-Badiano Aztec herbal of 1552. Translation and commentary by William Gates. Baltimore, Maya Society, 1939.

Cleland, Herdman Fitzgerald: Our Prehistoric Ancestors. New York, Coward-McCann, 1928.

Corbett, William Thomas: The Medicine Man of the American Indian and his Cultural Background. Springfield, Ill., Thomas, 1935.

Hewett, Edgar L.: Ancient Life in Mexico and Central America. Indianapolis, Bobbs, 1936.

Moll, Aristides A.: Aesculapius in Latin America. Philadelphia, Saunders, 1944.

Moodie, Roy L.: Paleopathology, An Introduction to the Study of Ancient Evidence of Disease. Urbana, Univ. Illinois Press, 1923.

Morley, Sylvanus G.: The Ancient Maya. Stanford Univ. Press, 1946.

Prescott, William H.: History of the Conquest of Peru. New York, Dutton, 1933.

Stone, Eric: Medicine among the American Indians. Clio Medica, New York, Hoeber, 1932.

MESOPOTAMIA

Contenau, Georges: La Civilisation d'Assur et de Babylonie. Paris, Payot, 1937.

————: La Médecine en Assyrie et en Babylonie. Paris, Maloine, 1938.

Harper, Robert Francis: The Code of Hammurabi, King of Babylon about 2250 B.C., Second Edition. Chicago, Univ. Chicago Press, 1904.

Jastrow, Morris, Jr.: Babylonian-Assyrian Medicine. Ann. Med. Hist., s. 1, I:231, 1917.

————: The Medicine of the Babylonians and Assyrians. Proc. Roy. Soc. Med., VII:Part II, p. 109, 1914.

Krause, Arlington C.: Assyro-Babylonian Opthalmology. Ann. Med. Hist., n.s., VI:42, 1934.

Thompson, R. Campbell: Assyrian Medical Texts. Proc. Roy. Soc. Med., XVII:1, 1923-24, XIX:29, 1925-26.

————: The Assyrian Herbal. London, Luzac, 1924.

————: The Reports of the Magicians and Astrologers of Nineveh and Babylon in the British Museum. London, Luzac, 1900.

Towend, B. R.: The Story of the Tooth-worm. Bull Hist. Med., XV:37, 1944.

Witzel, M.: Zur Inkubation bei Gudea. Ztschr. f. Assyriologie, XXX:101, 1913-16.

EGYPT

Breasted, James Henry: The Edwin Smith Surgical Papyrus, Chicago, University of Chicago Press, 1930.

————: A History of Egypt, London, Hodder and Stoughton, 1948.

Bryan, Cyril P.: The Papyrus Ebers, London, Bles, 1930.

Budge, Sir E. A. Wallis: The Rosetta Stone, London, Religious Tract Society, 1929.

Dawson, Warren: The Beginnings, Egypt and Assyria, Clio Medica, New York, Hoeber, 1930.

Durant, Will: The Story of Civilization. I. Our Oriental Heritage . . . , New York, Simon and Schuster, 1942, p. 199.

Ebers, Papyros, Das hermetische Buch über die Arzeneimittel der alten Ägypter von Georg Ebers, Leipzig, Engelmann, 1875.

Erman, Adolf: Aegypten und Aegyptisches Leben im Altertum, Neu bearbeitet von Hermann Ranke, Tübingen, J. C. B. Mohr (Paul Siebeck), 1922-1923.

Hamburger, Ove: Un Cas de Paralysie Infantile dans l'Antiquité, Bull. Soc. franç. d'hist. de méd., 1911, X:407-412.

Hurry, Jamieson B.: Imhotep, The Vizier and Physician of King Zoser, Oxford, Humphrey Milford, 1926.

Herodotus, The History of, translated into English by G. C. Macaulay, London, Macmillan, 1890, 2 vols., ii 84; iii 1, 129; ii 82; i 197.

Joachim, H.: Papyros Ebers, Berlin, Reimer, 1890.

Jonckheere, Frans: La Circoncision des anciens Égyptiens, III Congrès Nat. des Sciences, Bruxelles, 1950, I. Hist. du Congrès et Hist. des Sciences, 136.

————: La Circoncision des anciens Égyptiens, Centaurus, 1951, I:212-234.

————: Diagnostic ex arte de Pathologie pharaonique, Communication faite au Comité belge d'Histoire des Sciences, le 28 avril 1951.

————: Médecins de Cour et Médecine Palatine sous les Pharaons, Chronique d'Egypte, 1952, XXVII: 51-87.

Kellaway, Peter: The Part Played by Electric Fish in the Early History of Bioelectricity and Electrotherapy, Bull. Hist. Med., 1946, XX:112.

Krause, Arlington C.: Ancient Egyptian Ophthalmology, Bull. Hist. Med., 1933, I:258.

Leake, Chauncey D.: Ancient Egyptian Therapeutics, Ciba Symposia, 1940, I:311.

————: The Old Egyptian Medical Papyri, Lawrence, University of Kansas Press, 1952.

Montet, Pierre: La Vie Quotidienne en Égypte au Temps des Ramses, Paris, Hachette, 1946.

Murray, Margaret A.: The Splendor That Was Egypt, London, Sidgwick & Jackson, 1950.

Ranke, Hermann: Medicine and Surgery in Ancient Egypt, Bull. Hist. Med., 1933, I:237.

Reisner, George A.: The Hearst Medical Papyrus, Leipzig, J. C. Hinrichs, 1905.

Ruffer, Sir Marc Armand: Studies in the Paleopathology of Egypt, Chicago, University of Chicago Press, 1921.

Sarton, George: The Edwin Smith Surgical Papyrus, Isis, 1931, XV:355.

Temkin, Owsei: Recent Publications on Egyptian and Babylonian Medicine, Bull. Hist. Med., 1936, IV:247.

Weinberger, Bernhard W.: Ancient Dentistry in the Old and New World, Ann. Med. Hist., 1934, n.s., VI:264.

————: Further Evidence that Dentistry was Practiced in Ancient Egypt, Phoenicia and Greece, Bull. Hist. Med., 1946, XX:188.

Wilson, John A.: The Burden of Egypt, Chicago, University of Chicago Press, 1951.

Wreszinski, Walter: Der grosse medizinische Papyrus des Berliner Museums, Leipzig, Hinrichs, 1909.

————: Der Londoner medizinische Papyrus und der Papyrus Hearst, Leipzig, Hinrichs, 1912.

ANCIENT HEBREW MEDICINE

Brim, Charles J.: Medicine in the Bible. New York, Froben, 1936.

Hume, Edgar Erskine: The Military Sanitation of Moses in the Light of Modern Knowledge. Carlisle Barracks, Pennsylvania, Medical Field Service School, 1940.

Macht, David I: Pharmacological Appreciation of a Biblical Reference to Mass Poisoning. II Kings, IV:38-41, Bull. Johns Hopkins Hosp., XXX:38, 1919.

Preuss, Julius: Biblisch-talmudische Medizin. Berlin, Karger, 1921.

INDIA

Bhishagratna, K. K. L.: An English Translation of the Sushruta Samhita, Calcutta, 1907, 1911, 1916, 3.

Burgham, Edward: Die Gross-Monguln und ihre Aerzte, Ciba Zeitschrift, 1938, VI:2167.

Charaka-Samhita, Translated into English, Avinash Chandra Kaviratna, Calcutta, Charkravarti and Kaviratna, 1896, 1903, 1907, 1913, 4.

Esser, A. Albert M.: Die Ophthalmologie des Susruta, Studien zur Gesch. der Medizin, Leipzig, 1934.

————: Pathologie und Therapie der Lider bei Vāgbhata, Klin. Monatsbl. f. Augenh., 98:216, 1937.

Hammett, Frederick S.: The Anatomical Knowledge of the Ancient Hindus. Ann. Med. Hist., n.s., I:325, 1929.

Hoernle, A. F. Rudolf: The Authorship of the Charaka Samhita, Arch. f. Gesch. d. Med., I:29, 1908.

Jelliffe, Smith Ely: Charaka and his Times, Proc. Charaka Club, New York, Wood, II:21, 1906.

Jolly, J.: Grundriss der Indo-Arischen Philologie und Altertumskunde Medicin. Strassburg, Trübner, 1901.

Klebs, Arnold C.: Die Variolation im achtzehnten Jahrhundert, Giessen, Topelmann, 1914.

Marshall, Sir John: Mohenjo-Daro and the Indus Civilization, London, Probsthain, 1931.

————: Prehistoric Civilization of the Indies. London, Illustrated News, Jan. 7, 1928.

Müller, R. F. G.: Die Harnruhr der Alt-Inder, Sudhoffs Arch. f. Geschich. d. Med., XXXV:1, 1932.

Mukhopadhyaya, Girindranath: History of Indian Medicine, Calcutta, Univ. of Calcutta, 1923, 1926, 1929, 3.

Sachs, B.: On Hindoo Medicine, Proc. Charaka Club, New York, Wood, I:1, 1902.

Sarma, P. J.: The Art of Healing in Rigveda, Ann. Med. Hist., s.3, I:538, 1939.

————: Hindu Medicine and its Antiquity. Ann. Med. Hist., n.s., III:318, 1931.

Sudhoff, Karl: Aus der Geschichte des Krankenhauswesens in früheren Mittelalter in Morgenland und Abendland. Sudhoffs Arch. f. Gesch. d. Med. XX:164, 1928.

Vāgbhaṭa's Aṣṭāṅgahṛdayasaṃhita. Translated by Luise Hilgenberg and Willibald Kirfel. Leiden, E. J. Brill, 1941.

Wise, T. A.: Commentary on the Hindu System of Medicine. Calcutta, Thacker, Spink & Co., 1845.

CHINA

Cleyer, Andreas: Specimen Medicinae Sinicae. . . . Frankfurt, Zubrodt, 1682.

Dabry, P.: La Médecine chez les Chinois. Paris, Plon, 1863.

Hübotter, Fr.: Die Chinesische Medizin. Leipzig, Schindler, 1929.

Hume, Edward H.: The Chinese Way in Medicine. Baltimore, Johns Hopkins Press, 1940.

Maxwell, James L.: Leprosy. Chinese M. J., XLII:869, 1928.

Morse, William R.: Chinese Medicine. New York, Hoeber, 1938.

Stuart, G. A.: Chinese Materia Medica. Shanghai, Presbyterian Mission Press, 1928.

Veith, Ilza: Huang Ti Nei Ching Su Wên The Yellow Emperor's Classic of Internal Medicine. Baltimore, Williams & Wilkins, 1949.

Wong, K. Chimin: China's Contribution to the Science of Medicine. Chinese M. J., XLIII:1193, 1929.

————: Chinese Hospitals in Ancient Times. Chinese M. J., XXXVII:77, 1923.

Wong, K. Chimin and Wu, Lien Teh: History of Chinese Medicine. Tientsin, Tientsin Press, 1932.

Wong, K. Chimin: The Pulse Lore of Cathay. Chinese M. J., XLII:884, 1928.

GREEK MEDICINE

Adams, Francis: The Genuine Works of Hippocrates. New York, Wood, 1886.

Bauer, Wilhelm: Der ältere Pythagorismus, Berner Studien zur Philosophie und ihrer Geschichte, Bd. VIII. Bern, Steiger, 1897.

Beck, Theodor: Hippokrates Erkenntnisse. Jena, Diederichs, 1907.

Burnet, John: Early Greek Philosophy, London, Black, 1930.

Caton, Richard: The Temples and Ritual of Asclepios. London, Clay, 1900.

Cavvadias, A. P.: From Epidauros to Galenos. Ann. Med. Hist., n.s., III:501, 1931.

Daremberg, Ch.: État de la Médecine entre Homère & Hippocrate. Paris, Didier, 1869.

————: La Médecine dans Homère. Paris, Didier, 1865.

————: Oeuvres choisies d'Hippocrate. Paris, Labe, 1855.

Durant, Will: The Life of Greece. New York, Simon & Schuster, Inc., 1939.

Ebstein, Wilhelm: Die Pest des Thukydides. Stuttgart, Enke, 1899.

Edelstein, Emma and Ludwig: Asclepius. Baltimore, Johns Hopkins Press, 1945.

Edelstein, Ludwig: The Hippocratic Oath. Baltimore, Johns Hopkins Press, 1943.

Foës, Anutius: Magni Hippocratis mediocorum omnium facile principis opera omnia quae extant. Geneva, Chouët, 1657.

Fuller, B. G. A.: A History of Philosophy. New York, Holt, 1938.

Gask, G. E.: Early Medical Schools. Ann. Med. Hist., s.3, I:128, 1939; II:15, 1940; II:383, 1940; III:524, 1941.

Gerster, Arpad: On the Hippocratic Doctrine of the Injuries of the Cranium. Proc. Charaka Club, I:32, 1902.

Gordon, Benjamin Lee: Medicine Throughout Antiquity. Philadelphia, Davis, 1949.

Hamilton, Mary: Incubation. London, Simpkin, Marshall, Hamilton, Kent & Co., 1906.

Herzog, Rudolf: Die Wunderheilungen von Epidauros. Leipzig, Dieterich, 1931.

————: Kos, Ergebnisse der Deutschen Ausgrabungen und Forschungen. Berlin, Keller, 1932.

von Hovorka, O.: Altgriechische Heilvotive vom ärztlichen Standpunkte. Proc. XVII Internat. Congr. Med., Section XXIII, London, Frowde, p. 357, 1913.

Jayne, Walter A.: The Healing Gods of Ancient Civilizations. New Haven, Yale, 1925.

Jones, W. H. S.: The Doctor's Oath. London, Cambridge Univ. Press, 1924.

————: Hippocrates. New York, Putnam, 1923, 1931. 3 v.

————: Malaria and Greek History. Manchester, University Press, 1909.

————: Philosophy and Medicine in Ancient Greece. Baltimore, Johns Hopkins Press, 1946.

Kerényi, Karl: Der göttliche Arzt. Basel, Ciba, 1948.

Littré, É.: Oeuvres complètes d'Hippocrate. Paris, Ballière, 1839-1861. 10 v.

Lund, Fred B.: Greek Medicine. New York, Hoeber, 1936.

Major, Ralph H.: Hippocrates and the Isle of Cos. Bull. Soc. M. Hist. Chicago, V:328, 1946.

Marx, K. F. H.: Herophilus, ein Beitrag zur Geschichte der Medizin. Carlsruhe & Baden, Marx, 1838.

Meyer-Steineg, Theodor: Chirurgische Instrumente des Altertums, Jenaer medizin-historische Beiträge, Heft 1. Jena, Fischer, 1912.

————: Darstellungen normaler und krankhaft veränderter Körperteile in antiken Weihgaben, Jenaer medizin-historische Beiträge, Heft 2. Jena, Fischer, 1912.

Moon, R. O.: The Influence of Pythagoras on Greek Medicine. Proc. XVII Internat. Congr. Med., Section XXIII, London, Frowde, 55, 1913.

Moorman, Lewis J.: Francis Adams of Banchory. South. M. J., XXIX:435, 1936.

Petersen, William F.: Hippocratic Wisdom. Springfield, Ill., Thomas, 1946.

Petrequin, J. E.: Chirurgie d'Hippocrate. Paris, Imprimerie Nationale, 1877-78.

Pohl, Rudolf: De Graecorum medicis publicis. Janus, X:491, 1905.

Pohlenz, Max: Hippokrates und die Begründung der wissenschaftlichen Medizin, Berlin, de Gruyter, 1938.

Sarton, George: Introduction to the History of Science. Baltimore, Williams & Wilkins, 1927-47. 3 v. in 5.

Sudhoff, Karl: Zur Geschichte der Lehre von den kritischen Tagen im Krankheitsverlaufe. Wien. med. Wchnschr., LII:210, 322, 1902.

Thucydides: History of the Grecian Wars. Translated by Thomas Hobber. London, Clark, 1676.

Walton, Alice: The Cult of Asclepios, Cornell Studies in Classical Philology. Boston, Ginn, 1894.

Withington, E. T.: The Asclepiadae and the Priests of Asclepius. In: Singer, C. J.: Studies in the History and Method of Science, Vol. II, Oxford, Clarendon Press, p. 192, 1921.

———: Hippocrates. New York, Putnam, 1927.

ETRURIA

Cles-Reden, Sibylle: Das Versunkene Volk. Innsbruck-Wien, Rohrer, 1948.

Dennis, George: The Cities and Cemeteries of Etruria. London, Murray, 1878.

Ducati, Pericle: Le Problème Étrusque, Paris, Leroux, 1938.

Herodotos: The History of Herodotus. London, Macmillan, 1890, Vol. I, p. 49.

Körte, G.: Die Bronzeleber von Piacenza, Mitteil. a. d. Kaiser. deutsch. Archaeol. Inst. Roemische Abteilung, Rom, Loescher, 1905, XX:348.

Pallottino, M.: La Civilisation Étrusque. Paris, Payot, 1949.

Pazzini, A.: Storia della Medicina. Milano, Società Editrice Libraria, 1947, Vol 1, p. 148.

Wanscher, V.: La Langue Étrusque Renaît. Copenhagen, Munksgaard, 1951.

MEDICINE IN THE ROMAN EMPIRE

Alexander von Tralles, translated by Theodor Puschmann, Wien, Braumüller, 1878.

Broadbent, W. H.: The Pulse, London, Cussell, 1890.

Brock, Arthur J.: Greek Medicine, New York, Dutton, 1929.

Burr, C. W.: Galen, Ann. Med. Hist., n.s., III:209. 1931.

Celsus: De Medicina, translated by W. G. Spencer, Cambridge, Harvard, 3 v., 1935-38.

Choulant, Ludwig: Handbuch der Bücherkunde für die ältere Medicin, Leipzig, Voss, 1841.

Contenau, Georges: La Civilisation Phénicienne, Paris, Payot, 1949.

Durant, Will: Caesar and Christ, New York, Simon & Schuster, 1939.

Galeni librorum, Venice, Junta, 1576.

Gordon, Benjamin Lee: Medicine Throughout Antiquity, Philadelphia, Davis, 1949.

Gunther, Robert T.: The Greek Herbal of Dioscorides, Oxford, 1934.

Herschel, Clemens: The Two Books on the Water Supply of the City of Rome of Sextus Julius Frontinus, Boston, Esler, 1899.

Malloch, Archibald: Galen, Ann. Med. Hist., s.1, VIII:61-68, 1926.

Meunier, L.: Caelius Aurelianus, Janus, XI:129, 208, 1906.

Meyer-Steineg, Theodor: Kranken-Anstalten im griechisch-römischen Altertum, Jenaer medizin-historische Beiträge, Heft 3, Jena, Fischer, 1912.

———: Studien zur Physiologie des Galenus, Sudhoffs Arch. Gesch. d. Med., V:172, 1911-12.

Paulus Aegineta, The Seven Books of, translated by Francis Adams, London, Sydenham Society, 1844.

Payne, Joseph Frank: Harvey and Galen, Lancet, II:1133, 1896.

Pliny: The Natural History, translated by John Bostock and H. T. Riley, London, Bohn, 1856.

Pliny's Epistles and Panegyrick. Translated by several hands, London, Mears, 1724, 2 v.

Rufus d'Éphèse, Oeuvres de. Translated by Ch. Daremberg and Ch. Émile Ruelle, Paris, Imprimerie Nationale, 1879.

Theophrastus' Enquiry into Plants. Translated by Sir Arthur Hart, Loeb Classical Library, New York, Putnam, 1916, 2 vols.

von Vilas, Hans: Der Arzt und Philosoph Asklepiades von Bithynien, Wien & Leipzig, Braumüller, 1903.

Walsh, Joseph: Date of Galen's Birth, Ann. Med. Hist., n.s., I:378-382, 1929.

———: Galen's Discovery and Promulgation of the Function of the Recurrent Laryngeal Nerve, Ann. Med. Hist., s.l., VIII:176-184, 1926.

———: Galen's Studies at the Alexandrian School, Ann. Med. Hist., s.l, IX: 132-143, 1927.

———: Galen's Writings and Influences Inspiring Them, Ann. Med. Hist., n.s., VI:1-30, 143-149, 1934. n.s., VII:428-437, 570-589, 1935. n.s., VIII:65-90, 1936. n.s., IX:34-61, 1937. s.3, I:525-537, 1939.

———: Refutation of Ilberg as to the Date of Galen's Birth, Ann. Med. Hist., n.s., IV:126-146, 1932.

———: Refutation of the Charges of Cowardice Made against Galen, Ann. Med. Hist., n.s., III:195-208, 1931.

Wellman, Max: Asklepiades von Bithynien, Neue Jahrbücher für das klassische Altertum, Leipzig, Teubner, XI:684, 1908.

THE MIDDLE AGES—THE EARLIER PERIOD
ARABIC MEDICINE

Abd-Allatif: Relation de l'Égypt, traduit par M. Silvestre de Sacy. Paris, Treuttel et Würtz, 418-420, 1810.

Abhomeron Abynzohar: Colliget Averroys. Venice, Octavianus Scotus, 1496.

Abulcasis: La Chirurgie, traduite par le Dr. Lucien LeClerc. Paris, Ballière, 1861.

———: De Chirurgia Arabice et Latine cura Johannis Channing. Oxford, Clarendon Press, 1778.

Ali Ibn Isa: Erinnerungsbuch für Augenärzte. Translated by J. Hirschberg and J. Lippert. Leipzig, Veit, 1904.

Arnold, Thomas, and Guillaume, Alfred, editors: The Legacy of Islam. (Especially the chapter, "Science and Medicine," by Max Meyerhof). Oxford, Clarendon Press, 1931.

Browne, Edward G.: Arabian Medicine. Cambridge Univ. Press, 1921.

Campbell, Donald: Arabian Medicine. London, Kegan Paul, Trench, Trubner & Co., 1926.

Chatard, J. A.: Avicenna and Arabian Medicine. Bull. Johns Hopkins Hosp., XIX:157, 1908.

Elgood, Cyril: Jundi Shapur—A Sassanian University. Proc. Roy. Soc. Med., XXXII:1033, 1939.

————: A Medical History of Persia and the Eastern Caliphate. Cambridge Univ. Press, 1951.

————: Medicine in Persia. New York, Hoeber, 1934.

Fisher, George Jackson: Haly Abbas. Ann. Anat. & Surg., VII:208, 1883.

Friedenwald, Harry: Manuscript Copies of the Medical Works of Isaac Israeli. In: The Jews and Medicine. Baltimore, Johns Hopkins Press, p. 185, 1944.

————: Moses Maimonides the Physician. Bull. Inst. Hist. Med., III:555, 1935.

Galen: Sieben Bücher Anatomie. Translated by Max Simon from an Arabic translation 9th Century A.D. Leipzig, Hinrich, 1906. 2 v.

Gruner, O. C.: The Interpretation of Avicenna, Ann. Med. Hist., s.1, III:354, 1921.

Haddad, Sami Ibrahim: Arabian Contributions to Medicine, Ann. Med. Hist., s.3, III:60. 1941.

Haly filius Albas: Liber Aetius medicinae, Lyons, Jac. Myt, 1523.

Hitti, Philip K.: The Arabs, A Short History, Princeton, Princeton U., 1949.

————: History of the Arabs, London, Macmillan, 1949.

Jackson, A. W. W.: Persia Past and Present, New York, Macmillan, 1906.

Jensen, Deborah MacLurg: A History of Nursing, St. Louis, Mosby, 1943.

Khairallah, Amin A.: Arabic Contributions to Anatomy and Surgery, Ann. Med. Hist., s.3, IV: 409, 1942.

————: Outline of Arabic Contributions to Medicine and the Allied Sciences, Beirut, Lebanon, American Press, 1946.

LeClerc, Lucien: Histoire de la médecine arabe, Paris, Lerous, 1876.

Meyerhof, M.: Arabian Pharmacology, Ciba Symposia, VI:1847, 1944.

————: Ibn an Nafis (XIIIth cent.) and his theory of the lesser circulation, Isis, XXIII:100, 1935.

—— ——: Science and Medicine. In: The Legacy of Islam, Oxford, The Clarendon Press, p. 311, 1931.

Nidhami-i-'Arudi-i-Samargandi: The Chahar Maqala, translated into English by Edward G. Browne, J. Roy. Asiat. Soc., p. 817, 1899.

d'Ohsson, M. le Baron C.: Histoire des Mongols depuis Tchinguiz Khan jusqu'a Timour Bey ou Tamerlan, Amsterdam, Muller, I:VI, 1852.

Osler, Sir William: The Evolution of Modern Medicine. New Haven, Yale, 1921.

Ranking, George S. A.: The Life and Works of Rhazes (Abu Bakr Muhammad ben Zakaruja ar-Razi), Internat. Cong. Med., Section XXIII, History of Medicine, XVII:237, 1914.

Rhazes: (Muḥammad ibn Zakariyya al-Razi) 'Ali ibn al'Abbas et Ali ibn Sina: Trois Traites d'Anatomie Arabes, traduction de P. de Koning. Leyden, Brill, 1903.

Richter, Paul: Über die spezielle Dermatologie des 'Ali ibn al-'Abbās (Haly Abbas) aus dem 10. Jahrhundert unserer Zeitrechnung. Arch. f. Dermat. u. Syph., CXII:849, 1912.

Rihab, Mohammed: Der arabische Arzt At Tabari. Arch. f. Gesch. d. Med., XVIII:123, 1926.

Ruska, Julius: Al-Biruni als Quelle für das Leben und die Schriften al-Razis. Isis, V:26, 1923.

Sa'di, Lutfi M.: A Bio-Bibliographical Study of Hunayn ibn Is-Haq al-Ibadi (Johannitus) (809-877 A.D.). Bull. Inst. Hist. Med., II:409, 1934.

————: The Millennium of Ar-Razi (Rhazes) (850-932 A.D.), Ann. Med. Hist., n.s., VII:62, 1935.

Steinschneider, M.: Wissenschaft und Charlatanerie unter den Arabern im neun-ten Jahrhundert. Virchow's Archiv, XXXVI:570, 1866.

de Vaux, Baron Carra: Avicenne, Paris, Alcan, n.d.

Whipple, Allen O.: Role of the Nestorians as the Connecting Link between Greek and Arabic Medicine. Ann. Med. Hist., n.s., VIII:313, 1936.

Wüstenfeld, Ferdinand: Geschichte der Arabischen Aerzte und Naturforscher. Göttingen, Vanderhoech & Ruprecht, 1840.

Yellin, David, and Abrahams, Israel: Maimonides. Jewish Pub. Soc. of America, 1903.

THE MIDDLE AGES—THE LATER PERIOD

Adami, J. George: Sir John Harington. Bull. Johns Hopkins Hosp., XIX:285, 1908.

Allbutt, T. Clifford: The Historical Relations of Medicine and Surgery. London, Macmillan, 1905.

Antoine, Thomas M.: Jean Pitart Chirurgien et Poete. Janus, XXII:279, 1917.

Astruc, Jean: Mémoires pour servir a l'Histoire de la Faculté de Médecine de Montpellier. Paris, Cavelier, 1767.

Barbour, A. H. F.: Soranus on Gynaecological Anatomy. Proc. Intern. Congr. Med., London, Sect. XXIII, p. 269, 1913.

Bayon, H. P.: Trotula and the Ladies of Salerno. Proc. Roy. Soc. Med., XXXIII: 471, 1940.

Brennan, W. A.: Guy de Chauliac on Wounds and Fractures. Chicago, Translator, 1923.

Brown, Horace M.: De Venenis of Petrus Abbonus. Ann. Med. Hist., s.1, VI:25, 1924.

von Brunn, Walter: Die Stellung des Guy de Chauliac in der Chirurgie des Millelalters. Sudhoffs Arch. f. Gesch. d. Med., XII:85, 1920; XIII:65, 1921.

Castiglioni, Arturo: Bologna. Ciba Symposia, VII:70, 1945.

————: The Medical School at Padua and the Renaissance of Medicine. Ann. Med. Hist., n.s., VII:214, 1935.

————: The School of Salerno. Bull. Inst. Hist. Med., VI:883, 1938.

Cholmeley, H. P.: John of Gaddesden andd the Rosa Medicinae. Oxford, Clarendon Press, 1912.

Colle, Francesco Maria: Storia scientifico-letteraria dello Studio di Padova. Padua, Minerva, 1824.

Collins, Joseph: Medicine in England in Chaucer's Time. Proc. Charaka Club, IV:139, 1916.

Cooper, Sonoma: The Medical School of Montpellier in the Fourteenth Century. Ann. Med. Hist., n.s., II:163, 1930.

Corner, George W.: Anatomical Texts of the Earlier Middle Ages. Washington, Carnegie Inst., 1927.

―――: The Rise of Medicine at Salerno in the Twelfth Century. In: Lectures on the History of Medicine. Mayo Foundation Series. Philadelphia, Saunders, 1933, p. 371.

Crawford, Raymond: Plague and Pestilence in Literature and Art. Oxford, Clarendon Press, 1914.

Croke, Sir Alexander: Regimen Sanitatis Salernitanum. Oxford, Talboys, 1830.

Crummer, Le Roy: Copho's "Anatomia Porci." Ann. Med. Hist., s.1, IX:180, 1927.

Cushing, Harvey: Ercole Lelli and His Écorché. Yale J. Biol. & Med., IX:200, 1936-37.

Daremberg, Charles: Glossulae Quatuor Magistrorum super Chirurgiam, Rogerii et Roland. Naples, Filiatre-Sebezio; Paris, Baillière, 1854.

Diepgen, Paul: Studien zu Arnold von Villanova. Sudhoffs Arch. f. Gesch. d. Med., III:115, 188, 369, 1909-10; V:88, 1911-12; VI:380, 1912-13.

Dorveaux, Paul: L'Antidotaire Nicolas. Paris, Welter, 1896.

Gerster, Arpad G.: Surgical Manners and Customs in the Times of Henry de Mondeville. Proc. Charaka Club, III:70, 1910.

Handerson, Henry E.: Gilbertus Anglicus, Medicine of the Thirteenth Century. Cleveland, Cleveland Med. Library Assn., 1918.

Haven, Marc (Emmanuel Lalonde): La vie et les oeuvres de maître Arnaud de Villeneuve. Paris, Chamuel, 1896.

Hecker, J. F. C.: The Epidemics of the Middle Ages. Translated by B. G. Babington. London, Sydenham Society, 1844.

Henschel, A. W. E. Th.: Berühmte Wundärzte und Aerzte des XIII. and XIV. Jahrhunderts. Janus, II:375, 1853.

―――: Die Salernitanische Handschrift. Janus, I:40, 300, 1846.

Hitti, Philip K.: An Arab-Syrian Gentleman and Warrior. Memoirs of Usāmah ibn Munquidh. New York, Columbia Univ. Press, 1929.

Horine, Emmet F.: Episodes in the History of Anesthesia. J. Hist. Med., I:521, 1946.

Hume, Edgar Erskine: Medical Work of the Knights Hospitallers of Saint John of Jerusalem. Baltimore, Johns Hopkins Press, 1940.

Husemann, Th.: Die Schlafschwämme und andere Methoden des allgemeinen und örtlichen Anästhesie im Mittelalter. Deutsche. Ztschr. f. Chir., XLII:517, 1896.

―――: Weitere Beiträge zur chirurgischen Anästhesie im Mittelalter. Deutsche Ztschr. f. Chir., LIV:503, 1899.

d'Irsay, Stephen: The Life and Works of Gilles de Corbeil. Ann. Med. Hist., s.1, VII:362, 1925.

―――: Teachers and Textbooks of Medicine in the Medieval University of Paris. Ann. Med. Hist., s.1, 1926, VIII:234, 1926.

―――: The Teaching and Practice of Medicine in the Medieval University of Paris. Bull. Soc. M. Hist. Chicago, IV:41, 1928.

Jackson, A. W. Williams: Persia Past and Present. New York, Macmillan, 1906.

Joubert, Laurens: La Grande Chirurgie de M. Guy de Chauliac. Tournon, Michel, 1619.

Kristeller, Paul Oscar: The School of Salerno. Bull. Hist. Med., XVII:138, 1945.

van Leersum, E. C.: De "Cyrurgie" van Meester Jan Yperman. Leyden, Sijthoff, 1912.

————:Master Jan Yperman's Cyrurgia. Janus, XVIII:199, 1913.

————: Note concernant l'année de la mort de Jan Yperman. Janus, XIX:35, 1914.

————: Notes concerning the life of Jan Yperman. Janus, XVIII:1, 191.

Malgaigne, J.-F.: Introduction à Oeuvres Complètes d'Ambroise Paré. Paris, Baillière, 1840.

Martinotti, Giovanni: L'Insegnamento dell 'Anatomia in Bologna. Bologna, 1911.

Mason-Hohl, Elizabeth: The Diseases of Women by Trotula of Salerno. Los Angeles, Ward Ritchie Press, 1940.

Medici, Michele: Compendio Storico della Scuola Anatomica di Bologna. Bologna, Volpe e del Sassi, 1857.

Mercier, Charles Arthur: Astrology in Medicine. London, Macmillan, 1914.

Meyer, Ernst H. F.: Geschichte der Botanik, Königsberg. Bornträger, III:435, II Book, 1856.

Munro, Dana C. and Haagensen, Cushman D.: Arabian Medicine as Represented in Memoirs of Usāmah Ibn-Munquidh. Ann. Med. Hist., n.s., V:226, 1933.

Nicaise, E.: Chirurgie de Maître Henri de Mondeville. Paris, Alcan, 1893.

————: La Grande Chirurgie de Guy de Chauliac. Paris, Alcan, 1890.

Nohe, Johannes: Der schwarze Tod. Potsdam, Kiepenheuer, 1924.

Ordronaux, John: Regimen Sanitatis Salernitanum. Philadelphia, Lippincott, 1870.

Packard, Francis R.: History of the School of Salernum in "The School of Salernum" New York, Hoeber, 1920.

————: The School of Salernum. New York, Hoeber, 1920.

Pansier, P.: Les Maîtres de la faculté de médecine de Montpellier au Moyen age. Janus, IX:443, 499, 537, 1904.

Pifteau, Paul: Chirurgie de Guillaume de Salicet. Toulouse, Saint-Cyprien, 1898.

Pilcher, Louis Stephen: The Mondino Myth. Med. Lib. Hist .J., IV:311, 1906.

Power, Sir D'Arcy: De Arte Phisicali et de Cirurgia of Master John Arderne, Surgeon of Newark. New York, Wood, 1922.

de Renzi, Salvatore: Collectio Salernitana. Naples, Filiatre-Sebezio, 1852-1859. 5 v.

Riesman, David: A Physician in the Papal Chair. Ann. Med. Hist., s.l, V:29ı. 1923.

————: The Story of Medicine in the Middle Ages. New York, Hoeber, 1935.

Sa'di, Lufti M.: Reflection of Arabian Medicine at Salerno and Montpellier. Ann. Med. Hist., n.s., V:213, 1933.

Sigerist, Henry E.: An Elizabethan Poet's Contribution to Public Health: Sir John Harington and the Water Closet. Bull. Inst. Hist. Med., XIII:229, 1943.

Singer, Charles: The Evolution of Anatomy. New York, Knopf, 1925.

————: Science. In: Bailey, Cyril, ed.: The Legacy of Rome. Oxford, Clarendon Press, 1923.

————: The Scientific Views and Visions of Saint Hildegard (1098-1180). In: Singer, Charles, ed.: Studies in the History and Method of Science. Oxford, Clarendon Press, I:1, 1917-21. 2 v.

Soranus von Ephesus: Die Gynäkologie des, übersezt von H. Lüneburg. München, Lehmann, 1894.

Steinschneider, M.: Constantinus Africanus und seine arabischen Quellen. Virchows Arch. f. path. Anat., XXXVII:351, 1866.

Sudhoff, Karl: Beiträge zur Geschichte der Chirurgie im Mittelalter. Leipzig, Barth, 1918.

————: Die Salernitaner Handschrift in Breslau. Sudhoffs Arch. f. Gesch. d. Med., XII:101, 1920.

————: Ein Chirurgisches Manual des Jean Pitard. Sudhoffs Arch. f. Gesch. d. Med., II:189, 1908-09.

————: Salerno: A Mediaeval Health Resort and Medical School on the Tyrrhenian Sea. In: Sudhoff, Karl: Essays in the History of Medicine. New York, Med. Life Press, p. 229, 1926.

————: Schlafschwämme der Borgognoni. Sudhoffs Arch. f. Gesch. d. Med., XIII:127, 1921.

Thorndike, Lynn: History of Magic and Experimental Science. New York, Columbia Univ. Press, 1943.

Verrier, René: Études sur Arnaud de Villeneuve. Leiden, Brill, 1947.

Virchow, Rudolf: Zur Geschichte des Aussatzes, besonders in Deutschland. Virchows Arch. f. path. Anat., XVIII:138, 273; XIX:43: 1861, XX:166, 1860.

Walsh, James J.: Medieval Medicine. London, Black, 1920.

————: Old-Time Makers of Medicine. New York, Fordham Univ. Press, 1911.

Wellmann, Max: Die pneumatische Schule bis auf Archigenes. Berlin, Weidmann, 1895.

Wickersheimer, Er.: Nicolaus Prepositi, ein französischer Arzt ums Jahr 1500. Sudhoffs Arch. f. Gesch. d. Med., V:302, 1911.

Zaccagnini, Guido: La vita dei maestri e degli scholari nello Studio di Bologna nei secoli XIII e XIV. Geneva, Olschki, 1926.

THE RENAISSANCE

Astruc, Jean: A Treatise of Venereal Diseases (English translation). London, Innys & Richardson, 1754.

Baker, Frank: The Two Sylviuses. Bull. Johns Hopkins Hosp., XX:329, 1909.

Barlow, H. M.: Old English Herbals, 1525-1640. Proc. Roy. Soc. Med., VI, Part II, Sect. Hist. Med., p. 108, 1913.

Bartscherer, Agnes: Paracelsus Paracelsisten und Goethe's Faust. Dortmund, Ruhfus, 1911.

Basilio de Telepnef: Paracelsus. St. Gallen, Zollikofer, 1945.

Baumgartner, Leona and Fulton, John F.: A Bibliography of the Poem, Syphilis, sive Morbus Gallicus. New Haven, Yale, 1935.

Betschart, Ildefons: Theophrastus Paracelsus, Der Mensch an der Zeitenwende. Einsiedeln & Köln, Benziger, 1941.

Brown, Alfred: Old Masterpieces in Surgery. Omaha, priv. print., 1928.

Burggraeve, Ad.: Études sur André Vésale. Gand, C. Annoot-Braeckman, 1841.

Capitaine, P. A.: Un grand Médecin du XVIᵉ siècle, Jean Fernel. Paris, Librairie le Francois, 1925.

Capparoni, Pietro: Profili Bio-Bibliografici di Medici e Naturalisti Celebri Italiani. Roma, Istituto Naz. Medico Farmacologico "Serono," 1932.

Cardan, Jerome: The Book of My Life. Translated by Jean Stoner. New York, Dutton, 1930.

Castiglioni, Arturo: Fallopius and Vesalius. In: Cushing, Harvey: A Bio-Bibliography of Andreas Vesalius. New York, Schuman's, p. 182, 1943.

————: Il Volto di Ippocrate. Milan, Unitas, 1925.

Cushing, Harvey: A Bio-Bibliography of Andreas Vesalius. New York, Schuman's, 1943.

Doe, Janet: A Bibliography of the Works of Ambroise Paré: Premier Chirurgien & Conseiller du Roy. Chicago, Univ. Chicago Press, 1937.

Eckman, James: Jerome Cardan. Baltimore, Johns Hopkins Press, 1946.

Fiessinger, Ch.: La Thérapeutique des Vieux Maîtres. Paris, Soc. d'Edit. scientifiques, 1897.

Fracastorii Hieronymi de contagione et contagiosis morbis et eorum curatione, Libri III, translation and notes by Wilmer Cane Wright. New York, Putnam, 1930.

Frank, Mortimer and Frank, Ira: Gasparo Tagliacozzi and his Contribution to Rhinoplasty. Ann. Otol. Rhin. & Laryng., XXVIII:505, 1918.

Franklin, K. J.: De venarum ostiolis 1603 of Hieronymus Fabricius of Aquapendente (1535-1619). Springfield, Ill., Thomas, 1933.

Fuller, B. A. G.: A History of Philosophy. New York, Holt, 1938.

Gnudi, Martha Teach, and Webster, Jerome Pierce: The Life and Times of Gaspare Tagliacozzi. New York, Herbert Reichner, 1950.

Hartmann, Franz: The Life of Philippus Theophrastus, Bombast of Hohenheim, known by the name of Paracelsus. London, Redway, 1897.

Hemmeter, John B.: Master Minds in Medicine. New York, Med. Life Press, 1927.

Hendrickson, G. L.: The Syphilis of Girolamo Fracastoro. Bull. Inst. Hist. Med., II:515, 1934.

Holländer, Eugen: Marktschreizettel von Georg Bartisch. Deutsche med. Wchnschr., XLIII:1369, 1917.

Jaeckle, Erwin: Paracelsus, Seine Weltschau in Worten des Werkes. Zürich, Verlag, 1942.

Jeanselme, Edouard: Traité de la syphils, Tome I. Paris, Doin, 1931.

Johnson, John N.: The Life of Linacre. London, Lumley, 1835.

Keele, K. D.: Leonardo da Vinci on Movement of the Heart and Blood. Philadelphia, Lippincott, n.d., 1952.

Kocher, Paul H.: Paracelsan Medicine in England: The First Thirty Years (ca.1570-1600). J. Hist. Med., II:451, 1947.

Lienard, Réné-Albert: Paracelse sa Vie, son Oeuvre. Lyon, Basc. Rion, 1932.

MacCurdy, Edward: The Notebooks of Leonardo da Vinci. New York, Reynal, 1938.

Malgaigne, J.-F.: Oeuvres complètes d'Ambroise Paré, Paris, Baillière, I:CCXXIV, 1840.

McMurrich, J. Playfair: Leonardo da Vinci the Anatomist, Baltimore, Williams and Wilkins, 1930.

Morejon, Don Antonio Hernandez: Historia Bibliográfica de la Medicina Española, 7 vols. Madrid, Jordan, 1842-1852.

Morley, Henry: Jerome Cardan. London, Chapman & Hall, Ltd., 1854.

Morrison, Samuel Elliott: Admiral of the Ocean Sea, Boston, Little, Brown & Co., 1942. II: p. 193.

Netzhammer P. Raymond, O.S.B.: Theophrastus Paracelsus. Einsiedeln, Benziger, 1901.

O'Malley, Charles D., and Saunders, J. B. de C. M.: Leonardo da Vinci on the human body. New York, Schuman, 1952.

Osler, William: Fracastorius. Proc. Charaka Club, New York, Wood, II:5, 1906.

————: Thomas Linacre. Cambridge, Univ. Press, 1908.

Packard, Francis R.: Guy Patin and the Medical Profession in Paris in the Seventeenth Century. Ann. Med. Hist., s.l, IV:136, 215, 357, 1922.

————: Life and Times of Ambroise Paré. New York, Hoeber, 1926.

Paget, Stephen: Ambroise Paré and His Times. New York, Putnam, 1899.

Parker, G.: The Early History of Surgery in Great Britain. London, Black, 1920.

Peuckert, Will Erich: Theophrastus Paracelsus. Stuttgart, Kohlhammer, 1943.

Pilcher, Lewis Stephen: A Surgeon to the Pope. Proc. Charaka Club, New York, Wood, III:106, 1910.

Platt, Walter B.: Fabricius Guilhelmus Hildanus: The Father of German Surgery. Bull. Johns Hopkins Hosp., XVI:7, 1905.

Power, Sir D'Arcy: Certain Works of Chirurgerie by Thomas Gale, Maister in Chirurgerie. Brit. J. Surg., XV:177, 1927-28.

————: De Arte Phisical et de Chirurgia of Master John Arderne. New York, Wood, 1922.

————: John Halle. Brit. J. Surg., V:181, 1917-18.

————: Medicine in the British Isles. New York, Hoeber, 1930.

————: Selected Writings. Oxford, Clarendon Press, 1931.

————: Thomas Gale. Brit. J. Surg., VIII:145, 1920-21.

Proksch, J. K.: Die Geschichte der venerischen Krankheiten. Bonn, Hanstein. 1895.

Pusey, Wm. Allen: Syphilis as a Modern Problem. Chicago, A.M.A., 1915.

Putti, Vittorio: Berengario da Carpi. Bologna, Cappelli, 1937.

Raynaud, Maurice: Les médecins au temps de Molière. Paris, Didier, 1863.

Rosen, George: Some Recent European Publications Dealing with Paracelsus. J. Hist. Med., II:537, 1947.

Roth, M.: Andreas Vesalius Bruxellensis. Berlin, Reimer, 1892.

Saunders, J. B. de C. M., and O'Malley, Charles D.: Vesalius, the Illustrations from His Works. Cleveland and New York, World Publishing Co., 1950.

Sherrington, Sir Charles: The Endeavour of Jean Fernel. Cambridge, University Press, 1946.

Sigerist, Henry E.: Four Treatises of Theophrastus von Hohenheim, called Paracelsus. Baltimore, Johns Hopkins Press, 1941.

————: L'origine della silfilide. Arch. di Storia della Scienza, IV:163, 1923; VII:243, 1926.

Singer, Charles: The Evolution of Anatomy. New York, Knopf, 1925.

Singer, Charles and Robin, C.: A Prelude to Modern Science; being a discussion of the History, Sources and Circumstances of the 'Tabulae Anatomical Sex' of Vesalius. Cambridge, Univ. Press, 1946.

Singer, Charles and Dorothy: The Scientific Position of Girolamo Fracastoro. Ann. Med. Hist., s.1, I:1, 1917.

Spielmann, M. H.: The Iconography of Andreas Vesalius, London. Bale & Danielsson, 1925.

Spunda, Franz: Paracelsus. Wien u. Leipzig, König, 1925.

Stillman, J. M.: Paracelsus. Chicago, Open Court Co., 1920.

Stoddart, A. M.: The Life of Paracelsus. Philadelphia, McKay, 1911.

Streeter, Edward C.: Leoniceno and the School of Ferrara. Bull. Soc. Med. Hist., Chicago, I:18, 1916.

Sudhoff, Karl: Die medizinische Fakultät zu Leipzig im ersten Jahrhundert der Universität. Leipzig, Barth, 1909.

———: Guihelmus Fabricius Hildanus. München med. Wchnschr., LVII:1401, 1910.

Venn, John: The Works of John Caius, M.D. Cambridge, University Press, 1912.

Vesalius, The Epitome of: Translated by L. R. Lind. New York: Macmillan, 1949.

Vigo, John: The Most Excellent Workes of Chirurgerys. Translated by Traheron. London, Edward Whytchurch, 1543.

Waters, W. G.: Jerome Cardan. London, Lawrence & Bullen, 1898.

Wickersheimer, Ernest: Anatomies de Mondino dei Luggi et de Guido de Vigevano Paris, E. Droz, 1926.

Williams, Herbert U.: The Origin and Antiquity of Syphilis. Arch. Path., XIII: 779. 1932.

THE SEVENTEENTH CENTURY

Castiglioni, Arturo: La Vita e l'opera di Santorio Santorio Capodistriano MCLXI-MDCXXXVI. Bologna-Trieste, Cappelli, 1920.

Catchpole, Hubert R.: Regnier de Graaf. Bull. Hist. Med., VII:1261, 1940.

Clay, Reginald S. and Court, Thomas H.: The History of the Microscope. London, Griffin, 1932.

Dobell, Clifford: Antony van Leeuwenhoek and his "Little Animals." New York, Harcourt, 1932.

Dock, George: Robert Talbor, Madame de Sevigne and the Introduction of Cinchona. Ann. Med. Hist., s.1, IV:241, 1922.

Fulton, John F.: Aviation Medicine in its Preventive Aspects. London, Oxford, 1948.

———: A Bibliography of Two Oxford Physiologists, Richard Lower and John Mayow. Oxford, Univ. Press, 1935.

———: Robert Boyle and his Influence on Thought in the Seventeenth Century. Isis, XVIII:77, 1933.

Garrison, Fielding H.: Life as an Occupational Disease. Bull. New York Acad. Med., X:679, 1934.

Gotch, Francis: Two Oxford Physiologists. Oxford, Clarendon Press, 1908.

Haden, Russell L.: Early Microscopes and Early Microscopists. Tr. A. Am. Physicians, Philadelphia, LIV:343, 1939.

Hoff, Ebbe C. and Phebe M.: The Life and Times of Richard Lower, Physiologist and Physician. Bull. Inst. Hist. Med., IV:517, 1936.

Kopp, Hermann: Die Alchemie, Heidelberg. Winter, 1886.

Major, Ralph H.: Athanasius Kircher. Ann. Med. Hist., s.3, I:105, 1939.

————: Santorio Santorio. Am. Med. Hist., n.s., X:369, 1938.

Manni, Domenico Maria: Degli occhiali da naso inventati da Salvino Armati. Florence, Albizinni, 1738.

Patterson, T. S.: John Mayow in Contemporary Setting. Isis, XV:47, 504, 1931.

Payne, J. F.: Thomas Sydenham. London, Unwin, 1900.

Pierce, C. S.: Note on the Age of Basil Valentine. Science, n.s., VIII:169, 1898.

Power, Sir D'Arcy: Richard Wiseman, Brit. J. Surg., III:349, 1915-16.

————: Severall Chirurgical Treatises by Richard Wiseman, 1676. Brit. J. Surg., XVI:357, 1929.

Riesman, David: Thomas Sydenham. New York, Hoeber, 1926.

Rolleston, Sir Humphry: The Cambridge Medical School. Cambridge, Univ. Press, 1932.

————: History of Cinchona and its Therapeutics. Ann. Med. Hist., n.s., III:261, 1931.

Saunders, J. B. de C. M., and O'Malley, Charles Donald: Bernardino Montaña de Monserrate. J. Hist. Med., I:87, 1946.

Scott, H. Harold: A History of Tropical Medicine. Baltimore, Williams & Wilkins, 1939.

Stillman, John Maxson: Basil Valentine: A Seventeenth Century Hoax. Pop. Sc. Monthly, LXXXI:591, 1912.

Sudhoff, Karl: Bibliographia Paracelsica. Berlin, Reimer, 1894.

de Waele, Henri: J. B. Van Helmont. Brussels, Office de Publicité, 1947.

THE EIGHTEENTH CENTURY

Baron, John: The Life of Edward Jenner, M.D., LL.D., F.R.S. London, Colburn, 1838. 2 v.

Beer, Rüdiger Robert: Der Grosse Haller. Säckingen, Stratz, 1947.

Bettany, G. T.: Eminent Doctors. London, Hogg, 1885.

Burget, G. E.: Lazzaro Spallanzani. Ann. Med. Hist., s.1, VI:177, 1924.

Clar, D.: Leopold Auenbrugger. Groz, Leuscher & Lubensky, 1867.

Clark-Kennedy, A. E.: Stephen Hales. Cambridge, Univ. Press, 1929.

Comrie, John D.: History of Scottish Medicine. London, Ballière, Tindall & Cox, 1927.

Franchini, Guiseppe: Lazzaro Spallanzani. Ann. Med. Hist., n.s., II:56, 1930.

French, Sidney J.: Torch and Crucible, The Life and Death of Antoine Lavoisier. Princeton, Princeton, 1941.

Grimaux, Édouard: Lavoisier, 1743-1794. Paris, Alcan, 1888.

Guttmacher, Manfred S.: John Hunter, His Enemies and His Friends. Bull. Johns Hopkins Hosp., XLV:15, 1929.

Harvey-Gibson, R. J.: Outlines of the History of Botany. London, Black, 1919.

Herrick, James B.: A Short History of Cardiology. Springfield, Ill., Thomas, 1942.

Hoefer, Ferdinand: Histoire de la Chimie. Paris, Firmin Didot, 1869.

Inoculation and Vaccination, The History of. London, Burroughs Wellcome & Co., 1913.

Jarcho, Saul: Giovanni Battista Morgagni. Bull. Hist. Med., XXII:503, 1948.

Kiesewetter, Carl: Franz Anton Mesmer's Leben and Lebre. Leipzig, Spohr, 1893.

Lenard, Philipp: Grosse Naturforscher. Munich, Lehmann, 1937.

Meyer, Arthur W.: The Rise of Embryology. Stanford University, Stanford Univ. Press, 1939.

von Meyer, Ernst: A History of Chemistry. London, Macmillan, 1891.

Moore, James: The History and Practice of Vaccination. London, Callow, 1817.

Moore, Norman: The History of the Study of Medicine in the British Isles. Oxford, Clarendon Press, 1908.

Needham, Joseph: A History of Embryology. Cambridge, University Press, 1934.

Neuburger, Max: Leopold Auenbrugger's Inventum Novum. Vienna and Leipzig, Šafář, 1922.

Nordenskiöld, Erik: The History of Biology. New York, Tudor, 1936.

Oppenheimer, Jane: New Aspects of John and William Hunter. New York, Schuman, 1946.

Paget, Stephen: John Hunter. London, Unwin, 1897.

Peachey, George C.: A Memoir of William & John Hunter. Plymouth, Brendon, 1924.

Priestley, Joseph: Experiments and Observations on different Kinds of Air. London, Johnson, 1774.

————: The Memoirs of. London, Johnson, 1805.

Schönbauer, Leopold: Das Medizinische Wien. Vienna, Urban, 1947.

Tischner, Rudolf: Franz Anton Mesmer. Munich, Münchner Drucke, 1928.

Virchow, Rudolf: The Influence of Morgagni on Anatomical Thought. Lancet, I:843, 1894.

THE NINETEENTH CENTURY—THE FIRST HALF

Ameke, Wilhelm: History of Homeopathy, London, Gould, 1885.

Baumgartner, Leona, and Ramsey, Elizabeth M.: Johann Peter Frank and His "System einer vollständigen medicinischen Polizey," Ann. Med. Hist., n.s., V:525, 1933. VI:69, 1934.

Bright, Richard: Travels from Vienna through Lower Hungary, Edinburgh, Constable, 1818, p. 78.

Brown, Lawrason: The Story of Clinical Pulmonary Tuberculosis, Baltimore, Williams & Wilkins, 1941.

Coues, William: Guillaume Dupuytren, Boston M. & S. J., CLXXV:489, 1916.

Duclos, Henri: Laennec, Paris, Flammarion, 1932.

Fuller, B. A. G.: A History of Philosophy, New York, Holt, 1938.

Hahnemann, Samuel: Organon of the Rational Art of Healing, London, Dent., 1913.

Herrick, James B.: A Short History of Cardiology, Springfield, Ill., Thomas, 1942.

Hirschel, Bernhard: Compendium der Geschichte der Medicin, Vienna, Braumüller, 1862.

Holmes, Oliver Wendell: Medical Essays, Boston, Houghton, 1888.

Jonas, A. F.: Dupuytren and His Contemporaries, Nebraska M. J., 1919, IV:320.

Kirkpatrick, T. Percy: Abraham Colles, Irish J. M. Sc., VI:241, 1931.

———: The History of Doctor Steevens' Hospital. Dublin, Univ. Press, 1924.

Olmsted, J. M. D.: François Magendie, New York, Schuman's, 1944.

Ormsby, L. D.: Medical History of the Meath Hospital, Dublin, Fannin, 1888.

Osler, William: The Influence of Louis on American Medicine, Bull. Johns Hopkins Hosp., VIII:161, 1897.

Pagel, Julius: Einführung in die Geschichte der Medicin, Berlin, Karger, 1898.

Potain, C.: Clinique médicale de la Charité, Paris, Masson, 1894.

Rolleston, J. D.: F. J. V. Broussais (1772-1838), His Life and Doctrines. Proc. Roy. Soc. Med., XXXII:405, 1939.

———: Jean Baptiste Bouillaud (1796-1881), A Pioneer in Cardiology and Neurology, Proc. Roy. Soc. Med., XXIV:1253, 1931,

Saintignon, Henri: Laënnec, sa vie et son oeuvre. Paris, Baillière, 1904.

Spurzheim, J. C.: Outlines of Phrenology. London, Treuttel, Wurtz & Richter, 1827.

Stokes, William: William Stokes, His Life and Work. London, Unwin, 1898.

Temkin, Owsei: Gall and the Phrenological Movement. Bull. Hist. Med., XXI: 275, 1947.

Thayer, William S.: Osler and Other Papers. Baltimore, Johns Hopkins Press, p. 247, 1931.

Triaire, Paul: Bretonneau et ses correspondants, Paris, Alcan, 1892.

———: Dominique Larrey. Tours, Mame, 1902.

Wiese, E. Robert: Guillaume Dupuytren. Med. Life, XXXVIII:477, 1931.

Wilks, Samuel and Bettany, G. T.: A Biographical History of Guy's Hospital. London, Ward, Lock, Bowden & Co., 1892.

THE RISE OF AMERICAN MEDICINE

Boland, Frank Kells: The First Anesthetic; the Story of Crawford Long. Athens, Univ. Georgia Press, 1950.

Chavez, Ignacio: Mexico en la Cultura Medica. Mexico, D. F., Edicion de el Colegio Nacional, 1947.

De Jong, Russell N.: The First American Textbook on Psychiatry. Ann. Med. Hist., s.3, II:195, 1940.

Flexner, James T.: Doctors on Horseback. New York, Garden City, 1939.

Goodman, Nathan G.: Benjamin Rush. Philadelphia, Univ. Penn. Press, 1934.

Gordon, Maurice Bear: Aesculapius Comes to the Colonies. Ventnor, N.J., Ventnor Publishers, Inc., 1949.

Gross, Samuel D.: Autobiography. Philadelphia, Barrie, 1887.

———: Lives of Eminent American Physicians and Surgeons of the Nineteenth Century. Philadelphia, Lindsay & Blakiston, 1861.

Juettner, Otto: Daniel Drake and His Followers. Cincinnati, Harvey, 1909.

Kelly, Howard A.: A Cyclopedia of American Medical Biography, Philadelphia, Saunders, 1912.

Keys, Thomas E.: The History of Surgical Anesthesia. New York, Schuman's, 1945.

Middleton, W. S.: John Morgan, Father of Medical Education in North America. Ann. Med. Hist., s.l, IX:13, 1927.

———: Philip Syng Physick. Ann. Med. Hist., n.s., I:562, 1929.

———: William Shippen, Junior. Ann. Med. Hist., n.s., IV: 440, 538, 1932.

Miller, Joseph L.: Joyfull Newes out of the New-Found Worlde. Rochester, Mayo Foundation, 1929.

Miller, W. S.: William Beaumont. Ann. Med. Hist., n.s., V:28, 1933.

———: William Beaumont and His Book. Elisha North and His Copy of Beaumont's Book. Ann. Med. Hist., n.s., I:155, 1929.

Moll, Aristides A.: Aesculapius in Latin America. Philadelphia, Saunders, 1944.

Mumford, James G.: A Narrative of Medicine in America. Philadelphia, Lippincott, 1903.

Myer, Jesse S.: Life and Letters of Dr. William Beaumont. St. Louis, Mosby, 1912.

Packard, Francis R.: History of Medicine in the United States. New York, Hoeber, 1931. 2 v.

Randolph, J.: A Memoir on the Life and Character of Philip Syng Physick, M.D. Philadelphia, Collins, 1839.

Ruschenberger, W. S. W.: An Account of the Institution of the College of Physicians of Philadelphia. Philadelphia, Tr. Coll. Phys., 1887.

Rush, Benjamin: The Autobiography of Benjamin Rush. Edited by George W. Corner. Princeton, Princeton, 1948.

Schachner, August: Ephraim McDowell. Philadelphia, Lippincott, 1921.

Tucker, David A., Jr.: Practical Essays on Medical Education by Daniel Drake, M.D. Baltimore, Johns Hopkins, 1952.

Viets, Henry R.: A Brief History of Medicine in Massachusetts. Boston and New York, Houghton, 1930.

THE NINETEENTH CENTURY—THE SECOND HALF

Ackerknecht, Erwin H.: Rudolf Virchow. Madison, Univ. Press, 1953.

Ball, James M.: Samuel Thomson. Ann. Med. Hist., s.l, VII:144, 1925.

Baumgartner, Leona: Edwin Klebs. New England J. Med., CCXIII:60, 1935.

Behring, Emil: Die Geschichte der Diphtherie. Leipzig, Thieme, 1893.

Bullock, William: The History of Bacteriology. London, Oxford, 1938.

Celli, Angelo: Die Malaria in ihrer Bedeutung für die Geschichte Roms und der römischen Campagna. Leipzig, Thieme, 1929.

Chesney, Alan M.: The Johns Hopkins Hospital and The Johns Hopkins University School of Medicine. Baltimore, Johns Hopkins Press, 1943.

Cheyne, Sir William Watson: Lister and His Achievement. London, Longmans. 1925.

Clodd, Edward: Thomas Henry Huxley. New York, Dodd, 1902.

Conklin, Edwin G.: Predecessors of Schleiden and Schwann. Biological Symposia, Lancaster, 1940, p. 58.

Cushing, Harvey: The Life of Sir William Osler. Oxford, Clarendon Press, 1925.

Dakin, Edwin Franden: Mrs. Eddy. New York, Scribner's, 1929.

Darwin, Francis: Life and Letters of Charles Darwin. New York, Appleton-Century, 1888.

Descour, L.: Pasteur and His Work. New York, Stokes, n.d.

Duclaux, Émile: Pasteur, the History of a Mind. Philadelphia, Saunders, 1920.

Dukes, Cuthbert: Lord Lister. London, Parsons, 1924.

Fishbein, Morris: Fads and Quackery in Healing, New York, Covici, Friede, 1932.

Foster, Michael: Claude Bernard. New York, Longmans, 1899.

Glasser, Otto: Wilhelm Conrad Röntgen. Springfield, Ill., Thomas, 1934.

Godlee, Sir Rickman John: Lord Lister. London, Macmillan, 1918.

Gorgas, Marie D. and Hendrick, Burton J.: William Crawford Gorgas, New York, Doubleday Page, 1924.

Henry, William C.: Memoirs of the Life and Scientific Researches of John Dalton. London, Harrison, 1854.

Hulburt, R. G.: Osteopathy. Encyclopedia Britannica, XIV Edition, XVI; 956.

Hume, Edgar E.: Max von Pettenkofer's Theory of the Etiology of Cholera, Typhoid Fever and Other Intestinal Diseases. Ann. Med. Hist., s.1, VII:319, 1925.

Huxley, Leonard: Life and Letters of Thomas Henry Huxley. London, Macmillan, 1900.

Jones, Bence: The Life and Letters of Faraday. London, Longmans, 1870.

Karling, John S.: Schleiden's Contribution to the Cell Theory. Biological Symposia, Lancaster, 1940, p. 37.

Kelly, Howard A.: Walter Reed and Yellow Fever. New York, McClure, Phillips, 1907.

Koenigsberger, Leo: Hermann von Helmholtz. Oxford, Clarendon Press, 1906.

Lister and the Ligature. New Brunswick, Johnson & Johnson, 1925.

Lister and the Lister Ward. Glasgow, Jackson, 1927.

Löffler, Friedrich: Vorlesungen über die geschichtliche Entwickelung der Lehre von den Bacterien. Leipzig, Fogel, 1887.

Major, Ralph H.: Charles Edward Brown-Séquard. In: Evans, Herbert M., in honor of, written by his friends. Berkeley and Los Angeles, Univ. California Press, p. 369, 1943.

———: Karl Vierordt. Ann. Med. Hist., n.s., X:463, 1938.

Megros, R. L.: Ronald Ross. London, Allen & Unwin, 1931.

Metcalfe, Richard: Life of Vincent Priessnitz. London, Metcalfe's London Hydro., 1898.

Milmine, Georgine: The Life of Mary Baker G. Eddy and the History of Christian Science. New York, Doubleday Page, 1909.

Müller, Martin: Über die philosophischen Anschauungen des Naturforschers Johannes Müller. Leipzig, Barth, 1927.

Naunyn, B.: Erinnerungen Gedanken und Meinungen. Munich, Bergmann, 1925.

Olmsted, J. M. D.: Charles-Édouard Brown-Séquard. Baltimore, Johns Hopkins Press, 1946.

———: Claude Bernard, Physiologist. New York, Harper, 1938.

Pagel, J.: Rudolf Virchow, Leipzig, Feuer Verlag, 1906.

Paget, Stephen: Memoirs and Letters of Sir James Paget. London, Longmans, 1903.

Phisalix, Marie: Alphonse Laveran, sa Vie, son Oeuvre. Paris, Masson, 1923.
Rieux, J.: La vie et l'oeuvre de J-A Villemin. *Presse Méd.*, 1927, 35 1273.
Rosen, George: What is Social Medicine? Bull. Hist. Med., XXI:674, 1947.
Ross, Ronald: Memoirs. New York, Dutton, 1923.
Schönbauer, Leopold: Das Medizinische Wien. Vienna, Urban, 1947.
Scott, H. Harold: A History of Tropical Medicine. Baltimore, Williams & Wilkins, 1939. 2 v.
Sigerist, Henry: From Bismarck to Beveridge. Bull. Hist. Med., XIII:368, 1943.
Sigerist, Henry E.: Grösse Ärzte. München, Lehmann, 1932.
Simpson, Sir W. G.: Works of Sir J. R. Simpson. New York, Appleton-Century, 1872.
Sinclair, Sir William J.: Semmelweis, his Life and Doctrine. Manchester, Univ. Press, 1909.
Smith, Clifford, LL.B., C.S.B.: Christian Science. Encyclopedia Britannica, XIV Edition, V:638.
Stirling, William: Some Apostles of Physiology. London, Waterloo, 1902.
Vallery-Radot, Réné: The Life of Pasteur. New York, McClure, Phillips, 1906.
———: Pasteur, Images de sa Vie. Paris, Flammarion, 1947.
Virchow, Rudolf: Briefe an seine Eltern. Leipzig, Engelmann, 1906.
———: Gedächtnissrede an Joh. Lucas Schönlein. Berlin, Hirschwald, 1865.
———: Johannes Müller, Eine Gedächtnissrede. Berlin, Hirschwald, 1858.
White, Andrew D.: A History of the Warfare of Science with Theology. New York, Appleton-Century, 1897. 2 v.

THE TWENTIETH CENTURY

Babkin, B. P.: Pavlov. *Chicago Univ. Press,* 1947.
Bast, T. H., and Gardner, Weston D.: The Activity of the Embryonic Heart. J. Hist. Med. & Allied Sc., IV:289, 1949.
———: Wilhelm His, Jr. and the Bundle of His. J. Hist. Med. & Allied Sc., IV:170, 1949.
Blalock, Alfred: Walter Edward Dandy. Surgery, XIX:577, 1946.
British Medical Journal, Jan. 7, 1950, Fifty Years of Medicine. With articles by Sir Henry H. Dale, Geoffrey Jefferson, R. W. Johnstone, Sir Henry Cohen, Sir Lionel Whitby, Robert Cruikshank, John Rickman, J. S. K. Boyd, S. Cochrane Shanks, Sir Arthur MacNalty, Percy Stocks, Charles Singer, Sir Robert Hutchison, G. Grey Turner, Sir Robert Young, Alfred Cox and W. J. Bishop.
Brunel, Jules: Antibiosis from Pasteur to Fleming. J. Hist. Med., 1951, VI:287.
Ehrlich, Paul: Festschrift zum 60. Geburtstage des Forschers. Jena, Fischer, 1914.
Fairman, David: Evolution of Neurosurgery through Walter E. Dandy's Work. Surgery, XIX:581, 1946.
Fishbein, Morris: A History of The American Medical Association 1847 to 1947. Philadelphia & London, Saunders, 1947.
Flexner, Abraham: Medical Education. New York, Macmillan, 1925.
———: Medical Education in Europe. The Carnegie Foundation for the Advancement of Teaching, Bulletin Number Six, New York, 1912.

————: Medical Education in the United States and Canada. The Carnegie Foundation for the Advancement of Teaching, Bulletin Number Four, New York, 1910.

————: Universities, American, English, German, New York. Oxford, Oxford, 1930.

Fulton, John F.: Harvey Cushing. A Biography. Springfield, Ill., Thomas, 1946.

————: Science in the Clinic as exemplified by the life and work of Joseph Babinski. J. Nerv. & Ment. Dis., LXXVII:121, 1933.

Garrison, Fielding H.: Professor Karl Sudhoff and the Institute of Medical History at Leipzig. Bull. Soc. M. Hist. Chicago, III:1, 1923.

Ginzberg, Raphael: Three Years with Hans Berger. A Contribution to His Biography. J. Hist. Med., IV:361, 1949.

Hume, Edgar E.: Garrison and the Army Medical Library. Bull. Inst. Hist. Med., V:301, 1937.

Keefer, Chester S.: The Uses of Penicillin and Streptomycin. Lawrence, Univ. Kansas Press, 1949.

Long, Perrin H., and Bliss, Eleanor A.: The Clinical and Experimental Use of Sulfanilamide, Sulfapyradine and Allied Compounds. New York, Macmillan, 1939.

Napier, L. Everard: The Principles and Practice of Tropical Medicine. New York, Macmillan, 1946.

Rivers, Thomas M., and collaborators: Virus Diseases. Ithaca, Cornell Univ. Press, 1943.

Schoenbach, Emanuel: The Newer Antibiotics: Polymyxin, Chloromycetin and Aureomycin. J. Mt. Sinai Hosp., XVI:71, 1949.

Sington, Harold (quoted): Current Researches in Anesthesia & Analgesia. XXVIII, 1949.

Sketch of the History of the Mayo Clinic and the Mayo Foundation. Philadelphia, Saunders, 1926.

Stevenson, Lloyd: Sir Frederick Banting. Springfield, Illinois, Charles C Thomas, Publisher, 1947.

Stevenson, R. Scott, and Guthrie, Douglas: A History of Oto-Laryngology. Baltimore, Williams & Wilkins, 1949.

Strong, Richard P.: Stitt's Diagnosis, Prevention and Treatment of Tropical Diseases. Philadelphia, Blakiston, 1942.

Strümpell, Adolf: Aus dem Leben eines deutschen Klinikers. Leipzig, Vogel, 1925.

Wilder, Lucy: The Mayo Clinic, Minneapolis, printed by the McGill Lithograph Co., 1936.

Wilson, R. McNair: The Beloved Physician, Sir James Mackenzie. London, Murray, 1926.

Wolbach, S. Burt, Todd, John L., and Palfrey, Francis W.: The Etiology and Pathology of Typhus. Cambridge, Harvard, 1922.

Zilboorg, Gregory, and Henry, George W.: A History of Medical Psychology. New York, Norton, 1941.

Index of Names

Numbers in regular type indicate mention in text.
Numbers in **heavy type** indicate biography.
Number in *italics* indicate illustration.

on properties of tissues, 577
publications of, 576
scientific work of, 575
on sensibility, 577
Halsted, William Stewart, *854*, 855, 858, **913**
block-anesthesia, 859, 913
"cigarette drain," 913
re-infusion, 913
rubber gloves, 914
thyroid studies of, 914
Haly Abbas, 240, 263
Hamburger, Ove, 1061
Hamilton, Archbishop John, 380
Hamilton, Mary, 1064
Hamman, Carl A., 954
Hammer, Adam, **771**
Hammett, Frederick S., 1062
Hammurabi, *24*, 26
Hamusco, Juan Valverde di, 472
Handerson, Henry E., 1069
Hansen, Armauer, 842
Hare, Hobart A., 955
Harington, Sir John, 286, *295*
Hārith, al, ibn Kalada al Thakesi, 229, 262
Harley, George, **893**
Harper, Robert Francis, 1060
Harris, Walter, 561
Hart, Sir Arthur, 1066
Hartman, Franz, 1072
Harun-al-Rashid, Caliph, 230, 262
Harvey, Gideon, 560
Harvey, William, **494**, *495*, 552
De generatione animalium, 498
De motu cordis, 497
circulation, discovery of, 497
stemma, **499**
Harvey-Gibson, R. J., 1058, 1075
Hashinger, Edward H., 955, 1030
Haven, Marc, 1069
Havers, Clopton, 543
Hawks, Ellison, 1058
Hayem, Georges, 967, 1035
Haygarth, John, **637**
Hayyan, Jabir ibn, **234**, 235
Heberden, William, **598**, *599*, 634
Commentaries, 598
angina pectoris, 598
chicken-pox, 598
"Heberden's nodes", 598

nyctalopia, 598
Hebra, Ferdinand, **783**, 786, 883
Hecker, A. F., viii
Hecker, Justus Friedrich Karl, **711**, 1069
Hegel, G. W. F., 565
Heister, Lorenz, **631**
on appendicitis, 631
Hektoen, Ludvig, 951
Heidenhain, Rudolf Peter Heinrich, **897**
Helmholtz, Henry F., 998
Helmholtz, Hermann von, **802**, *803*, 887, 1020
Erhaltung der Kraft, 804
on color, 805
ophthalmoscope, invention of, 804
on optics, 805
on sound, 805
on velocity of nerve impulse, 804
Helmont, Jean Baptiste van, **500**, *502*, 552
Ortus Medicinae, 501
on asthma, 503, **941**
experiments of, 501
on ferments, 501
medical theories of, 503
on specific gravity of urine, 503
Hemmeter, John B., 1072
Hench, Philip, 998, 1056
Henderson, Lawrence Joseph, 978, **1035**
Henderson, Yandell, **1035**
Hendrick, Burton J., 1097
Hendrickson, G. L., 1072
Henle, Friedrich Gustav Jacob, **797**, *799*, 881
Von den Miasmen und Contagien, 798
Henoch, Eduard, **886**
Henri de. Mondeville, **319**, *320*, 354
Henry, George W., 1081
Henry, William C., 1079
Henschel, August Wilhelm Eduard Theodor, **708**
Herakleides, 149, 161
d'Hérelle, Félix-Hubert, 968
Hernández, Francisco, 12
Herodotos, 26, 27, 33, 53, 115, 1065
Herodotos the physician, 220
Herophilos, 116, **143**, 161
anatomy of, 143

Index of Subjects

Numbers in regular type indicate mention in text.
Numbers in **heavy type** indicate biography.
Numbers in *italics* indicate illustration.

Anesthesia
　block, 913
　cyclopropane, 1018
　cyprome, 1018
　divinyl oxide, 1018
　endotrachial, 1019
　evipan, 1019
　hypnotism, 710
　intravenous, 925, 1019
　local, 930
　new methods, 1019
　rectal, 176, 1018, 1019
　spinal, 925 1019
Anesthesia, local
　Dioskorides, 176
　Halsted, 913
　Koller, 930
　Salernus, Magister, 275
　Schleich, 1020
　Tagault, 425
　William of Saliceto, 298
Anesthesia, rectal
　Dioskorides, 176
　Pirogoff, 1019
Anesthesia, surgical
　discovery of, 751
　first demonstration of, *755*
Aneurysm
　Antyllos, 204
　Baccelli, 972
　Galen, 199
　Lancisi, 542
　Matas, 959
　Moragni, 587
　Mott, 734
　Papyrus Ebers, 51
　Paré, 431
Aneurysm and syphilis
　Lancisi, 542
　Morgagni, 587
　Paré, 431
Aneurysmorrhaphy, 959
Angina pectoris
　Brunton, 905
　Caelius Aurelianus, 206
　Fothergill, 635
　Heberden, 598
　Hunter, J., 605
　Jenner, 607
　Papyrus of Ebers, 51
　Parry, 600
Angina pectoris, nitrites in, 905

Angioeurotic edema, 904
Aniline dye stains, 906
Animal electricity, 637
Animal spirit, 149, 195
Animism, 566
Ankylostomiasis, 51, 914
Annals of Medical History, x, 995
"Anoci-association," 959
Ant sutures, 71, 75, 251, 330
Anthelminthics
　Aetios, 212
　China, 97
　Papyrus of Ebers, 50
　Theophrastos, 140
Anthrax
　bacillus of, 829
　spores (discovery of), 838
　vaccination against, 833
Anthropology
　Broca, 888
　Huxley, 813
　Quatrefages, 881
　Toldt, 1050
　Virchow, 808, 881
Antibiosis, 1010
Antibiotics, 1010
Antidotaria magna, 274
Antidotaria parva, 274
Antidotarium, 274
Antidotarium of Nicholas, 274
Antimony
　Triumphal Chariot of Antimony, 457
　war over, 457
Antisepsis, 821
　v. Bergman, 826
　Billroth, 895
　Halsted, 855
　Lister, 824
　Lucas-Champonnière, 969
　Pringle, 594
　Semmelweis, 786
　Thiersch, 825, 888
　Volkmann, 825
Antitoxin
　diphtheria, 845, 915
　tetanus, 845, 915
Aorta, abdominal, ligation of, 694
Aorta, coarctation of, 587
Aortic insufficiency
　Corrigan, 685
　Cowper, 629

A HISTORY OF MEDICINE

Orthopedic surgery (cont'd)
 Lorenz, 927, 1041
 Paré, 430, 430
 Pott, 635
 Putti, 1073
 Scarpa, 639
Osiris, 995
Osler's disease, 910
Osler's nodes, 910
Osmosis, 961, 1049
Ospedale del Cappo, Pistoia, 363
Ossicles of ear, discovery of, 395
Osteitis deformans, 818
Osteitis fibrosa cystica, 897
Osteomalacia, 765
Osteosis of femur in Pithecantropus
 erectus, 4
Osteopathy, 873
Oswaldo Cruz Institute, 1003
Otolaryngology
 Bárány, 1021
 Czermak, 1021
 Garcia, 1021
 Holmgren, 1021
 Lempert, 1021
 Sourdille, 1021
 Türck, 1021
 Valsalva, 622
Ovarian follicles, discovery of, 535
Ovariotomy, first, 741
Ovum, mammalian, discovery of, 710
Oxford Physiologists, 513
Oxford University, medieval, 322
Oxidation, 617
Oxygen, discovery of
 Lavoisier, 617
 Mayow?, 521
 Priestley, 615
 Scheele, 616

Pa Kua, 84
Pacchonian bodies, 628
Padua, 327
 dissection at, 327
 foundation of, 327
 Jews, 328
 organization, 329
 professors, famous, 330-333
 Protestants, 328
 tolerance, 328
 University of, 327, 497
Paget's disease, 818

Paludrine, 1022
Panama Canal, construction of, 915
Pancreas, extirpation of, 563
Pancreas, first named, 183
Pancreatic fistula, d. Graaf, 534, 535
Pancreatitis, 905
Pantegri, 270
Papilla of Vater, 631
Papyrus
 Berlin, 44
 Brugsch, 335
 Ebers, 42, 44, 49
 Edwin Smith, 44, 45
 Hearst, 44
 Kahun, 44
 London, 44
Paracelsus Society, Swiss, 392
Parathyroid extract, 1001
Parathyroid, relation to tetany, 927
Paresis
 malarial therapy, in 928
 Spirochaeta pallida in, 980
Paris
 foundation of, 312
 organization, 313
 professors, famous, 313-318
 study, course of, 313
 University of, medieval, 312
Paris in 1528, 416
Paris School, 644, 772
Parkinson's disease, 701
Parotitis
 see Mumps
Paroxysmal, tachycardia, 912
Pasteur Institute, 833, 835
Patent medicines, 874
Pathology
 Addison, 690
 Aschoff, 1026
 Baillie, 702
 Baillou, 423
 Benivieni, 371
 Bennett, 882
 Bonet, 536
 Bowman, 883
 Bright, 689
 Cannon, 951
 Cohnheim, 901
 Cruveilhier, 674
 Davis, 951
 Ehrlich, 935
 Ewing, 955, 1033

THIS BOOK

A HISTORY OF
MEDICINE

By Ralph H. Major, M.D.

was set, printed and bound by The Collegiate Press of Menasha, Wisconsin. The type face is Linotype Baskerville, set 10 point on 12 point. The type page is 25 x 41 picas. The text paper is 60-lb. White Winnebago Enamel. The binding is Bancroft Natural Finish Buckram 3521.

With THOMAS BOOKS careful attention is given to all details of manufacturing and design. It is the publisher's desire to present books that are satisfactory as to their physical qualities and artistic possibilities and appropriate for their particular use. THOMAS BOOKS will be true to those laws of quality that assure a good name and good will.